# Dilemmas in Abdominal Surgery

T0136306

# Dilemmas in Abdominal Surgery

## A Case-Based Approach

Edited by

**Savio George Barreto, MBBS, MS, FRACS, PhD**

Division of Surgery and Perioperative Medicine
Flinders Medical Centre
and
SA Portfolio Advisor, Advanced Studies & Senior Lecturer
College of Medicine and Public Health
Flinders University
Adelaide, Australia

**Shailesh V. Shrikhande, MBBS, MS, MD**

Deputy Director
Gastrointestinal and Hepato-Pancreato-Biliary Surgical Services
Department of Surgical Oncology
Tata Memorial Center
Mumbai, India

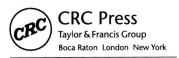

CRC Press
Taylor & Francis Group
Boca Raton London New York

CRC Press is an imprint of the
Taylor & Francis Group, an **informa** business

First edition published 2021
by CRC Press
6000 Broken Sound Parkway NW, Suite 300, Boca Raton, FL 33487-2742

and by CRC Press
2 Park Square, Milton Park, Abingdon, Oxon, OX14 4RN

© 2021 Taylor & Francis Group, LLC

CRC Press is an imprint of Taylor & Francis Group, LLC

---

*Library of Congress Cataloging-in-Publication Data*

---

Names: Barreto, Savio George, editor. | Shrikhande, Shailesh V. (Shailesh Vinayak), 1971- editor.
Title: Dilemmas in abdominal surgery : a case-based approach / edited by Savio George Barreto, Shailesh V. Shrikhande.
Description: First edition. | Boca Raton, FL : CRC Press, 2020. | Includes bibliographical references and index. | Summary: "This book approaches a surgical disease or its management by providing an evidence-based approach to a specific clinical dilemma. The chapters take the reader through a step-by-step 'decision-making' approach to commonly encountered, but difficult to manage, situations where the editors share their rationale behind the process"-- Provided by publisher.
Identifiers: LCCN 2020037676 (print) | LCCN 2020037677 (ebook) | ISBN 9780367187699 (paperback) | ISBN 9780367559014 (hardback) | ISBN 9780429198359 (ebook)
Subjects: MESH: Gastrointestinal Diseases | Digestive System Surgical Procedures--methods | Clinical Decision-Making--methods | Case Reports
Classification: LCC RD540 (print) | LCC RD540 (ebook) | NLM WI 980 | DDC 617.4/3--dc23
LC record available at https://lccn.loc.gov/2020037676
LC ebook record available at https://lccn.loc.gov/2020037677

---

ISBN: 9780367559014 (hbk)
ISBN: 9780367187699 (pbk)
ISBN: 9780429198359 (ebk)

Typeset in Palatino
by Deanta Global Publishing Services, Chennai, India

*To our patients*
*&*
*Merlyn, Gina, and Ian*

Savio George Barreto


*To my two excellent teams – at home and at work*

Shailesh V. Shrikhande

# Contents

# Preface

Surgical diseases affecting abdominal organs are among the most common conditions managed on a day-to-day basis around the world. The abdominal cavity with the organs and vessels contained within it constitute a field of work shared by generalists and specialists, including general surgeons, esophagogastric and hepato-pancreato-biliary surgeons, colorectal surgeons, vascular surgeons, gastroenterologists, radiologists, intensivists, and general practitioners. Among the myriad of surgical problems to affect these structures there remain situations in their management that can challenge even the most seasoned and experienced of surgeons. The aim of this book was to bring together an experienced team of authors, who are regarded as experts in their field, to present their approach to various situational dilemmas encountered when dealing with surgical conditions of the abdomen. These chapters are designed to provide the reader with an erudite and evidence-based approach. The chapters are also practical, taking a step-by-step approach to real-world issues in patient care. All those providing care to patients with these diseases will find value in these pages.

We are sincerely grateful to the individual authors who have contributed to this book. They have been excellent to work with, and responsive to the demands of both editors and the publisher. And, as expected, we have gained new knowledge and perspectives, which has made this an enriching experience for us. This project would not have been possible without the sterling support of Ms. Shivangi Pramanik, Ms. Himani Dwivedi, and Ms. Mouli Sharma, from CRC Press/Taylor & Francis, through the entire process of bringing you this book.

Surgical diseases of the abdomen continue to be our collective clinical interest and we hope you will be inspired to provide the very best of care for your patients as you read and apply all that is contained here.

**Savio George Barreto**
*Adelaide, Australia*

**Shailesh V. Shrikhande**
*Mumbai, India*

# Editors

**Savio George Barreto, MBBS, MS, FRACS, PhD,** is a gastrointestinal and hepato-pancreato-biliary (GI and HPB) surgeon and a senior lecturer in surgery at Flinders University, Australia. He is a surgeon–scientist whose research interests include the pathophysiology and surgical management (including outcomes) of the diseases of the stomach, pancreas, and biliary tree. He has published a carcinogenesis model in gallbladder cancer to aid in the understanding of the development of the cancer and to guide future therapy-directed research. Together with Professor John Windsor, he has proposed the first evidence-based definition of early stomach cancer. He has made numerous presentations and has published more than 200 articles in his field of research. He is the editor of the book, *Surgical Diseases of the Pancreas and Biliary Tree* (Springer, 2018). He serves on the editorial boards of surgical journals as well as the Indian Council of Medical Research, a task force group for the development of guidelines for the management of stomach, pancreatic, and neuroendocrine cancers for India. He also serves as the South Australia Profile Advisor for the MD Advanced Studies Programme at Flinders University, South Australia.

**Shailesh V. Shrikhande, MBBS, MS, MD,** is deputy director at the Tata Memorial Center in Mumbai, India. He is professor and head of gastrointestinal and hepato-pancreato-biliary (GI and HPB) service and also heads the division of cancer surgery. He was the first Asian to be awarded the Kenneth Warren Fellowship of the International Hepato-Pancreato-Biliary Association (IHPBA) in 2005. He was awarded the title of Doctor of Medicine (magna cum laude) by Heidelberg University, Germany for his original clinical and basic research on chronic pancreatitis and pancreatic cancer in 2006. He has been invited to over 500 lectures and orations all over India and other parts of the world. As well as having published over 230 clinical and basic science research papers in leading peer-reviewed journals (including a series of 1200 Whipple resections), Professor Shrikhande has also performed 49 live operative teaching demonstrations on pancreatic, gastric, gallbladder, and colorectal cancers across India to promote modern gastrointestinal cancer surgery. He has contributed over 60 book chapters and is the chief editor of the books *Surgery of Pancreatic Tumors* (BI Publications, 2008), *Pancreatic Cancer: Current Understanding* (Elsevier, 2011), and *Modern Gastrointestinal Oncology* (Elsevier, 2015). He is the associate editor of *Langenbeck's Archives of Surgery* (Springer, 2018). He is the chairman of the Indian Council of Medical Research (ICMR), a committee for developing guidelines for the management of pancreatic and gastric cancer in India. He is also on the editorial boards of many international journals dealing with GI and HPB surgery. He is the current president of the Indian Chapter of IHPBA. He is the chairman of the Scientific Committee of the International Hepato-Pancreato-Biliary Association (2018–2020) and treasurer of the Asia-Pacific Hepato-Pancreato-Biliary Association (2019–2021). In recognition of his work on pancreatic cancer and digestive cancer surgery in India, he was awarded Honorary Fellowship of the Royal College of Surgeons of England in 2014 (FRCS – Ad Eundem).

# Contributors

**René Adam**
AP-HP Hôpital Paul Brousse
Centre Hépato-Biliaire
Université Paris Sud
Villejuif, France

**N. Ananthakrishnan**
Department of Surgery
Mahatma Gandhi Medical College and
    Research Institute
Sri Balaji Vidyapeeth
Pondicherry, India

**Valentina Andreasi**
Pancreatic Surgery Unit
Pancreas Translational and Clinical Research
    Center
San Raffaele Scientific Institute
Vita-Salute San Raffaele University
Milan, Italy

**Shun-ichi Ariizumi**
Department of Surgery
Institute of Gastroenterology
Tokyo Women's Medical University
Tokyo, Japan

**Apurva Ashok**
Division of Thoracic Surgery
Department of Surgical Oncology
Tata Memorial Hospital
Homi Bhabha National Institute
Mumbai, India

**Atef Baakza**
MIMER Medical College
Mumbai, India

**Gayatri Balachandran**
Institute of Digestive and HPB Sciences
Sakra World Hospital
Bangalore, India

**Savio George Barreto**
Hepatobiliary and Oesophagogastric Unit
Division of Surgery and Perioperative Medicine
Flinders Medical Centre
and
College of Medicine and Public Health,
    Flinders University
Adelaide, Australia

**Courtney E. Barrows**
Beth Israel Deaconess Medical Center
Harvard Medical School
Boston, Massachusetts

**Sofia Battisti**
Department of Radiology
Ospedale "M. Bufalini"
Cesena, Italy

**Onur Bayram**
Department of Visceral, Vascular and
    Endocrine Surgery
Halle University Hospital
Martin-Luther-University Halle-Wittenberg
Halle (Saale), Germany

**Anu Behari**
Department of Surgical Gastroenterology
Sanjay Gandhi Postgraduate Institute of
    Medical Sciences
Lucknow, India

**Manish S. Bhandare**
Gastrointestinal and Hepato-Pancreato-Biliary
    Surgical Services
Department of Surgical Oncology
Tata Memorial Hospital
Mumbai, India

**Sarah Bormann**
Division of Surgery and Perioperative
    Medicine
Flinders Medical Centre
Adelaide, Australia

**Ibrahim Büdeyri**
Department of Visceral, Vascular and
    Endocrine Surgery
Halle University Hospital
Martin-Luther-University Halle-Wittenberg
Halle (Saale), Germany

**Tim Bright**
Oesophagogastric Unit
Division of Surgery and Perioperative
    Medicine
Flinders Medical Centre
and
College of Medicine and Public Health
Flinders University
Adelaide, Australia

**Vikram A. Chaudhari**
Gastrointestinal and Hepato-Pancreato-Biliary
    Surgical Services
Department of Surgical Oncology
Tata Memorial Hospital
Mumbai, India

**Jacob Chisholm**
Oesophagogastric Unit
Division of Surgery and Perioperative Medicine
Flinders Medical Centre
Adelaide, Australia

**Federico Coccolini**
General, Emergency and Trauma Surgery
    Department
Pisa University Hospital
Pisa, Italy

**Michael Cox**
Nepean Hospital Clinical School
University of Sydney
Sydney, Australia

**Murtaza Dadla**
Department of General Surgery
Topiwala National Medical College and B.Y.L.
    Nair Ch. Hospital
Mumbai, India

**Dayan de Fontgalland**
Colorectal Surgery Unit
Division of Surgery and Perioperative
    Medicine
Flinders Medical Centre, Bedford Park
Adelaide, Australia

**Marco Del Chiaro**
Department of Surgery
University of Colorado
Anschutz Medical Campus
Denver, Colorado

**Massimo Falconi**
Pancreatic Surgery Unit
San Raffaele Scientific Institute
Vita-Salute San Raffaele University
Milan, Italy

**Nisar Hamdani**
Department of Surgical Gastroenterology
    (GI & HPB Oncosurgery)
Government Medical College
Srinagar, India

**Jakob R. Izbicki**
Department of General, Visceral and Thoracic
    Surgery
University Medical Center Hamburg-Eppendorf
Hamburg, Germany

**Sabita Jiwnani**
Division of Thoracic Surgery
Tata Memorial Hospital
Homi Bhabha National Institute
Mumbai, India

**Rajeev M. Joshi**
Department of General Surgery
Topiwala National Medical College and B.Y.L.
    Nair Ch. Hospital
Mumbai, India

**R. Kalayarasan**
Department of Surgical Gastroenterology
Jawaharlal Institute of Post-Graduate Medical
    Education and Research (JIPMER)
Pondicherry, India

**V.K. Kapoor**
Department of Surgical Gastroenterology
Sanjay Gandhi Postgraduate Institute of
    Medical Sciences
Lucknow, India

**George Karimundackal**
Division of Thoracic Surgery
Tata Memorial Hospital
Homi Bhabha National Institute
Mumbai, India

**Vikram Kate**
Department of  General & Gastrointestinal
    Surgery
Jawaharlal Institute of Post-Graduate Medical
    Education and Research (JIPMER)
Pondicherry, India

**Mufaddal Kazi**
Department of Surgical Oncology
Tata Memorial Hospital
Mumbai, India

**Tara S. Kent**
Beth Israel Deaconess Medical Center/Harvard
    Medical School
Boston, Massachusetts

**Charles W. Kimbrough**
Department of Surgery
The Ohio State University Wexner Medical
    Center
Columbus, Ohio

**Yuki Kitano**
AP-HP Hôpital Paul Brousse
Centre Hépato-Biliaire
Université Paris Sud
Villejuif, France
and
Department of Gastroenterological
    Surgery
Graduate School of Medical Sciences
Kumamoto University
Kumamoto, Japan

**Jörg Kleeff**
Department of Visceral, Vascular and
    Endocrine Surgery
Halle University Hospital
Martin-Luther-University Halle-Wittenberg
Halle (Saale), Germany

**Paul Kolarsick**
Department of Colorectal Surgery
Cleveland Clinic Florida
Weston, Florida

**Lilian Kow**
Hepatobiliary and Oesophagogastric Unit
Division of Surgery and Perioperative Medicine
Flinders Medical Centre
Adelaide, Australia

**Kaushal Kundalia**
Kings College
London, UK

**Kailash Kurdia**
Post Graduate Institute of Medical Education
    and Research (PGIMER)
Chandigarh, India

**S.M. Lagarde**
Department of Surgery
Erasmus University Medical Center
Rotterdam, the Netherlands

**Divya Manikandan**
Department of Biology
University of Michigan – Ann Arbor
Ann Arbor, Michigan

**Varughese Mathai**
Apollo Health City
Hyderabad, India

**Christoph W. Michalski**
Department of Visceral, Vascular and
    Endocrine Surgery
Halle University Hospital
Martin-Luther-University Halle-Wittenberg
Halle (Saale), Germany

**Arindam Mondal**
Division of GI and HPB Surgery
Department of Surgical Oncology
Tata Memorial Centre
Mumbai, India

**Takanori Morikawa**
Department of Surgery
Tohoku University Graduate School of
    Medicine
Sendai, Japan

**Francesca Muffatti**
Pancreatic Surgery Unit
Pancreas Translational and Clinical Research
    Center
San Raffaele Scientific Institute
Vita-Salute San Raffaele University
Milan, Italy

**Ganesh Nagarajan**
PD Hinduja Hospital and Medical Research
    Centre
Mumbai, India

**Govind Nandakumar**
Columbia Asia Hospitals
Bangalore, India
and
Courtesy Faculty Weill Cornell Medical
    College
New York, New York

**Michael F. Nentwich**
University Medical Center Hamburg-
    Eppendorf
Department of General, Visceral and Thoracic
    Surgery
and
Department of Intensive Care Medicine
Hamburg, Germany

**Alain Nguyen**
Division of Surgery and Perioperative
    Medicine
Flinders Medical Centre, Bedford Park
Adelaide, Australia

**Devayani Niyogi**
Division of Thoracic Surgery
Department of Surgical Oncology
Tata Memorial Hospital
Homi Bhabha National Institute
Mumbai, India

**Atsushi Oba**
Department of Surgery
Division of Surgical Oncology
University of Colorado
Anschutz Medical Campus
Denver, Colorado
and
Department of Hepatobiliary and Pancreatic
    Surgery
Cancer Institute Hospital
Japanese Foundation for Cancer Research,
    Ariake
Tokyo, Japan

**W.K. Ooi**
Department of Surgery
Queen Elizabeth Hospital I
Sabah, Malaysia
and
Department of Surgery
Erasmus University Medical Center
Rotterdam, the Netherlands

**Rajesh Panwar**
Department of GI Surgery and Liver
  Transplantation
All India Institute of Medical Sciences
New Delhi, India

**Stefano Partelli**
Pancreatic Surgery Unit
Pancreas Translational and Clinical
  Research Center
San Raffaele Scientific Institute
Vita-Salute San Raffaele University
Milan, Italy

**Timothy M. Pawlik**
Department of Surgery
The Ohio State University Wexner
  Medical Center
Columbus, Ohio

**C.S. Pramesh**
Division of Thoracic Surgery
Tata Memorial Hospital
Homi Bhabha National Institute
Mumbai, India

**Peush Sahni**
Department of GI Surgery and Liver
  Transplantation
All India Institute of Medical Sciences
New Delhi, India

**Inian Samarasam**
Upper GI Surgery Unit
Christian Medical College Hospital
Vellore, India

**Sandeep Sangale**
Department of General Surgery
Topiwala National Medical College and
  B.Y.L. Nair Ch. Hospital
Mumbai, India

**Richard D. Schulick**
Department of Surgery
Division of Surgical Oncology
University of Colorado
Anschutz Medical Campus
Denver, Colorado

**K. Senthilnathan**
Upper GI Surgery Unit
Christian Medical College Hospital
Vellore, India

**Parvez Sheikh**
Department of Colorectal Surgery
Saifee Hospital
Mumbai, India

**Jon Shenfine**
Oesophagogastric Unit
Division of Surgery and Perioperative
  Medicine
Flinders Medical Centre
Adelaide, Australia

**Shailesh V. Shrikhande**
Gastrointestinal and Hepato-Pancreato-Biliary
  Surgical Services
Department of Surgical Oncology
Tata Memorial Hospital
Mumbai, India

**Maria Grazia Sibilla**
Department of Surgery and Department
  of Morphology
Surgery and Experimental Medicine
S. Anna University Hospital and University
  of Ferrara
Ferrara, Italy

**Sadiq S. Sikora**
Institute of Digestive and HPB Sciences
Sakra World Hospital
Bangalore, India

**Rajneesh Kumar Singh**
Sanjay Gandhi Post Graduate Institute of
  Medical Sciences
Lucknow, India

**Richard Smith**
General Surgery and Surgical Oncology
The Royal Adelaide Hospital
Adelaide, Australia

**Virendra Kumar Tiwari**
Department of Surgical Oncology
Tata Memorial Hospital
Homi Bhabha National Institute
Mumbai, India

**Robert J. Torphy**
Department of Surgery
University of Colorado
Anschutz Medical Campus
Denver, Colorado

**Edward Travers**
Department of Vascular and Endovascular
   Surgery
Flinders Medical Centre and Flinders
   University
Adelaide, Australia

**Maxwell T. Trudeau**
Department of Surgery
University of Pennsylvania Perelman School
   of Medicine
Philadelphia, Pennsylvania

**Lohith Umapathi**
Columbia Asia Hospitals
Bangalore, India

**Michiaki Unno**
Department of Surgery
Tohoku University Graduate School of
   Medicine
Sendai, Japan

**Charles M. Vollmer**
Department of Surgery
University of Pennsylvania Perelman
   School of Medicine
Philadelphia, Pennsylvania

**David I. Watson**
Flinders University Discipline of Surgery
Flinders Medical Centre
Adelaide, Australia

**Steven D. Wexner**
Department of Colorectal Surgery
Cleveland Clinic Florida
Weston, Florida

**B.P.L. Wijnhoven**
Department of Surgery
Erasmus University Medical Center
Rotterdam, the Netherlands

**John A. Windsor**
Auckland District Health Board
Faculty of Medical and Health Sciences
University of Auckland
Auckland, New Zealand

**Masakazu Yamamoto**
Department of Surgery
Institute of Gastroenterology
Tokyo Women's Medical University
Tokyo, Japan

# PART 1

# ESOPHAGUS

# 1 Acute Presentation (Boerhaave's Syndrome)

*Jon Shenfine*

## CONTENTS

## CASE SCENARIO

A 48-year-old man presented to the emergency department with severe, excruciating chest pain. He had spent the day with his family, drinking alcohol and eating a large dinner. At 21:00 he felt nauseated and vomited. There was a tearing sensation in his chest and he collapsed in agony on the floor. He presented in severe pain despite opioid analgesia. He was pale, short of breath, and peripherally shutdown. His voice was weak and high pitched; he was distressed with pain and sweat. He had subcutaneous emphysema over the chest wall, but his abdomen was soft to palpate. His pulse rate was 120 bpm and his blood pressure was 100/60. His electrocardiogram was normal and his chest radiograph confirms subcutaneous emphysema.

## BACKGROUND OF THE PATHOLOGY

This is a classical presentation of a "spontaneous perforation of the esophagus" or Boerhaave's syndrome which is a barogenic, esophageal injury [1]. Although various degrees of damage and contamination are possible, spontaneous perforation of the esophagus is most accurately defined as a full-thickness disruption of the esophageal wall occurring in the absence of pre-existing pathology, and typically leads to immediate and gross gastric content contamination of the mediastinal and pleural cavities. This progresses rapidly to a life-threatening chemical and septic mediastinitis.

The injury is nearly always associated with a sudden rise in intra-abdominal pressure, most usually as a result of retching or vomiting, hence the term "barogenic". Vomiting is commonplace but spontaneous esophageal perforation is not, which suggests that there may be unidentified anatomical or perhaps pathological abnormalities that underlie the injury. An underlying pathology, such as malignancy, peptic ulceration, infectious, or eosinophilic esophagitis is identified in only 10–20% of cases and these cases do not truly represent spontaneous perforations. Another common misconception is that Mallory–Weiss tears are a lesser but related injury. However, it is more likely that these mucosal injuries reflect "shearing" rather than "barogenic" trauma.

Spontaneous perforations are invariably single, longitudinal, between 1–8 cm long, and with the mucosal injury being longer than the muscular tear. They tend to occur in the left posterolateral position just above the esophagogastric junction. Pleural perforation can be immediate or delayed and transgression of esophagogastric contents is exacerbated by the negative intrathoracic pressure. Men are more often affected, in a ratio of 4:1, which may reflect a tendency to overindulge in alcohol and vomit rather than a gender difference.

## APPROACH TO MANAGEMENT

### Clinical findings (symptoms and signs)

Patients with Boerhaave's syndrome classically present with sudden onset of chest pain following vomiting, and the subsequent development of subcutaneous emphysema. The associated pain is constant, retrosternal, severe, exacerbated by movement, and poorly relieved by opioid analgesia. Patients are usually tachycardic and tachypnoeic. Mediastinal emphysema develops rapidly and can be seen on a plain chest radiograph, as can a hydropneumothorax once the pleura is breached. There is an early low-grade pyrexia due to the chemical pleuro-mediastinitis, worsening as the systemic inflammatory response gives way to sepsis. Within 24–48 hours, bacterial mediastinitis and systemic circulatory collapse supervene; survival is dependent on the removal of the contamination from the mediastinal and pleural cavities at the earliest opportunity.

However, classical is not the same as typical, since patients with spontaneous perforation of the esophagus can present in many ways. The temporal relationship of the barogenic event to the development of the chest pain is frequently overlooked due to the severity and associated cardiopulmonary collapse. The pathognomonic development of subcutaneous emphysema takes time to evolve, and abdominal pain and tenderness are also not uncommon and can lead to a negative laparotomy. The combination of chest pain and shock commonly lead to an early cardiology opinion and significant diagnostic delay. The diagnosis becomes more obscure as time passes due to circulatory collapse. As a result, the diagnostic error is high and only 5% of cases are diagnosed at presentation, with delay being the norm rather than the exception. Some cases may not even be correctly diagnosed pre-mortem.

The most important factor in making the diagnosis is a high index of suspicion in someone with severe chest pain following an episode of violent vomiting.

### Investigations: To arrive at a diagnosis and plan treatment

*Computed tomography (CT) (Figure 1.1)*

CT chest and abdomen with intravenous and oral contrast is the first choice in diagnostic imaging for stable patients. In an intubated patient, a nasogastric tube can be placed in the proximal esophagus to run a small amount of water-soluble contrast in to increase the sensitivity of detecting a leak. CT also plays a significant role post-therapy to assess ongoing leakage and healing and guide

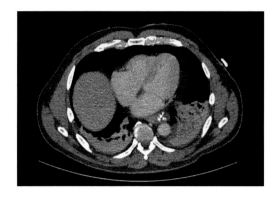

**Figure 1.1**  Axial section of a CT scan of the chest demonstrating contrast leak, pneumomediastinum and lung changes.

the need for further intervention with serial studies.

*Plain radiography (chest X-ray)*

The commonest associated findings on plain radiography are of pleural effusion, pneumomediastinum, subcutaneous emphysema, hydropneumothorax, pneumothorax and lung consolidation or collapse. However, these can be subtle and develop over time.

*Contrast radiography*

Water-soluble oral contrast radiography has been superseded by CT since the logistics of their performance are frequently limited in patients who are in shock. However, their dynamic nature gives information about the degree of containment and the degree of drainage of the perforation. They also remain useful post-treatment to assess progress of healing.

*Upper gastrointestinal endoscopy*

Endoscopy was previously avoided due to the perceived risk of insufflation and increase in size of the perforation. However, this has not borne out and can be performed in the most unwell of patients, preferably "on table", safety being enhanced by being performed by a highly experienced endoscopist under a general anesthetic with the patient intubated (Figure 1.2). Endoscopy can influence management if underlying pathology is discovered and allows the placement of a nasojejunal tube or adjunctive therapies such as clipping a defect, lavage of a perforation cavity, or the placement of a "vacuum" endo-sponge as a potential therapeutic option in contained perforations

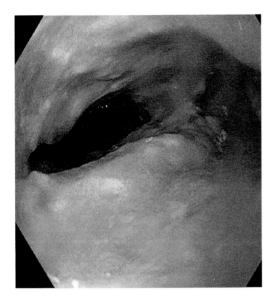

**Figure 1.2** Endoscopic image of esophageal perforation demonstrating a clean esophageal defect above the esophagogastric junction.

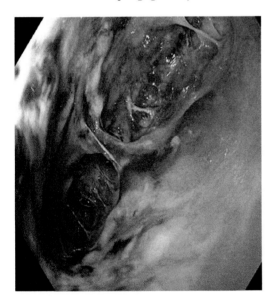

**Figure 1.3** Endoscopic image of mediastinal cavity in a case of a contained perforation.

with no gross contamination (see treatment) (Figure 1.3).

### Treatment options with benefits and risks

All patients with an esophageal perforation are critically ill. The immediate priority is resuscitation: establishing a secure airway, stabilising the cardiovascular system, relieving pain, and administering broad-spectrum antibiotics,

antifungals and anti-secretory medication (see Box 1.1). An initially stable patient can rapidly decompensate, and early anesthetic review is strongly recommended. Ultimately, patients will benefit from a multidisciplinary approach with input from intensive care, radiology, physiotherapy, dieticians, and rehabilitation services. Hospitals lacking these specialists or the expertise necessary to deal with esophageal surgery should transfer the patients as soon as possible after initial stabilisation. Survival is dependent on controlling sepsis, so prompt surgery remains obligatory when there is significant contamination. Non-operative treatment is sometimes feasible when contamination is limited and there has been minimal delay.

> **BOX 1.1 INITIAL RESUSCITATION IN SPONTANEOUS ESOPHAGEAL PERFORATION**
>
> - Control of airway and administration of supplementary oxygen
> - Early anesthetic involvement
> - Large-bore intravenous access and intravenous fluid resuscitation
> - Central venous access and arterial line monitoring ± inotropic support
> - Urethral catheterization and close monitoring of fluid balance
> - Broad-spectrum antibiotic and antifungal agents
> - Intravenous antisecretory agents (H-receptor antagonists or proton pump inhibitors)
> - Strictly nil by mouth
> - Large-bore intercostal chest drainage – possibly bilaterally
> - Nasogastric tube (only to be placed under endoscopic vision or radiological guidance)

*Non-operative management*

Non-operative management may be possible in carefully selected patients (see Box 1.2) and in those with a delayed diagnosis who have demonstrated "tolerance" where despite no intervention, the patient has not become overwhelmingly septic. This has become increasingly conceivable with advances in radiological intervention, antibiotics, and enteral nutritional supplementation. However, in contrast to iatrogenic esophageal injuries, these criteria are rarely met in spontaneous esophageal perforations, and non-operative management should therefore be viewed as a "radical" therapeutic option.

The criteria must *all* be met [2]. Non-operative management comprises observation in intensive care or a high-dependency unit with patients kept nil oral and fed enterally, if necessary, via a surgically placed feeding jejunostomy. A nasogastric tube should be placed under endoscopic and/or radiological assistance past the perforation to decompress the stomach and to limit reflux. An alternative is a surgical venting gastrostomy placed at the same time as a formal feeding jejunostomy. Where pleural perforation has occurred, chest drainage should be instituted and repeated contrast radiology, endoscopy and CT performed to monitor the status of the perforation – all collections should be drained. Serial contrast or CT studies can be used to monitor progress until sufficient healing has occurred. All patients should be given broad-spectrum intravenous antibiotics, antifungal, and a proton pump inhibitor. A low threshold for operative intervention is maintained.

*Adjuncts to non-operative management*
Endoscopic therapies such as clips, stents, sealants, and vacuum sponge dressings as a primary treatment to seal a spontaneous perforation are limited in the face of gross contamination. In addition, these approaches are technically difficult and should not be attempted by inexperienced operators unable to deal with the consequences of their actions. However, in the absence of contamination, small perforations may be treated with these adjuncts in addition to ongoing non-operative management. In these situations, the author has found that repeated endoscopic lavage of contained mediastinal perforations or endoscopic placement of a vacuum sponge drainage system are the most useful of these interventions. Self-expanding stents may also be used

to seal the intraluminal defect allowing oral nutrition during the healing phase, but again do not deal with any underlying contamination [3]. Beware that stent placement may extend the defect, trauma can be sustained on stent removal and migration rates are high. The author advises using a removable, softer material stent, such as the Polyflex™ with planned removal at six weeks to minimize these risks.

*Operative management*
Surgery is advocated if the patient has overt signs of sepsis, shock, gross contamination, or has failed non-operative management. The objectives are to restore integrity, clear contamination, and prevent further soiling. Thorough debridement, drainage, lavage, and irrigation are probably more important for survival than the type of repair utilized. A feeding jejunostomy should be fashioned to facilitate enteral feeding and a venting gastrostomy can obviate the need for prolonged nasogastric tube placement.

Based on the site, a posterolateral thoracotomy is used, most commonly through the left seventh or eighth intercostal space. Solid debris is removed and the pleural cavity cleaned. The mediastinal pleura is widely incised to expose the injury, and necrotic, devitalized tissue debrided (Figure 1.4). A longitudinal myotomy is made as the mucosal injury is commonly longer than the muscular one [4]. A primary suture repair is one option, using 2/0 or 3/0 interrupted absorbable sutures as a single- or two-layer closure. A small esophageal bougie or nasogastric tube can facilitate this repair. There is a high leak rate and many advocate reinforcement of the

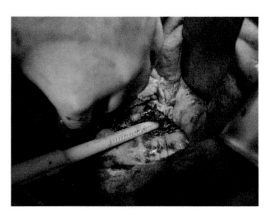

**Figure 1.4**   Intraoperative left thoracotomy view with lung retracted demonstrating dirty mediastinal pleural defect through into esophagus.

suture line with an onlay patch of nearby tissue: omentum, pleura, lung, pedicled intercostal muscle, gastric fundus, pericardium, or diaphragm. The author would suggest that, assuming the repair will leak, all primary repairs should at the very least be "covered" by placing drains around the repair.

An alternative, given the high leak rate, is to form a controlled esophagocutaneous fistula with a T-tube [5]. A large-diameter (6–10 mm) T-tube is placed through the tear with the limbs lying beyond the boundaries of the perforation and the esophageal wall closed loosely around the tube with interrupted, absorbable sutures. The tube is externalized and secured at the skin, a further drain is placed down to the repair, and apical and basal intercostal chest drains are sited. Healing is monitored by serial radiology. The T-tube is left until a defined tract is established, with the majority removed around six weeks.

Surgeons have also combined surgical drainage with endoscopic stent placement to reduce leakage from repair. The stent can be endoscopically sutured into place to prevent migration. This could help to expedite a return to enteral nutrition. Although, this leaves a foreign body within a septic field.

There may also be a role for a minimally invasive surgical approach, either laparoscopically or thoracoscopically, in cases where there is limited contamination that can be cleared in this fashion. This is obviously not the case in an unstable patient with gross soiling. This also requires advanced laparoscopic skills in specialist centres with appropriate facilities.

Our 48-year-old male patient with Boerhaave's syndrome had a CT which demonstrated significant contamination of his left pleural cavity. He was resuscitated and urgently underwent a left thoracotomy with washout and debridement, and as the tissues were unhealthy a T-tube repair was fashioned with drains placed nearby. He then underwent a laparotomy where a feeding jejunostomy and a venting gastrostomy were placed. He made a slow but steady recovery. He was eventually discharged three weeks after admission. At six weeks, in the outpatient clinic, his T-tube was removed. A month later, his feeding jejunostomy was removed after a contrast swallow and endoscopy showed complete resolution.

### KEY MESSAGES

- Spontaneous perforation of the esophagus (Boerhaave's syndrome) is a rare but rapidly fatal event.
- Diagnostic error and diagnostic delay are high.
- Flexible video endoscopic and CT scanning are the diagnostic investigations of choice.
- Criteria can be applied to guide management.
- Non-operative management is more "radical" than operative management and surgery remains the mainstay of treatment.
- Washout, debridement, and drainage are probably more important than the type of surgical repair.

### CONFLICTS OF INTEREST
None to declare.

### REFERENCES

1. Derbes VJ, Mitchell RE Jr. Hermann Boerhaave's Atrocis, nec descripti prius, morbi historia, the first translation of the classic case report of rupture of the esophagus, with annotations. *Bull Med Libr Assoc* 1955;43(2):217–240.
2. Shenfine J, Dresner SM, Vishwanath Y et al. Management of spontaneous rupture of the oesophagus. *Br J Surg* 2000;87(3):362–373.
3. Schweigert M, Beattie R, Solymosi N et al. Endoscopic stent insertion versus primary operative management for spontaneous rupture of the esophagus (Boerhaave syndrome): An international study comparing the outcome. *Am Surg* 2013 Jun;79(6):634–640.
4. Carrott PW Jr, Low DE. Advances in the management of esophageal perforation. *Thorac Surg Clin* 2011 Nov;21(4):541–555.
5. Naylor AR, Walker WS, Dark J et al. T tube intubation in the management of seriously ill patients with oesophagopleural fistulae. *Br J Surg* 1990;77(1):40–42.

## 2 Endoscopic Biopsy Demonstrating High-Grade Dysplasia in Barrett's Esophagus

*David I. Watson*

## CONTENTS

## CASE SCENARIO

A 56-year-old man with no significant comorbidities presented with a 25-year history of intermittent heartburn symptoms consistent with gastroesophageal reflux disease. Seven years earlier he sought medical care for increasingly severe heartburn and underwent a gastroduodenoscopy for the first time. At that endoscopy, Barrett's esophagus was identified, and measured to be 6 cm in maximal length with 5 cm of circumferential Barrett's esophagus and 1 cm of Barrett's "tongues" (C5M6). Biopsies from the distal esophageal mucosa confirmed Barrett's esophagus by demonstrating columnar mucosa with intestinal metaplasia, but no dysplasia. He was commenced on a program of regular surveillance endoscopy, and his reflux symptoms were managed with a proton pump inhibitor (pantoprazole 40 mg daily).

Recently, he underwent further surveillance endoscopy at which four quadrant biopsies were taken from the Barrett's esophagus segment at 2 cm intervals (three levels) commencing 1 cm above the gastroesophageal junction. The reporting pathologist identified high-grade dysplasia in two of four biopsies taken 1 cm above the gastroesophageal junction, and low-grade dysplasia in the other two biopsies at that level, and two of four from the next level – 3 cm above the gastroesophageal junction. High-grade dysplasia was confirmed by a second pathologist.

Gastroduodenoscopy was repeated four weeks later, and the Barrett's esophagus segment was carefully inspected using narrow band imaging and a high-resolution endoscope (Figures 2.1 and 2.2). No visible lesions or nodules suitable for endoscopic mucosal resection were seen. Four quadrant biopsies were collected at 1 cm intervals across the Barrett's esophagus segment, and high-grade dysplasia was confirmed in biopsies taken 1 cm and 2 cm above the gastroesophageal junction.

The patient's situation was discussed at the local multidisciplinary team meeting, and ablation of the mucosa demonstrating dysplasia using radiofrequency ablation was recommended. He was treated with radiofrequency ablation on three occasions to achieve complete eradication of the entire Barrett's esophagus segment, and resolution of the dysplasia. Follow-up endoscopies have been scheduled every three months for the next year, and six-monthly after that.

## BACKGROUND AND PATHOLOGY

Barrett's esophagus is present when the normal distal esophageal squamous mucosa is replaced by a metaplastic columnar mucosa containing goblet cells (intestinal metaplasia). This is visible at esophagoscopy by the characteristic "salmon-pink" appearance and confirmed by mucosal biopsy. It is identified at endoscopy performed to investigate suspected gastroesophageal reflux symptoms in approximately 10% of individuals and is present in 1–2% of all adults in many Western countries. Barrett's esophagus is a significant issue as it is the only known precursor to esophageal adenocarcinoma. Esophageal cancer can be of two subtypes (squamous and adenocarcinoma), with squamous cell cancer more common in Asia and many parts of the world. Esophageal adenocarcinoma is an increasingly important problem, mainly in Western developed countries, where its incidence has increased more than six-fold over the last four decades. It now accounts for 70–80% of esophageal cancers diagnosed in Australia, UK, and the United States. Barrett's esophagus is the identifiable

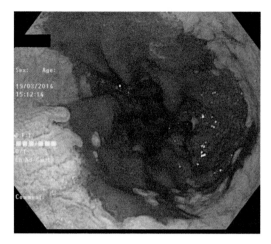

**Figure 2.1** Barrett's esophagus. The photograph shows the proximal margin of the Barrett's esophagus, below which are some islands of squamous mucosa.

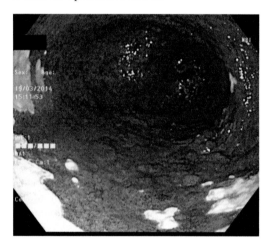

**Figure 2.2** Narrow band imaging view of the same segment of Barrett's esophagus.

intermediate step in the development of esophageal adenocarcinoma.

Barrett's esophagus was previously defined by the length of metaplastic mucosa requiring a minimum length of 3 cm. However, in recent times, even shorter lengths are considered to be Barrett's esophagus. In published guidelines from Australia and the United States, the presence of intestinal metaplasia is required for diagnosis, whereas UK guidelines do not require this.

Non-dysplastic Barrett's esophagus can progress to low-grade dysplasia, high-grade dysplasia, and then to esophageal adenocarcinoma in a stepwise fashion, or it can sometimes bypass the low-grade dysplasia or high-grade dysplasiastep and progress

directly to cancer. As progression to cancer generally takes years, current management entails surveillance endoscopy to identify dysplasia or early cancer when endoscopic treatment options are likely to be feasible and effective. Progression to cancer is more likely in men (risk doubled), individuals with longer segments of Barrett's esophagus, and in those who develop dysplasia [1]. Barrett's esophagus and progression to cancer is also more likely in obese individuals and in those with poorly controlled reflux symptoms [2]. The annual risk of progression from high-grade dysplasia to cancer is estimated to be approximately 8–10%/year. Some form of intervention is indicated in most individuals in whom high-grade dysplasia is identified. The significance of low-grade dysplasia is less clear, partly due to difficulties with pathological diagnosis resulting from significant differences in opinion between different pathologists. When low-grade dysplasia is diagnosed in a community setting, the risk of progression appears to be between 1.5–2%/year. However, in the control arm from a Dutch randomized trial of ablation vs surveillance for low-grade dysplasia, the rate of progression to early cancer in the surveillance arm was 9% [3]. In this trial, though, confirmation of low-grade dysplasia was required from a panel of three pathologists, and the majority of community diagnoses of low-grade dysplasia were not confirmed by that panel, and not included in the trial.

## APPROACH TO MANAGEMENT

Most individuals diagnosed with high-grade dysplasia should be offered treatment which aims to remove or destroy (ablate) the Barrett's esophagus mucosal segment, and thereby prevent progression to cancer. Almost all individuals will be fit for endoscopic therapies. However, if surgical resection is to be considered, and it is occasionally appropriate, additional consideration then needs to be given to the individual patient's age, fitness, and comorbidities.

Prior to intervention, accurate estimation of the Barrett's esophagus segment is warranted coupled with the diagnosis of high-grade dysplasia confirmed by two pathologists on two consecutive biopsies obtained at the time of endoscopy or endoscopic mucosal resection. The Barrett's esophagus segment should be carefully examined for its mucosal pattern, any mucosal irregularities, and nodules, and suspicious areas should be targeted for additional biopsies or endoscopic mucosal resection (Figure 2.3). Before proceeding to definitive therapy, review and discussion in an upper

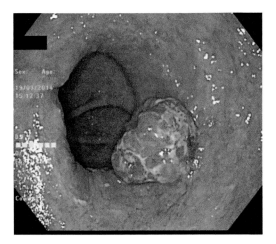

**Figure 2.3**  Barrett's esophagus with nodule. This nodule was excised by endoscopic mucosa resection and pathology confirmed stage T1a adenocarcinoma.

gastrointestinal cancer multidisciplinary team meeting is advised.

### Symptoms and signs

There are no specific clinical signs or symptoms that are pathognomonic of Barrett's esophagus or high-grade dysplasia. Clinical trials are underway evaluating an alternative diagnostic strategy that can be applied in the community setting, namely, the Cytosponge. At the present time, Barrett's esophagus is identified incidentally in patients who undergo endoscopy, usually in the context of investigation of symptoms of gastroesophageal reflux disease (heartburn and/or regurgitation). Barrett's esophagus is usually present at the first endoscopy, and in most individuals its length is relatively stable over time, suggesting that the metaplastic change occurs early in susceptible individuals.

### Investigations

Endoscopy underpins diagnosis. Once diagnosed patients are usually enrolled in regular endoscopic surveillance programs. Published guidelines from Australia, UK, and the United States describe standard surveillance programs [4–6]. Some guidelines stratify for risk and recommend less frequent surveillance in low-risk individuals. Generally, for individuals with longer (≥3 cm) segments of Barrett's esophagus a surveillance interval of 2–3 years is recommended, with a longer interval of 3–5 years reserved for those with shorter segments (≤2 cm). These intervals are based on expert opinion rather than high-level evidence. If low-grade dysplasia is diagnosed, most

endoscopists recommend a repeat endoscopy in six months. However, guidelines now allow for ablation in higher-risk individuals within the low-grade dysplasia cohort.

Irrespective of the endoscopy surveillance interval, it is important to apply a structured strategy to inspection of the Barrett's esophagus segment and collection of mucosal biopsies. Narrow band imaging and high-resolution endoscopy, coupled with thorough inspection, facilitate the identification of suspicious areas within the segment. The Seattle protocol, or a modified version, is recommended. This entails careful inspection with targeted biopsy of any suspicious areas within the Barrett's esophagus segment, followed by four quadrant (i.e. 3, 6, 9, and 12 o'clock) biopsies commencing 1 cm above the gastroesophageal junction and extending proximally at 2 cm intervals for the full length of the Barrett's esophagus segment. A lot of biopsies will be collected from long segments. For example, at least 20 biopsies should be collected from a 10 cm length. The endoscopist must avoid cutting corners in these patients, as those with the longer segments are at a higher risk of cancer. The aim of surveillance is to identify individuals in whom the mucosa demonstrates high-grade dysplasia or, worse still, stage T1a cancer, when endoscopic therapy is likely to be curative.

### Treatment options

Traditionally, the treatment for Barrett's esophagus entailed an esophagectomy for individuals with high-grade dysplasia or early stage cancer. However, comorbidities and advancing age have limited esophagectomy to a subset of younger and fitter individuals. The development of endoscopic interventions over the last two decades offers the option of lower risk interventions which can be applied to a wider population, including elderly and less fit patients. Current management now prioritizes endoscopic therapy as the first choice in patients diagnosed with high-grade dysplasia.

The principle underpinning endoscopic treatments is that destruction of the metaplastic columnar mucosa, in the absence of gastroesophageal reflux, is usually followed by healing with a neosquamous epithelium, and this is associated with a much lower risk of progression to cancer. Ablation can be achieved by thermal destruction using radiofrequency ablation, cryotherapy, and argon plasma coagulation, or by endoscopic excision using endoscopic mucosal resection or endoscopic submucosal dissection. In general, excision is used to fully ablate shorter (<3 cm) lengths of Barrett's esophagus, or to remove areas of concern within longer lengths for pathological analysis, before applying thermal ablation to the remaining segment.

Complete ablation of longer segments is best achieved by thermal ablation. radiofrequency ablation is the most commonly applied technique. It uses proprietary single use equipment to burn and destroy the mucosa, but not submucosa, of the distal esophagus. Devices can be used to treat the full circumference of the esophagus or targeted areas. Generally, 2–3 treatment sessions are required to ablate the Barrett's segment. Argon plasma coagulation is sometimes used as a cheaper alternative to radiofrequency ablation to deal with smaller residual areas of Barrett's esophagus following initial circumferential ablation.

Endoscopic mucosal resection entails targeting an area of concern, creation of a pseudopolyp, and using a snare and electocautery to excise a 1–2 cm diameter piece of the esophageal mucosa. Multiple excisions can be performed in a piecemeal fashion to excise larger areas of Barrett's esophagus. Endoscopic submucosal dissection can be used to excise larger areas *en bloc*. However, endoscopic submucosal dissection is operator-dependent, and has a longer learning curve than endoscopic mucosal resection. Hence, it is less commonly applied in the context of Barrett's esophagus.

A randomized trial has demonstrated the efficacy of radiofrequency ablation for ablation and prevention of progression to cancer [7]. This trial demonstrated a reduction in disease progression (high-grade dysplasia to cancer, or low-grade dysplasia to high-grade dysplasia) from 16.3 to 3.6% at 12 months following radiofrequency ablation ablation. However, the risk of development of cancer still remains, and lifelong endoscopic surveillance is recommended following ablation. Endoscopic mucosal resection also appears to be effective for short segments of Barrett's esophagus, and has the advantage of providing specimens which can be analysed by a pathologist for the presence of cancer and completeness of excision. In some patients, where a very early cancer is identified at endoscopic mucosal resection, endoscopic excision is likely to be curative. If confined to the mucosa (T1a), and not exhibiting any high-risk features (e.g. poor differentiation), the risk of metastasis to lymph nodes and beyond is very low. However, if invading into the submucosa or showing high risk features, lymph node metastases will be present in at least 20% of individuals, and more than 50% in some subsets. These patients need to be considered for alternative treatments such as esophagectomy, radiotherapy, and chemotherapy.

As endoscopic therapies preserve the intact esophagus, they are believed to offer a better quality of life compared to an esophagectomy. However, they are not without the risk of complications. Although uncommon, mucosal excision can be complicated acutely by bleeding and esophageal perforation. Esophageal strictures have been reported following circumferential excision of the Barrett's segment in a single treatment session. While these strictures generally respond to serial endoscopic dilations, they contribute to the morbidity of endoscopic therapy. Quite rarely, thermal ablation may be complicated by stricture formation and perforation, albeit less frequently than following endoscopic resection.

Important to the success of ablation is control of the gastroesophageal reflux associated with Barrett's esophagus. Ablation destroys the metaplastic columnar mucosa and allows regeneration of a new mucosa, probably from stem cells in the submucosal layer. The environment in which this new epithelium arises is likely to drive the direction of mucosal differentiation, and good control of reflux appears to improve the likelihood of development of a neosquamous mucosa. High-dose proton pump inhibitor therapy is generally the minimum required (e.g. pantoprazole 40 mg twice daily). In patients in whom reflux is difficult to control and ablative therapies seem less effective, a fundoplication is occasionally needed to adequately control reflux and facilitate successful ablation. Rarely, in individuals with very long Barrett's esophagus segments or in whom ablation has been unsuccessful, the performance of an esophagectomy merits consideration. Surgical resection will cure the Barrett's esophagus and eliminate the risk of recurrent high-grade dysplasia or subsequent cancer but is associated with significant morbidity and the risk of mortality, so can no longer be recommended as the first-line treatment for high-grade dysplasia.

To manage the risk of recurrence (noted in case reports and some large case series), ongoing surveillance is required following ablation. The timing of this follow-up is essentially guided by expert opinion. There are a few long-term outcome studies available and the risk of recurrence of Barrett's esophagus with high-grade dysplasia or T1a cancer is unknown, especially beyond five years. At the present time, expert consensus recommends follow-up for life. Initial endoscopy at three monthly intervals is standard, but with time this can almost certainly be lengthened. The author currently arranges endoscopy six monthly after the first year, and then yearly from five years. However, there is little evidence to support this protocol, or any protocol that advocates more frequent or less frequent endoscopy.

At follow-up endoscopy, the ablated segment should be carefully inspected, and any abnormality biopsied. Most recurrences occur below the new squamo-columnar junction, in areas of residual Barrett's esophagus, or in islands of residual metaplastic columnar mucosa, and these areas should be targeted for surveillance biopsies. Any significant lesions should be treated on their merits. The author's experience is that radiofrequency ablation ablation can "weld" the distal esophageal mucosa to the esophageal muscle and render subsequent endoscopic mucosal resection procedures difficult or even impossible. In these patients, treatment might need to proceed down a surgical or radiotherapy pathway.

## KEY MESSAGES

- Barrett's esophagus progresses to adenocarcinoma via dysplasia, with high grade dysplasia being the last step before invasive cancer.
- To identify high-grade dysplasia, individuals with known Barrett's esophagus must undergo endoscopic surveillance in a structured program with an appropriate biopsy protocol (e.g. Seattle protocol).
- Individuals diagnosed with high-grade dysplasia are usually offered endoscopic treatment to prevent progression to cancer. This entails ablation of the Barrett's esophagus segment by either thermal ablation, endoscopic resection, or a combination of both.

- Ablation can occasionally be followed by complications such as stricture formation or perforation, and a risk of recurrence or cancer remains, albeit a lower risk than if not ablated. To address this, lifetime endoscopic follow-up is required after ablation of high-grade dysplasia.

## REFERENCES

1. Lindblad M, Bright T, Schloithe A et al. Toward more efficient surveillance of Barrett's esophagus: Identification and exclusion of patients at low risk of cancer. *World J Surg* 2017;41(4):1023–1034.
2. Smith KJ, O'Brien SM, Smithers BM et al. Interactions among smoking, obesity, and symptoms of acid reflux in Barrett's esophagus. *Cancer Epidemiol Biomarkers Prev* 2005;14(11 Pt 1):2481–2486.
3. Phoa KN, van Vilsteren FG, Weusten BL et al. Radiofrequency ablation vs endoscopic surveillance for patients with Barrett esophagus and low-grade dysplasia: A randomized clinical trial. *JAMA* 2014;311(12):1209–1217.
4. Whiteman DC, Appleyard M, Bahin FF et al. Australian clinical practice guidelines for the diagnosis and management of Barrett's Oesophagus and Early Oesophageal Adenocarcinoma. *J Gastroenterol Hepatol* 2015;30(5):804–820.
5. Fitzgerald RC, di Pietro M, Ragunath K et al. British Society of Gastroenterology guidelines on the diagnosis and management of Barrett's esophagus. *Gut* 2014;63(1):7–42.
6. Wang KK, Sampliner RE. Updated guidelines 2008 for the diagnosis, surveillance and therapy of Barrett's esophagus. *Am J Gastroenterol* 2008;103(3):788–797.
7. Shaheen NJ, Sharma P, Overholt BF et al. Radiofrequency ablation in Barrett's esophagus with dysplasia. *NEJM* 2009;360(22):2277–2288.

# 3 Dysphagia Six Weeks Following Accidental Corrosive Ingestion

*Vikram Kate, R. Kalayarasan, and N. Ananthakrishnan*

## CONTENTS

## CASE SCENARIO

A 25-year-old man presented to the emergency ward due to accidental ingestion of approximately 100 ml of toilet cleaner under the influence of alcohol. Post-ingestion, the patient had retrosternal pain and odynophagia. He did not report difficulty in breathing, induced vomiting, or hematemesis. On examination, there was mild erythema of the posterior pharyngeal wall and there were no signs of peritonitis on abdominal examination. He was managed conservatively with parenteral antibiotics, proton pump inhibitors, and intravenous fluids. He did not undergo endoscopy during the acute phase (as this is the practice in the authors' unit) and no nasogastric tube was placed. Five days following admission the patient was allowed high-protein oral liquids which he tolerated with difficulty due to odynophagia. He was discharged one week after admission with a planned follow-up. Post-discharge, the patient was able to tolerate oral liquids with difficulty but had dysphagia to solids. Four weeks after corrosive ingestion, the patient began to notice a progressive increase in dysphagia to liquids, and at six weeks, he presented to the outpatient department with absolute dysphagia to oral liquids.

## BACKGROUND

The two important factors that determine the extent of the injury following corrosive ingestion are the nature (acid versus alkali) and the amount of substance ingested. Alkalis, by producing liquefaction necrosis, increase the likelihood of transmural injuries often accompanied by periesophageal injury with damage to adjacent organs such as the respiratory tract. Acids, except for hydrofluoric acid, usually cause coagulation necrosis and the transmural spread is limited by the coagulum formed in response to acid ingestion thereby reducing the incidence of full-thickness injury.

The clinical outcome of corrosive ingestions depends upon the extent of the initial injury. While mild injuries involving only the mucosa usually heal without any sequelae, moderate injuries extending beyond mucosa results in esophageal stricture. Perforation in the acute phase or dense undilatable stricture in the recovery phase is a common manifestation of severe transmural injuries. Following ingestion of corrosive substances, the tissue injury goes through three phases. The acute necrotic phase (phase 1) characterized by cell necrosis which lasts for 24–72 hours, followed by the second phase of ulceration and granulation that lasts for three to twelve days. The stricture formation that results in cicatrisation and scarring (phase 3) begins approximately three weeks after the initial injury and can continue for three to six months or longer in some instances. As the esophagus is at its weakest point during the ulceration and granulation phase (phase 2), invasive diagnostic (endoscopy), and therapeutic (dilation or stenting) procedures should be avoided during this phase. Injury to the small bowel is uncommon after corrosive ingestion as reflex pyloric spasm limits the passage of the corrosive substance into the small bowel. However, this protective mechanism is lost in patients with ingestion of a large quantity of corrosive substance or those with a history of prior gastric surgeries, such as pyloroplasty or gastroenterostomy, which may result in damage to the small bowel.

## APPROACH TO MANAGEMENT
### Clinical features

The clinical features depend upon the phase and severity of injury. In the acute phase, patients present with odynophagia, drooling of saliva due to dysphagia, ulceration of the lips, tongue, and oral cavity mucosa. Airway involvement can result in stridor requiring emergency tracheostomy. Intent of ingestion of corrosive substances also determines the clinical presentation. In suicidal ingestion, patients have an idea of what they are taking that often produces initial hesitancy resulting in extensive damage to the upper aerodigestive tract. Accidental ingestion is associated with intake of a relatively large quantity of corrosive substance as the patients are unaware of what they are taking resulting in esophageal and gastric injury. Vomiting, common with gastric injury, aggravates esophageal damage due to regurgitated corrosives. Hematemesis, although rare, is a manifestation of gastric injury. Chest pain, pleural effusion, and mediastinitis suggest esophageal perforation while peritonitis indicates transmural gastric injury with perforation.

Patients with moderate and severe injuries develop strictures in the chronic phase. Dysphagia is a typical feature of esophageal stricture and gastric outlet obstruction is a manifestation of an isolated gastric stricture. However, it is important to understand that typical symptom of gastric outlet obstruction may not be present in patients with a coexistent gastric and esophageal stricture. It has been observed that patients who develop strictures within six to eight weeks of corrosive ingestion progress rapidly compared to those who develop later strictures.

## Investigations

A barium or water-soluble (Gastrografin) contrast study would be the initial investigation in the patient described above since he presented with dysphagia six weeks after corrosive ingestion. In the acute setting, if there is no clinical suspicion of esophageal perforation (no fever, tachypnea, or subcutaneous crepitus) barium is preferred over water-soluble contrast as it allows better delineation of the location and extent of the stricture. Furthermore, even if the patient aspirates the contrast, barium does not cause aspiration pneumonitis commonly seen with water-soluble contrast agents. A barium study provides a roadmap for diagnostic and therapeutic endoscopy. Important points to note in the barium study that can influence further management are the upper extent of esophageal stricture, number of strictures, length of esophageal stricture, presence of sacculation, or tracheoesophageal fistula. The presence of these features predicts poor response to endoscopic dilation. The limitations of a barium study are that it cannot determine the extent of esophageal involvement in patients with pharyngeal stricture and it cannot reliably rule out gastric stricture if the patient cannot swallow enough contrast due to coexistent esophageal stricture.

If the barium study shows evidence of pharyngeal stricture, computed tomography (CT) of the neck and chest after air swallowing with sagittal and coronal reconstruction is a useful investigation to document the length of the stricture and the presence of patent distal esophageal lumen [1]. The presence of a patent distal esophageal lumen facilitates anastomosis below crico-pharynx after appropriate management of pharyngeal stricture with a good long-term outcome.

At six weeks, a transnasal flexible fiberoptic laryngoscopy evaluation by the otolaryngologist is essential to evaluate the mobility of epiglottis, aryepiglottic folds, pyriform sinus, and false and true vocal cords. The presence of pharyngeal adhesions indicates the need for adhesiolysis, and extensive airway involvement increases the chance of permanent tracheostomy.

An erect abdominal X-ray after overnight fasting is a simple investigation to determine gastric stricture in the present patient with a coexistent esophageal stricture [2]. The presence of gastric fluid level is diagnostic of gastric stricture with gastric outlet obstruction. Diagnosis of coexistent gastric stricture has important therapeutic implications.

At six weeks, an upper gastrointestinal endoscopy is primarily used to assess the degree of inflammation of esophageal mucosa and the feasibility of dilation.

Complete blood count, serum electrolytes, and serum albumin should be performed to assess the current nutritional and hydration status.

## Management

The management of the patient described focussed on nutritional optimization as well as management of the stricture, per se.

The need for an enteral feeding access depends upon the feasibility of endoscopic dilation. In the presence of a dilatable esophageal stricture without a coexistent gastric stricture, the patient can be managed on high-protein, high-calorie oral nutritional supplements till the stricture stabilizes with endoscopic dilation. However, if the stricture is not dilatable, then the patient needs enteral feeding access as no definitive surgical procedure can be performed at six weeks after corrosive ingestion. Feeding jejunostomy is preferred over feeding gastrostomy as a coexistent gastric stricture is not uncommon. Even in the absence of a gastric stricture, a feeding gastrostomy is avoided as it makes the use of the stomach as a conduit for esophageal bypass very difficult, if required in the future.

In corrosive stricture, definitive surgery is usually delayed from six months to one year to allow for the inflammation to settle and the stricture to stabilize. Hence, at six weeks, the management of the stricture is primarily non-operative in the form of endoscopic dilation. Specially designed biodegradable stents made of poly(L-lactide) or polydioxanone, although theoretically appealing, are not routinely used in view of cost, limited success rate (<50%), and high incidence of stent migration (10–25%). Endoscopic dilation can be done using either bougies (like Savary-Gilliard dilators) or through-the-scope balloon dilators. Dilation using Savary-Gilliard dilators under fluoroscopic guidance is ideal for long strictures as they offer the physician the advantage of a tactile feeling of dilation occurring in real time. The through-the-scope balloon dilators allow easy manipulation and enable dilation under vision. If repeated, endoscopic dilatation at two to three week intervals can achieve an esophageal lumen size of approximately 15 mm. With symptomatic relief of dysphagia, it becomes a definitive treatment option. However, in a significant number of patients, especially those with high pharyngeal strictures, endoscopic dilation is used as a bridge procedure to facilitate definitive surgical management. Synechiolysis under laryngoscopic guidance might be required before endoscopic dilation to identify the esophageal lumen. As endoscopic dilation for high cricopharyngeal strictures can cause airway compression and respiratory compromize during dilatation, a right neck exploration and esophagostomy might be required to perform repeated dilation using Savary-Gilliard dilators [3].

If the endoscopic dilatation is not feasible, then definitive surgical treatment is performed after six to twelve months depending upon the level of stricture, with a longer delay preferred for pharyngeal stricture. The colon is the preferred conduit, and the use of the ascending branch of the left colic artery-based mid-colon conduit has many advantages [4]. It has a consistent and good vascular supply and can accommodate anatomical variations as it is not based on preconceived vascular pedicles. Also, there is no problem of length even for high pharyngeal strictures.

The retrosternal route is the preferred route as the native esophagus is generally not resected. Large series have shown that the risk of malignancy in the native esophagus and esophageal mucocele are negligible. Patients with pharyngeal strictures refractory to dilation usually require a staged procedure in the form of pectoralis major or sternocleidomastoid myocutaneous flap to create a neocervical esophagus followed by a colonic bypass [3].

Similarly, patients with a coexistent gastric stricture require a staged procedure [5]. In patients with a distal gastric stricture, Billroth I gastrectomy is preferred over gastrojejunostomy as the first stage procedure as gastrojejunostomy can make future colonic bypass difficult. If gastrojejunostomy must be performed, the retrocolic route should be avoided as it can interfere with the colonic vascular arcade and preclude future colonic bypass. In patients with high gastric or total gastric stricture, jejunum is used for distal colonic anastomosis instead of the stomach. Total gastrectomy can be performed in relatively well-preserved patients while the stomach can be left in situ without major long-term sequences in patients with poor general condition.

The feasibility of laparoscopic Billroth I gastrectomy and laparoscopic colon bypass have been reported in the literature. However, these procedures, especially colonic bypass, is technically challenging, and a small technical error can have a devastating effect on the viability of colon conduit. Hence, minimally invasive approaches should be restricted to centers with extensive experience in advanced laparoscopic procedures. An algorithmic approach to the surgical management of corrosive esophageal stricture is depicted in Figure 3.1. In addition to the surgical management, patients with a history of ingestion with suicidal intention need a comprehensive psychological evaluation and appropriate treatment to prevent future suicidal attempts.

## KEY MESSAGES

- A barium swallow study is the important investigation in patients presenting with dysphagia secondary to corrosive stricture.
- Coexistent gastric stricture should be ruled out in patients with esophageal stricture.
- In the early chronic phase, endoscopic dilatation and establishing feeding access is the mainstay of treatment. Leaving a nasogastric tube in the esophagus after dilatation ensures that there is a residual passage to permit future dilation.
- The ascending branch of left colic artery-based mid-colon conduit is the preferred conduit for esophageal bypass.
- Patients with pharyngeal and coexistent gastric stricture usually required a staged treatment.

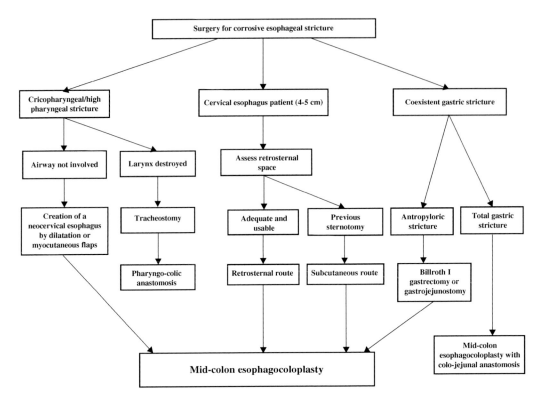

**Figure 3.1**  Algorithmic approach for the surgical management of corrosive stricture of the esophagus and stomach.

## REFERENCES

1. Ananthakrishnan N, Parthasarathy G, Kate V. Use of spiral CT to demonstrate esophageal lumen in corrosive strictures. *Indian J Gastroenterol* 2007;26(2):101.
2. Ananthakrishnan N, Parthasarathy G, Kate V. Gastric fluid level after overnight fast: Test to diagnose gastric outlet obstruction in corrosive esophageal stricture. *Indian J Gastroenterol* 2006;25(5):269–270.
3. Ananthakrishnan N, Kate V, Parthasarathy G. Therapeutic options for management of pharyngoesophageal corrosive strictures. *J Gastrointest Surg* 2011;15(4):566–575.
4. Ananthakrishnan N, Subbarao KSVK, Parthasarathy G et al. Long term results of esophageal bypass for corrosive strictures without esophageal resection using a modified left colon esophagocoloplasty—A report of 105 consecutive patients from a single unit over thirty years. *Hepatogastroenterology* 2014;61(132):1033–1041.
5. Ananthakrishnan N, Parthasarathy G, Kate V. Chronic corrosive injuries of the stomach—A single unit experience of 109 patients over thirty years. *World J Surg* 2010;34(4):758–764.

# 4 Symptomatic Giant Hiatal Hernia with Intrathoracic Stomach

*Tim Bright*

## CONTENTS

## CASE SCENARIO

A 75-year-old woman presented to the emergency department with severe chest pain and retching. After an electrocardiogram and blood tests ruled out a cardiac cause, a chest X-ray was performed and a large retrocardiac air-fluid level was noted, consistent with a hiatal hernia. On further history, the patient reported that on several occasions she had experienced milder episodes of a similar chest pain after eating, which lasted up to 30 minutes. The patient noted some mild dysphagia to solids over the last 12 months, and her spouse noted that she appeared to be eating more slowly and only consuming smaller meal portions. She was otherwise fit and well, with a proton pump inhibitor as her only regular medication. She had no history of previous abdominal surgery. The patient remembered having had an endoscopy some years ago which noted a "large" hiatal hernia.

## BACKGROUND OF THE PATHOLOGY

A hiatal hernia is an abnormal protrusion of some, or even all, of the stomach into the thoracic cavity via the esophageal hiatus. Hiatal herniae are subcategorized into four types. The overwhelming majority of hiatal herniae are type I (sliding), which involves displacement of the gastroesophageal junction above the esophageal hiatus but the fundus remaining in the abdomen. Type II (paraesophageal) involves herniation of the gastric fundus through the esophageal hiatus while the gastroesophageal junction remains at the level of the hiatus. Type III (mixed) is a combination of type I and type II herniae where both the gastroesophageal junction and the fundus have herniated into the chest. Type IV herniae can be any of the above but occur when other structures, such as colon or small bowel, are found in the hernia sac [1]. While generally presenting de novo, a proportion may be recurrent following previous attempted hiatal hernia repair or anti-reflux surgery.

Gastric volvulus is a rare complication of a hiatal hernia (Figure 4.1) and involves rotation or twisting of the stomach along either its long axis (organo-axial volvulus) or its short axis (mesentero-axial volvulus). A "giant hiatal" hernia suggests at least 30–50% of the stomach is in an intrathoracic position, with the author favoring >50% to be the definition. Other definitions include an endoscopic length of 6 cm for the hernia or an intercrural defect of 5 cm at the time of surgery.

## CLINICAL FINDINGS

### Symptoms and signs

Typically, patients with large hiatal herniae have symptoms related to reflux and/or symptoms related to mechanical obstruction, and only occasionally symptoms related to an acute volvulus. A surprising number of patients with large herniae will have noted minimal, if any, symptoms.

A history of reflux typically involves volume reflux and heartburn. Atypical symptoms of reflux, such as cough, sore throat, hoarse voice, or dental pathology, are very unreliably improved with hiatal hernia repair and should not be used as indications for surgery.

Large hiatal herniae often cause a degree of obstruction. Patients describe dysphagia and/

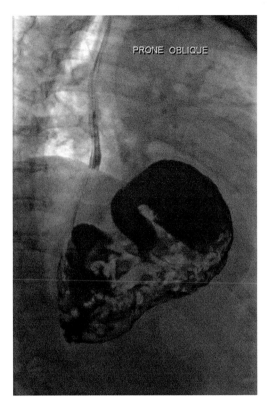

**Figure 4.1** Gastrografin swallow demonstrating an intrathoracic stomach with volvulus.

or odynophagia. As a result, patients modify their diet to avoid solids like bread or meat, and chew their food more thoroughly. They eat smaller meals and eat them more slowly. This is associated with early satiety, but rarely weight loss. Because these dietary changes are often subtle and long term, patients require direct questioning to elucidate these symptoms.

While patients often ascribe shortness of breath and breathing difficulties to their hernia, even very large herniae have little impact on respiratory function. Shortness of breath may be related to cardiac compression secondary to gastric distension in the hiatal hernia [2]. It is important to determine whether the shortness of breath is specifically post-prandial in nature, rather than more continual/chronic. Shortness of breath/fatigue are occasionally reproduced by the patient bending forward, again presumably via cardiac compression.

Patients often note a low retrosternal pain (like a ball or a fist in their chest) during a meal which causes them to stop eating while they wait for it to pass. Patients may belch to relieve the pain, but occasionally vomiting will be

required to resolve the symptoms. If the pain is severe or lasts greater than 30 minutes it is very concerning that the patient has a significant gastric volvulus.

Clinical signs with a giant hiatus hernia are often lacking. A minority of patients will have epigastric tenderness on deep palpation, but most will have no signs at all. In those patients presenting emergently with a gastric volvulus, epigastric tenderness is more common. These patients may also have signs of dehydration secondary to vomiting or poor oral intake and occasionally systemic toxicity if there is significant gastric ischemia. They may be retching in an attempt to relieve the volvulus.

As part of the routine patient examination, it is important to assess the patient's general body habitus and the presence of abdominal surgical scars as this may alter the surgical access approach.

## INVESTIGATIONS

Often, patients will present with radiology performed to investigate other problems that incidentally noted a large hiatal hernia. However, all patients require an up-to-date endoscopy prior to deciding on surgical repair. This enables an accurate assessment of the size of the hiatal hernia, the type, and any pathology associated with the hernia, such as reflux esophagitis, Barrett's esophagus, or a Cameron lesion. It is important to rule out any other coexisting significant pathology given that herniae are often long standing, and the presenting complaint of dysphagia or anemia may be relatively recent.

A barium swallow is a useful, although not mandatory, investigation. It enables accurate assessment of the size of the hernia and often provides a degree of functional assessment in that poor emptying, or actual partial volvulus, of the hiatal hernia may be noted.

In patients with severe shortness of breath, formal pulmonary function testing is recommended to assist both pre-anesthetic assessment and deciding how likely the hernia is contributing to the patient's symptoms. Similarly, in patients with chest pain, a cardiac assessment to rule out cardiac causes needs to be considered.

Patients with giant hiatal herniae rarely present with isolated reflux symptoms. However, for those who do, and in whom no objective signs of reflux are seen at endoscopy, formal esophageal pH studies should be undertaken to confirm pathological reflux before recommending surgical repair. Manometry is rarely contributory in patients with giant hiatal hernia as a cardiopexy or partial fundoplication only are used in the surgical repair.

For patients fully investigated with endoscopy, colonoscopy, and pill camera where no other cause for iron deficiency can be found, surgical repair of a large hiatal hernia can resolve iron deficiency in around 40% of patients. While Cameron lesions are a likely source of chronic blood loss, they do not have to be seen at endoscopy before proceeding to repair.

## TREATMENT OPTIONS

Emergency and elective presentations dictate different approaches.

### In the emergency setting

The first step is to achieve gastric decompression. This can generally be achieved at the bedside with the help of a nasogastric tube. Successful venting of the stomach should be confirmed both by a chest X-ray demonstrating the nasogastric tube within the stomach, and resolution of the acute chest pain and/or retching. If this cannot be achieved at the bedside, then an endoscopy is required to decompress the stomach, accompanied by the placement of a nasogastric tube under vision. Close liaison with an anesthetist is mandatory as these patients are at high risk of an aspiration event at the time of sedation or endotracheal tube placement. This procedure should be undertaken urgently, as would be appropriate for any other condition involving the likelihood of ischemia of the bowel.

For patients in whom an emergency decompression has been achieved, it is recommended that surgical repair of the hiatal hernia not be undertaken immediately but be deferred for a period of several days to up to two weeks. This will allow the patient to recover from the acute event and be fully optimized. It will allow edema of the hernia to settle, making subsequent surgery safer. In obese patients, this period of waiting may allow them to be started on a very low calorie diet in an attempt to shrink the left lobe of the liver, thereby improving surgical access. This period will also permit a more considered discussion with the patient and family as to the risks and benefits of surgery, given that a number of these patients will be very elderly and may not be fit for surgical repair. This group may be better managed with dietary modification (vitamized diet) and instructions to return to their nearest emergency department for placement of a nasogastric tube should their volvulus symptoms return.

### In the elective setting

Most patients being assessed electively will have symptoms. In the truly asymptomatic herniae, the risks of an elective repair must be weighed up against the risks of a future presentation with gastric volvulus requiring emergency repair. In patients under the age of 65 who are otherwise fit, elective repair of an asymptomatic giant hiatal hernia can probably be justified compared to the more conservative "watch and wait" approach in older patients [3]. All patients need to understand the potential for wind (bloating, increased flatulence, and diminished ability to belch) and dysphagia-related side effects after hiatal hernia repair, as well as a 5% rate of future revisional surgery. They can, however, be reassured that >90% of patients at five years postoperatively are highly satisfied with the results of surgery [4].

### Principles of surgical repair

Surgical repair in either the emergency or elective situation is performed the same way. A laparoscopic approach is preferred whenever feasible, with a low rate (2%) of conversion to open surgery expected. The hernial sac must be excised from the hiatal pillars before being reduced entirely with its contents. The sac does not need to be excised from the stomach. An interrupted non-absorbable (e.g. 2/0 Novafil®) suture repair of the hiatal defect posteriorly should then occur. If greater than five hiatal repair sutures are required posteriorly, care should be taken to avoid anterior angulation of the esophagus over the repair, and anterior sutures may need to be placed if further hiatal closure is required. A 52- or 54-Fr bougie can be used to calibrate the repair. There is no evidence that the addition of either absorbable or non-absorbable mesh to the hiatal crural repair reduces long-term revisional surgery rates [5]. While the "short esophagus" has been described historically, the author has never encountered the situation where the gastro-esophageal junction cannot be easily situated in the abdominal cavity. Theoretically, a Collis gastroplasty can be used if such a situation were ever encountered. Once the hiatal repair is appropriately snug around the esophagus, the gastroesophageal junction is secured in the abdominal cavity. This can be done with a combination of esophagopexy sutures to the hiatal rim, and either an anterior cardiopexy or partial fundoplication. Formal fundoplication is only required for those with significant reflux symptoms.

Postoperatively, patients can be started on free fluids. Perioperative antiemetics should be prescribed routinely to avoid postoperative nausea and retching. A water-soluble contrast study should be performed on day one after surgery to confirm the intra-abdominal position of the stomach. While only 1–2% of patients are likely to have an acute asymptomatic failure of the repair, it is much easier and safer to repair this in the first few days postoperatively than if diagnosed later.

## CASE SCENARIO

The patient described in the Case Scenario had a nasogastric tube placed with immediate venting of gastric contents and symptomatic relief. She was commenced on free fluids the following day and the nasogastric tube was clamped. Having demonstrated the ability to tolerate free fluids, the nasogastric tube was removed, the patient commenced on a vitamized diet, and was discharged home. She was readmitted electively for a laparoscopic hiatal hernia repair (Figure 4.2) with fundoplication (Figure 4.3) which was performed uneventfully. A day one postoperative contrast study confirmed an intact fundoplication in a subdiaphragmatic location (Figure 4.4). She was commenced on a vitamized diet and discharged the following day with instructions to remain on a vitamized diet until review in the outpatient clinic in one month.

### SALIENT POINTS

- Giant hiatal herniae are increasingly encountered in the elderly population with the general increase in radiological investigations performed.
- If a thorough history is taken, very few giant hiatal herniae will truly be asymptomatic.

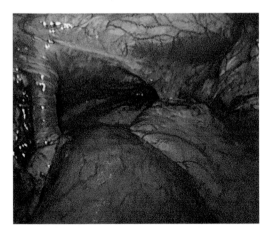

**Figure 4.2** Intraoperative photograph of a large hiatal hernia.

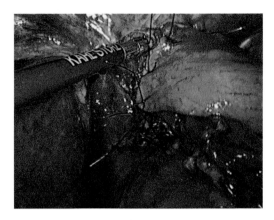

**Figure 4.3** Intraoperative photograph of completed repair.

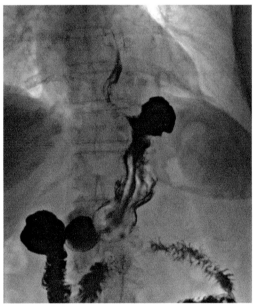

**Figure 4.4** Day one postoperative contrast study with a subdiaphragmatic intact fundoplication.

- Acute presentation with gastric volvulus is a surgical emergency and requires urgent decompression with a nasogastric tube to avoid gastric ischemia.
- A laparoscopic approach with suture repair of the hiatus is ideal.
- A day one postoperative contrast swallow to confirm the integrity of the repair is worthwhile.

## CONFLICTS OF INTEREST

None to declare.

## REFERENCES

1. Kohn GP, Price RR, DeMeester SR et al. Guidelines for the management of hiatal hernia. *Surg Endosc* 2013 Dec;27(12):4409–4428.
2. Naoum C, Falk GL, Ng AC et al. Left atrial compression and the mechanism of exercise impairment in patients with a large hiatal hernia. *J Am Coll Cardiol* 2011 Oct 4;58(15):1624–1634.
3. Stylopoulos N, Gazelle GS, Rattner DW. Paraesophageal hernias: Operation or observation? *Ann Surg* 2002 Oct;236(4):492–500; discussion - 1.
4. Parker DR, Bright T, Irvine T et al. Long-term outcomes following laparoscopic repair of large hiatus hernias performed by trainees Versus consultant surgeons. *J Gastrointest Surg* 2019 Apr 22.
5. Watson DI, Thompson SK, Devitt PG et al. Laparoscopic repair of very large hiatus hernia with sutures versus absorbable mesh versus nonabsorbable mesh: A randomized controlled trial. *Ann Surg* 2015 Feb;261(2):282–289.

# 5 Non-Metastatic Esophageal Cancer with Enlarged Carinal Lymph Nodes with Previous Sleeve Gastrectomy

*Apurva Ashok, Devayani Niyogi, Sabita Jiwnani, George Karimundackal, and C.S. Pramesh*

## CONTENTS

## CASE SCENARIO

A 55-year-old man had a body mass index (BMI) of 42 kg/m² (weight = 120 kg; height = 1.70 m) and associated comorbidities of type 2 diabetes mellitus, dyslipidemia, and hypertension. He also had a 20 pack-year history of smoking and no previous gastroesophageal reflux disease symptoms. Preoperative upper gastrointestinal endoscopy did not reveal a hiatus hernia, esophagitis, or *Helicobacter pylori* infection. He underwent an uneventful laparoscopic sleeve gastrectomy followed by an uneventful recovery. In the follow-up period, he lost 70% of his excess weight. Two years after surgery, he complained of new onset reflux symptoms. On evaluation with upper gastrointestinal endoscopy, intestinal metaplasia without atypia was seen at the gastroesophageal junction. He was started on proton pump inhibitors and surveillance endoscopy was advised. However, the patient failed to follow-up. Four years later, he presented with dysphagia and weight loss. An upper gastrointestinal endoscopy revealed an ulcero-proliferative growth in the lower esophagus and gastroesophageal junction, the biopsy of which revealed moderately differentiated adenocarcinoma. A staging positron emission tomography computed tomography (CT) scan confirmed a bulky lower third esophageal malignancy involving the gastroesophageal junction with evidence of gastrohepatic and subcarinal lymphadenopathy.

## BACKGROUND OF THE PATHOLOGY

Obese patients with gastroesophageal reflux disease are at increased risk of reflux symptoms, esophagitis, Barrett's esophagus, and subsequent possibility of developing an esophagogastric cancer. The effect of bariatric surgery on pre-existing gastroesophageal reflux disease, mainly after sleeve gastrectomy, is variable and the chance of progressing to adenocarcinoma of esophagus is a rare event. Isolated case reports have been published in literature linking bariatric surgery to esophageal cancer. After bariatric surgery, a total of 33 cases of esophageal adenocarcinoma and one case of squamous cell carcinoma have been reported in a systematic review in 2013 [1]. However, only four cases have been reported to date in patients who have undergone sleeve gastrectomy.

Development of esophageal cancer post-bariatric procedures may be purely coincidental. However, case reports have suggested an association, possibly due to the predisposing factors of obesity, smoking, and also due to impact of surgery on the anatomic structure and physiology of the gastroesophageal junction. The main pathophysiologic factors which can increase cancer risk are chronic gastroesophageal reflux disease and stasis of gastric acid and food in the pouch causing chronic mucosal irritation leading to changes such as intestinal metaplasia, mucosal atrophy, and development of Barrett's esophagus. While long-standing gastroesophageal reflux disease could contribute to development of adenocarcinoma, chronic stasis and other etiological factors like smoking, alcohol, dietary and genetic factors could predispose to squamous cell carcinoma.

The association of sleeve gastrectomy with gastroesophageal reflux disease is controversial. Some studies have shown that sleeve gastrectomy improves anti-reflux symptoms;

however, several others report worsening or development of de novo gastroesophageal reflux disease with restrictive bariatric procedures. DuPree and colleagues [2] found that 84% of patients with pre-existing gastroesophageal reflux disease persisted to have gastroesophageal reflux disease symptoms after sleeve gastrectomy and 8.6% of them developed de novo gastroesophageal reflux disease postoperatively. The mechanisms attributable to an increased risk of gastroesophageal reflux disease after sleeve gastrectomy are anatomic and physiologic variationsm such as a loss of the angle of His, hypotony of the lower esophageal sphincter, increased intragastric pressure, dysmotility, and hiatal hernia. The progression of persistent gastroesophageal reflux disease to metaplasia to dysplasia to neoplasia is well established and these patients carry a higher risk of developing esophageal adenocarcinoma compared to the general population.

There have been no reports of increased risk of squamous cell carcinoma post sleeve gastrectomy. Hence the risk factors remain the same as those carried by the general population, including tobacco/smoking, alcohol, caustic injury, consumption of hot beverages, smoked food, and genetic alterations.

## APPROACH TO THE PATIENT
### Clinical signs and symptoms
Progressive dysphagia and unintentional weight loss are the most common presenting complaints of esophageal cancer. However, in patients who have undergone bariatric procedures, the diagnosis could be delayed as the symptoms get attributed to the desired sequelae of surgery. Patients assume that the persistent reflux symptoms, vomiting, and weight loss are due to the surgery and hence present late for medical evaluation.

### Investigations
#### Upper gastrointestinal endoscopy
When patients who have had weight loss operations develop reflux symptoms or dysphagia, it is important to evaluate these symptoms with an upper gastrointestinal endoscopy. As a sleeve gastrectomy entails stapling of the stomach along its greater curvature and the fundus, the endoscopist needs to be aware of the altered anatomy and possible sequalae of the prior surgery. A minimum of six to eight biopsies from irregular mucosal areas or brush cytology from stricturous lesions are needed for adequate diagnosis. A complete study of the upper gastrointestinal tract with dilatation

of any post-surgery strictures is necessary to assess the whole stomach. It is advisable that patients undergoing bariatric surgery undergo a preoperative screening upper gastrointestinal endoscopy to rule out pre-existing conditions like *Helicobacter pylori* infection, mucosal metaplasia, or, rarely, esophagogastric neoplasms. A systematic review [1] noted that patients with preoperative screening endoscopy seemed to develop cancer at a longer follow-up time than those without preoperative upper gastrointestinal endoscopy (93 versus 25 months), although this was not statistically significant.

Endoscopic ultrasound further helps to delineate the T-stage accurately (T4 better than T1). However, endoscopic ultrasound will not be technically feasible in stenotic lesions.

### Imaging
The radiological imaging test recommended to stage esophageal cancer is [18]Fluorodeoxyglucose positron emission tomography combined with CT scan since the accuracy increases to 92% when the two modalities are combined. A contrast-enhanced CT scan may be an alternative initial modality in the absence of positron emission tomography imaging facilities. However, while it is useful in T-stage assessment, it is less accurate for assessing nodal and distant metastases. In patients after bariatric surgery, CT with oral contrast can be used to evaluate distension of the stomach remnant, but mucosal abnormalities and smaller, early lesions would be missed.

### Laparoscopy
Staging laparoscopy would be indicated in esophageal adenocarcinoma extending to involve the gastroesophageal junction and proximal cardia to detect advanced disease and peritoneal metastases.

## MANAGEMENT
The patient presented in the Case Scenario was labeled as having locally advanced disease in view of non-metastatic esophageal cancer with subcarinal nodes (bulky primary disease and lymph nodal involvement).

A multimodal approach is the standard of care for locally advanced esophageal cancers, with integration of chemotherapy (with or without radiation) and surgical resection.

The treatment options for the present Case Scenario would entail

■ Neoadjuvant therapy followed by surgery

■ Definitive chemoradiation

*Neoadjuvant therapy followed by surgery*

In locally advanced esophageal cancer (T1-T4a, N+), neoadjuvant chemotherapy or neoadjuvant chemoradiotherapy has been shown to have superior outcomes when compared to surgery alone [3,4]. However, controversy revolves around the optimal neoadjuvant treatment regime. The Chemoradiotherapy for Oesophageal Cancer followed by Surgery Study (CROSS) trial [5] and the recently published NEOCRTEC trial [6] showed significant survival benefit, improved pathological response, and R0 resection rates with neoadjuvant chemoradiotherapy followed by surgery, compared to surgery alone, in the management of esophageal cancer. However, it was the patients with squamous cell carcinoma who appeared to derive the maximum benefit from neoadjuvant chemoradiotherapy, while those with adenocarcinoma had no difference in survival. With respect to the neoadjuvant chemotherapy trials, the Medical Research Council Adjuvant Gastric Infusional Chemotherapy (MAGIC) [7] and the FLOT4 studies [8] established the superiority of perioperative chemotherapy (3/4 cycles presurgery and 3/4 cycles postsurgery) over surgery alone in esophageal and gastroesophageal junction adenocarcinoma, with the latter showing superior outcomes over the former. However, head-to-head comparisons of neoadjuvant chemotherapy with neoadjuvant chemoradiotherapy through randomized control trials have not demonstrated conclusive superiority of one over the other, especially for adenocarcinoma. Based on these trials, most clinicians favor neoadjuvant chemoradiotherapy or neoadjuvant chemotherapy for esophageal SCC and neoadjuvant chemoradiotherapy or perioperative chemotherapy for adenocarcinoma.

In this case, where the patient has a lower third adenocarcinoma with subcarinal nodes, we would first perform a staging laparoscopy, and if found to be non-metastatic, would consider neoadjuvant chemotherapy using the docetaxel, oxaliplatin, 5-fluorouracil, and leucovorin regimen. After completion of four cycles of two weekly docetaxel, oxaliplatin, 5-fluorouracil, and leucovorin, we would perform a positron emission tomography CT scan to assess response, rule out interval distant metastases, and plan surgery. We would routinely perform a functional evaluation and pulmonary rehabilitation in preparation for radical multimodality treatment.

Surgery would entail resection of the primary with a standard two-field lymphadectomy. For the resection of the primary lesion, we prefer a transthoracic approach – either McKeown or Ivor Lewis esophagectomy. Both procedures comprise of *en bloc* subtotal esophageal resection with a radical mediastinal and abdominal lymphadenectomy through a right posterolateral thoracotomy and laparotomy. However, they differ in their site of anastomosis. In a McKeown procedure, the anastomosis would be in the neck, whereas in an Ivor Lewis operation, the anastomosis is intrathoracic. A standard two-field lymphadenectomy involves resection of the infra-carinal thoracic nodes and abdominal D2 nodes. During the planning of the esophagectomy, it may be prudent to be in communication with the bariatric surgeon who performed the prior bariatric procedure.

Once the specimen has been resected, reconstruction is of prime importance which determines the quality of life following esophagectomy. An ideal conduit would need (i) adequate length to reach up to the normal cervical or upper thoracic esophagus, (ii) good vascular supply along its entire length, and (iii) intrinsic motility to minimize reflux. Usually, the stomach is the preferred conduit by most surgeons for its good blood supply, adequate reach, and requirement of a single anastomosis to restore continuity. However, in the present Case Scenario where the patient had undergone a previous sleeve gastrectomy, the stomach would no longer be available for use, as the gastroepiploic arcade would have been sacrificed during that surgery. Alternative options for a conduit include the right and left colon or jejunum, although there is no consensus on the best option [9,10].

Colonic interposition has the advantages of providing a sufficient length, reasonable vascularity, and resistance to acid. However, redundancy of the colon and the possibility of development of disease in the colon, like polyps or inflammatory diseases, are its disadvantages. Either the right or left colon may be used along with the transverse colon. The vascularity is based on the ileocolic artery on the right, and arcade of left colic and middle colic for the left colon. The colonic conduit may be placed through the posterior mediastinal or retrosternal route. If a retrosternal conduit is planned, the thoracic inlet might need widening. The colo-esophageal anastomosis in the neck or thorax is performed using a hand-sewn method or staplers. In the abdomen, the colon is anastomosed to the gastric remnant or roux loop of jejunum, and a third colocolic anastomosis completes the reconstruction. Larger case series report anastomotic leak rates of 12% and long-term stricture rates of 0–32%. Many studies also report high re-operation rates for conduit necrosis, anastomotic leak, and redundancy.

A jejunal conduit, on the other hand, has a reliable blood supply and intrinsic peristalsis which impacts the quality of life. However, its disadvantages are that it may require a complex microvascular anastomosis and vascular augmentation (supercharging), and in certain instances, the length maybe insufficient. The first and fourth jejunal arterial branches are preserved, while dividing the second and third branch. The jejunum, like the colonic conduit, can be positioned in the posterior mediastinum or retrosternal. The second jejunal artery and vein are anastomosed to a suitable inflow and outflow vessel, such as the internal thoracic artery/vein while supercharging in the neck. The jejunum is then anastomosed to the esophagus. Anastomotic leaks and re-operation rates reported are high (0–36%), but it has a similar mortality rate to colonic interposition. Overall, an isoperistaltic left colon may be a preferable choice of reconstruction when the stomach is unavailable. It is not dependent on microvascular anastomosis and is our preferred choice.

*Definitive chemoradiation*

If the patient refuses surgery, is medically unfit for surgery, or the tumor is unresectable, definitive chemoradiation is a good curative option. Numerous studies have established its efficacy over radiation alone, though results are more favorable when the histology is squamous cell carcinoma. Patients with esophageal adenocarcinoma treated with definitive chemoradiation have modest survival outcomes (five year survival of 15–20%) [11]. A dose of 60–64 Gy/30–32 fractions of external beam radiation to the primary lesion and draining lymph-nodal area, and concomitant chemotherapy with cisplatin/5-fluorouracil is one of the standard regimens followed.

## KEY MESSAGES

- Esophageal cancer after sleeve gastrectomy is a rare event and may be predisposed due to obesity and surgery-induced structural variations of the gastroesophageal junction.
- The diagnosis is delayed due to overlapping symptoms.
- Management of patients presenting with esophageal cancer can be daunting, and the surgery is technically challenging and complex due to previous adhesions and altered anatomy.

- The standard of care in locally advanced esophageal cancer would be multimodal – either neoadjuvant chemoradiotherapy or perioperative chemotherapy with surgery or definitive chemoradiation.
- Surgical reconstruction using alternative conduit options, such as the colon or jejunum, plays an important role in reconstruction and on the quality of life after esophageal resection.

## REFERENCES

1. Scozzari G, Trapani R, Toppino M et al. Esophagogastric cancer after bariatric surgery: Systematic review of the literature. *Surg Obes Relat Dis* 2013;9(1):133–142.
2. DuPree CE, Blair K, Steele SR et al. Laparoscopic sleeve gastrectomy in patients with preexisting gastroesophageal reflux disease: A national analysis. *JAMA Surg* 2014;149(4):328–334.
3. Sjoquist KM, Burmeister BH, Smithers BM et al. Australasian Gastro-Intestinal Trials Group. Survival after neoadjuvant chemotherapy or chemoradiotherapy for resectable oesophageal carcinoma: An updated meta-analysis. *Lancet Oncol* 2011;12(7):681–692.
4. Gebski V, Burmeister B, Smithers BM et al. Australasian Gastro-Intestinal Trials Group. Survival benefits from neoadjuvant chemodiotherapy or chemotherapy in oesophageal carcinoma: A meta-analysis. *Lancet Oncol* 2007;8(3):226–234.
5. Shapiro J, Van Lanschot JJ, Hulshof MC et al. Neoadjuvant chemoradiotherapy plus surgery versus surgery alone for oesophageal or junctional cancer (CROSS): Long-term results of a randomised controlled trial. *Lancet Oncol* 2015;16(9):1090–1098.
6. Yang H, Liu H, Chen Y et al. Neoadjuvant chemoradiotherapy followed by surgery versus surgery alone for locally advanced squamous cell carcinoma of the esophagus (NEOCRTEC5010): A phase III multicenter, randomized, open-label clinical trial. *J Clin Oncol* 2018;36(27):2796.
7. Cunningham D, Allum WH, Stenning SP et al. Perioperative chemotherapy versus surgery alone for resectable gastroesophageal cancer. *N Engl J Med* 2006;355(1):11–20.
8. Al-Batran SE, Homann N, Pauligk C et al. Perioperative chemotherapy with fluorouracil plus leucovorin, oxaliplatin, and docetaxel versus fluorouracil or capecitabine plus cisplatin

and epirubicin for locally advanced, resectable gastric or gastro-oesophageal junction adeno-carcinoma (FLOT4): A randomised, phase 2/3 trial. *Lancet* 2019;393(10184):1948–1957.

9. Marino KA, Weksler B. Esophagectomy After weight-reduction surgery. *Thorac Surg Clin* 2018;28(1):53–58.

10. Bakshi A, Sugarbaker DJ, Burt BM. Alternative conduits for esophageal replacement. *Ann Cardiothorac Surg* 2017;6(2):137.

11. Tougeron D, Scotte M, Hamidou H et al. Definitive chemoradiotherapy in patients with esophageal adenocarcinoma: An alternative to surgery? *Jsurgoncol* 2012;105(8):761–766.

# 6 Post-Esophagectomy Mediastinal Leak

*Devayani Niyogi, Virendra Kumar Tiwari, Apurva Ashok,*
*Sabita Jiwnani, George Karimundackal, and C.S. Pramesh*

## CONTENTS

## CASE SCENARIO

A 59-year-old diabetic man with a middle third squamous cell carcinoma of the esophagus underwent an open trans-thoracic esophagectomy with a three-field nodal dissection and a cervical stapled triangulating anastomosis with a linear stapler. He had received three cycles of neo-adjuvant chemotherapy prior to surgery. He had an uneventful intraoperative and postoperative course in the intensive recovery unit after surgery. On postoperative day three, he was found to have tachycardia, hypotension, and respiratory insufficiency suggestive of mediastinitis. Clinically, he was suspected to have a mediastinal leak and was shifted to the critical care unit. His electrocardiogram showed atrial fibrillation, and arterial blood gas results revealed a pH of 7.3 with a lactate of 4.9. After initial resuscitation and stabilization, a complete laboratory profile was sent and a contrast-enhanced CT scan of the neck, thorax, and upper abdomen was performed with on-table oral and intravenous contrast. It revealed a single large mediastinal collection with extravasation of contrast into it, confirming the diagnosis of an anastomotic leak (Figure 6.1).

## BACKGROUND OF PATHOLOGY

Esophagectomy alone, or as a part of multimodality treatment, is the mainstay of treatment for localized and locoregional esophageal cancer in medically fit patients [1]. Esophagectomy can be performed by various open and minimally invasive approaches. Depending on the level of the tumor and surgeon preference, the anastomosis can be sited in the neck or chest. It can be hand sewn or stapled. Putting together all these variations in the type of surgery, the overall anastomotic leak rate post-esophagectomy is between 3.8–11.7% [1]. The 30-day mortality for esophageal surgery after a clinically significant leak is as high as 13–35% [1,2]. Hence there is a need for early identification, a standardized definition, and clear management algorithms to deal with this dreaded complication.

The Esophagectomy Complications Consensus Group (ECCG) has defined anastomotic leaks as full-thickness defects involving the esophagus, anastomosis, staple line, or conduit, irrespective of the presentation or method of identification [1]. Leaks are divided into three types, depending on management strategy:

- Type I: No change in therapy, medical management or dietary modification

- Type II: Requires interventional, but not surgical therapy

- Type III: Requires surgical intervention [1]

Table 6.1 provides an overview of the perceived risk factors for anastomotic leaks. Low hospital procedural volumes and pulmonary and cardiovascular complications are factors associated with higher risk for anastomotic leaks [7]. Published guidelines mention that anastomotic leak rate should be less than 5% in high volume centers [2].

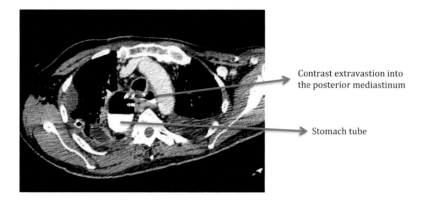

Contrast extravastion into the posterior mediastinum

Stomach tube

**Figure 6.1** Axial section of a contrast-enhanced CT scan of the thorax demonstrating a posterior mediastinal collection with evidence of oral contrast extravasation.

## CLINICAL FINDINGS

Most clinically significant leaks present on postoperative day five to seven. However, leaks may manifest as early as day one, to delayed leaks beyond day ten (range: 1–58 days) [3].

Anastomotic leaks may present with one or more of the following clinical signs:

- Tachycardia
- Fever
- Hypotension
- Respiratory distress
- Tachyarrhythmias
- Altered mental status
- Enteric content in intercostal drain
- Neck crepitus or emphysema

## INVESTIGATIONS

Investigating a patient with suspected leak should be with two intentions:

1) Confirming and mapping the leak

2) Estimating the magnitude of systemic insult

### Laboratory tests

- Arterial blood gas: Degree of metabolic acidosis and lactate levels
- Complete blood count: Leukocytosis/ leukopenia
- Renal and liver function tests
- Coagulation profile: If any intervention planned
- Drain fluid amylase can help confirm a leak if suspicious
- Fluid chylomicrons can help differentiate a chyle leak
- Drain fluid cultures to help guide antibiotic selection

### Imaging

An air-fluid level or new onset pleural effusion or pneumothorax on chest X-ray raises the suspicion of an anastomotic leak.

A computed tomography (CT) scan of the neck, thorax, upper abdomen with oral

## Table 6.1 Perceived Risk Factors for Anastomotic Leaks

| Risk Factor | Outcome |
| --- | --- |
| Type of neoadjuvant therapy | No difference in leak rates between neoadjuvant chemotherapy, neoadjuvant chemoradiation, or surgery alone [3]. |
| Transthoracic vs transhiatal approach | Transhiatal esophagectomy associated with higher leak rates (12% vs 9.8%) [4]. |
| Open vs total minimally invasive approach | Higher leak rate in the total minimally invasive approach in one series [3]. |
| Cervical vs chest anastomosis | Higher leak rate associated with cervical anastomosis (12.3% vs 9.3%) [5]. |
| Stapled vs hand-sewn anastomosis | No difference in leak rates. Stricture rate higher with circular stapler, less with triangulating anastomosis with linear staplers [6]. |
| Two-field vs three-field lymphadenectomy | No difference [2]. |
| Gastric outlet drainage procedure | Decreases leak rates by 61% [2]. |

contrast/contrast through the nasogastric tube in intubated patients, as well as intravenous contrast is used in most centers to investigate suspected leaks. It has a sensitivity of 58.8%, negative predictive value of 87%, and accuracy of 78.8% in detecting leaks.

As compared to a standard esophagogram, a CT scan was found to be more useful because it can help identify undrained mediastinal collections and guide drainage. Both modalities picked up all clinically significant leaks. Routine dye studies in asymptomatic post-esophagectomy patients, once a standard of care, are no longer recommended.

### Endoscopy

A timely endoscopy not only confirms the presence of a leak or conduit necrosis, but also helps map the exact location and extent of the leak and the feasibility of any endoscopic intervention. Endoscopy should be performed early in suspected conduit necrosis and large anastomotic dehiscence, especially in compromised patients. Endoscopy can be done as a bedside procedure in hemodynamically unstable patients [1].

## TREATMENT

The first step in the management of mediastinal leaks is resuscitation and stabilization. Intubation, mechanical ventilation, and vasopressor supports might be required in certain cases depending upon the magnitude of systemic insult. Broad-spectrum antibiotics should be started which can then be tailored as per the culture reports.

The management principles of mediastinal leaks can be broadly divided into three approaches:

1) Conservative management

2) Endoscopic management

3) Surgical management

The type of intervention depends on the etiology and size of the leak, degree of contamination, and the magnitude of systemic insult [1]. Other factors that influence management include the performance status of the patient, availability of interventional radiology support, endoscopic support, and the individual surgical unit protocol.

### Conservative management

This involves nasogastric decompression along with wide (and satisfactory) drainage of all mediastinal/ pleural collections with image-guided wide bore pigtails or intercostal drains.

More than one drain might be required to drain all pockets. It also involves the choice of antibiotic cover guided by culture reports along with the maintenance of nutrition. Enteral nutrition provided via a nasojejunal tube or intraoperatively placed feeding jejunostomy is the preferred strategy. If the anastomosis was performed in the neck with the leakage draining into the mediastinum, removing the neck sutures with a lavage can help in draining any local collection (please refer to Chapter 7, Post-Esophagectomy (for Esophageal Cancer) Neck Leak.

The most important aspect of this approach is periodic reassessment: clinical and laboratory. Any significant worsening of parameters should prompt repeat imaging to look for undrained pockets or widespread contamination. Clinical deterioration on conservative management, or recurrent loculated collections, are indications for surgical intervention [1,2].

### Endoscopic management

An increasing number of centers are using endoscopically placed stents to manage small, controlled anastomotic leaks [9]. Both self-expanding metal stents and covered stents have been used. Nguyen et al. have described their successful experience with the use of an endoscope to negotiate the leak and drain the mediastinal collection, placing a covered stent to bypass the leak, and retrieving the stent after six weeks in nine patients with no procedural complications [8].

Endoscopic stenting in this setting works by diverting contents away from the site of the leak, giving the mucosa a chance to heal. This mandates an adequate seal. Therefore, stenting may work well for small anastomotic leaks and leaks where an intrathoracic anastomosis has been performed using a circular stapler, but has not been found to be of benefit in leaks from the conduit staple line. The gastric tube is too wide to provide an adequate seal in such cases [9].

Endoscopic treatment options also include vacuum-assisted closure devices like the Eso-SPONGE®. This is an open pore polyurethane sponge with an attached drainage tube designed to sit in the leak site and when connected to a vacuum device, drain and cleanse the cavity. The vacuum also assists in early granulation and closure of the defect. This procedure needs to be repeated every three to four days to replace the sponge. Early reports look promising but as of now, there is no strong evidence to support its use [5].

The review by Fumagalli et al. reported endoscopic measures to have the highest retreatment rate (17.2%) but lowest mortality

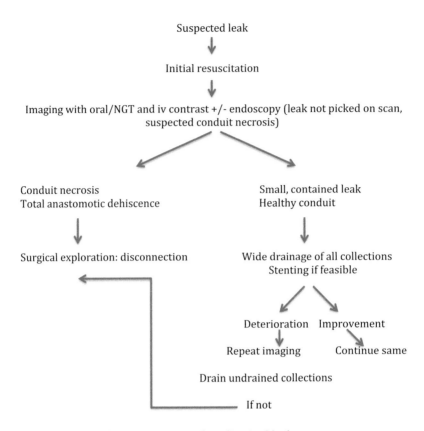

Suspected leak

↓

Initial resuscitation

↓

Imaging with oral/NGT and iv contrast +/- endoscopy (leak not picked on scan, suspected conduit necrosis)

Conduit necrosis
Total anastomotic dehiscence

Small, contained leak
Healthy conduit

Surgical exploration: disconnection

Wide drainage of all collections
Stenting if feasible

Deterioration   Improvement

Repeat imaging          Continue same

Drain undrained collections

If not

**Figure 6.2**  Algorithm for the management of mediastinal leaks.

rate (6.9%) [3]. The low mortality could reflect a selection bias, considering the smallest and most contained leaks are amenable to stenting.

### Surgical management

The main indications for a surgical exploration are gastric conduit necrosis, large circumference of anastomotic dehiscence causing extensive contamination, and clinical deterioration on conservative management [1,2].

The principles of surgical intervention involve taking down the anastomosis, a diverting esophagostomy, excision of the devitalized conduit, decompressing gastrostomy, and establishing an enteral feeding access, preferably a feeding jejunostomy, if one is not already in place. A few technical details to be kept in mind during this procedure are: adequate washes in the posterior mediastinum with the placement of a right intercostal drain (if one is not already in place), closure of the hiatus to prevent herniation of intra-abdominal contents, fashioning the gastrostomy with due consideration to facilitate a future anastomosis of the colon on the anterior wall, and performing a tracheostomy if prolonged ventilatory support is anticipated.

Restoring esophagogastric continuity should be considered after six to eight weeks, once the patient has completely recovered from the systemic insult, or after the patient has completed adjuvant treatment, if indicated. The usual choice for reconstruction is a left colonic conduit. A re-staging positron emission tomography, contrast-enhanced CT (triple phase), not only to reassess the disease but also study the colonic vascular anatomy, is preferred. The patient will also need a colonoscopy prior to reconstruction to rule out any colonic disease.

Some series have described a minimally invasive technique for surgical intervention in mediastinal leaks. This involves a thoracoscopic approach on the right side, retraction of the lung, thorough washes, and drainage of all collections. Insufflation through a simultaneous gastroscopy helps identify the site of leak. A T-tube drainage is then achieved through the leak site using combined endoscopic and thoracoscopic approach, which is then exteriorized, creating a controlled fistula [9].

### IMPLICATIONS OF MEDIASTINAL LEAKS

Apart from considerably increasing the mortality, morbidity, and hospital stay, anastomotic leaks also impact oncological outcomes. Patients with anastomotic leaks undergo significant nutritional depletion, affecting their ability to tolerate adjuvant therapy.

Significant esophageal anastomotic leaks have shown to be independently associated with a decreased over and disease-free survival (54.8 months vs 35.8 months, p<0.002 and 47.9 months vs 34 months, p<0.005 respectively). Patients with a clinically significant leak have a 28% higher likelihood of death due to disease. At a follow-up of five years, overall, locoregional and mixed recurrences were higher in patients with Clavien Dindo grade 3 leaks. However, it did not have a significant impact on distant failure. Clavien Dindo grade 1 and 2 leaks had no impact on survival outcomes or recurrence [9]. Grade 1 and 2 leaks have no impact on survival outcomes or recurrence [7].

## CASE SCENARIO (CONTINUED)

The posterior mediastinal collection was drained under CT guidance. Gradually, the cardio-respiratory parameters improved. The patient was kept nil by mouth, with nutrition being maintained through a nasojejunal tube. He received a course of antibiotics as per the culture sensitivity results. Once the pigtail stopped draining, he was gradually started on oral feeds and discharged on postoperative day 12.

### KEY MESSAGES

- Early diagnosis is the key.
- Extent of contamination and systemic response: key determinants of need for surgical exploration.
- Surgical intervention is the exception rather than the rule in mediastinal leaks without conduit necrosis.
- Early disconnection in conduit necrosis.
- Serial reassessment in patients on non-operative management is imperative.
- Routine postoperative screening with imaging prior to starting orals is not recommended.

## REFERENCES

1. Dent B, Griffin SM, Jones R et al. Management and outcomes of anastomotic leaks after oesophagectomy. *B J Surg* 2016;103(8):1033–1038.
2. Junemann-Ramirez M, Awan MY, Khan ZM et al. Anastomotic leakage post esophago-gastrectomy for esophageal carcinoma: Retrospective analysis of predictive factors, management and influence on longterm survival in a high volume centre. *Eur J Cardio Thor Surg* 2005;27(1):3–7.
3. Fumagalli U, Baiocchi GL, Celotti A et al. Incidence and treatment of mediastinal leakage after esophagectomy: Insights from the multicenter study on medistinal leaks. *World J Gastroenterol* 2019;25(3):356–366.
4. Ryan CE, Paniccia A, Meguid RA et al. Transthoracic anastomotic leak after esophagectomy: Current trends. *Ann Surg Oncol* 2017;24(1):281–290.
5. Verstegen MH, Bouwense SA, van Workum F et al. Management of intrathoracic and cervical anastomotic leakage after esophagectomy for esophageal cancer: A systematic review. *World J Emerg Surg* 2019;14(1):17.
6. Honda M, Kuriyama A, Noma H et al. Hand-sewn versus mechanical esophagogastric anastomosis after esophagectomy: A systematic review and meta-analysis. *Ann Surg* 2013;257(2):238–248.
7. Markar S, Gronnier C, Duhamel A et al. The impact of severe anastomotic leak on long-term survival and cancer recurrence after surgical resection for esophageal malignancy. *Ann Surg* 2015;262(6):972–980.
8. Nguyen NT, Rudersdorf PD, Smith BR et al. Management of gastrointestinal leaks after minimally invasive esophagectomy: Conventional treatments vs. endoscopic stenting. *J Gastrointest Surg* 2011;15(11):1952–1960.
9. Dindo D, Demartines N, Clavien PA. Classification of surgical complications: a new proposal with evaluation in a cohort of 6336 patients and results of a survey. *Ann Surg* 2004;240(2):205–213.

# 7 Post-Esophagectomy (for Esophageal Cancer) Neck Leak

*W.K. Ooi, S.M. Lagarde, and B.P.L. Wijnhoven*

## CONTENTS

## CASE SCENARIO

A 59-year-old man presented to the outpatient clinic with difficulty of swallowing solid food for a six-month duration. He gave a history of gastroesophageal reflux which was treated with proton pump inhibitors. His late father had succumbed to esophageal cancer. The patient himself did not smoke, but he consumed two units of alcohol a day. Physical examination was unremarkable. Esophagogastroscopy revealed a 10 cm segment of Barrett's esophagus with a malignant ulcer at the gastroesophageal junction. Biopsies from this region came back as moderately differentiated adenocarcinoma. Endoscopic ultrasound of the esophagus revealed a T2 tumor. Computed tomography (CT) scan of the chest demonstrated thickening of the distal esophagus with no enlarged lymph nodes or distant metastases. Positron emission tomography (PET) confirmed these findings and the tumor was staged cT2N0M0. The patient received neoadjuvant chemoradiotherapy and underwent a thoraco-laparoscopic esophagectomy with a cervical anastomosis. There were no intraoperative complications.

## BACKGROUND OF THE PATHOLOGY

### Post-esophagectomy anastomotic leak

Esophagectomy is a complex surgical procedure associated with considerable morbidity [1,4]. Following esophagectomy, the join between the conduit and proximal esophagus can be created in the neck (cervical

anastomosis) or in the chest (intrathoracic anastomosis). An anastomotic leakage is considered a major complication as this is associated with significant morbidity [1,2]. The anastomotic leak rate ranges from 6–40%. The leak rate of a cervical anastomosis leakage is higher (8–35%) than an intrathoracic anastomosis (9–21%) although cervical leaks are easier to manage. This is due to the belief that a cervical leak will likely be confined to the neck, and mediastinal contamination is limited therefore preventing a potentially life-threatening mediastinitis. However, cervical anastomotic leakage still carries a 50% risk of intrathoracic manifestations and they are associated with prolonged hospital stay and mortality [3]. Several perioperative factors are associated with the risk for anastomotic leakage. Proximally located tumors, patient with American Society of Anesthesiologists (ASA) grade 3 or higher, history of cardiac arrhythmia, chronic obstructive pulmonary disease, and diabetes mellitus are preoperative risk factors for an anastomotic leak. Meanwhile, lower intraoperative pH and mean arterial pressure are also known to be associated with anastomotic leakage. Postoperative complications that are associated with anastomotic leakage include cardiac arrhythmia, pneumonia or acute respiratory distress syndrome, empyema, sepsis, and renal failure. However, whether the anastomotic leak is a result of these signs/symptoms, or if a leak induces these sequelae remains unclear. In addition, tension on the anastomosis due to an inadequately mobilized, small, and/or dilated and fluid-filled gastric conduit joined with the esophageal remnant may impair the vascularity of the anastomosis and increase the risk for a leak. Esophagogastric anastomosis closure technique in the neck can either be end to side or side to side. Cervical anastomosis was mainly hand sewn until the 1990s when the linear stapled technique was developed. The stapled technique of anastomosis has a similar leak rate as compared to a hand-sewn technique. However, the larger anastomotic cross-sectional area leads to fewer anastomotic strictures when compared with a linear side-to-side stapled technique.

## CLINICAL FEATURES OF AN ANASTOMOTIC LEAK

*The immediate postoperative course was uneventful. On day four after surgery, the patient developed dyspnea. He was febrile (38.1°C) and tachycardic (120 beats per minute). The cervical neck wound looked normal. Blood investigations showed a raised white cell count and serum C-reactive protein. He developed a new onset atrial fibrillation with hypotension that required pharmacological cardioversion. Radiograph of the chest showed right basal opacification.*

Early diagnosis and management of an esophageal anastomotic leakage depends largely on the recognition of signs and symptoms associated with a leak. The clinical manifestations of a leak can range from a patient being asymptomatic to someone who has severe sepsis. Even subtle signs and a clinical suspicion (mild fever, difficulty swallowing, mild dyspnea, and arrythmias) should initiate further diagnostic modalities. These signs, when present, can be specific or non-specific for a cervical anastomotic leak. Obvious signs of a cervical esophageal anastomotic leakage include redness and swelling with discharge of pus/saliva/enteric content from the neck wound. An intrathoracic manifestation of a cervical anastomotic usually presents non-specific signs, including fever, cardiac arrhythmias, undefined leukocytosis, and respiratory distress which may be indistinguishable from postoperative pneumonia, pulmonary embolism, and sepsis. Diagnostic tests should immediately be ordered.

## APPROACH TO INVESTIGATIONS

*A CT scan of the thorax with oral water-soluble contrast on postoperative day five did not demonstrate a leak. Gastroscopy revealed a healthy gastric conduit with no sign of anastomotic dehiscence or mucosal ischemia. Despite that, the fever and dyspnea persisted. A follow-up CT scan on postoperative day*

*eight revealed minimal mediastinal free air with a collection.*

Ideally, diagnostic tests should be able to assess the viability of the conduit, the integrity of the anastomosis, as well as other possible causes for the patient being unwell. These diagnostic tests should be ordered when there is presence of physical signs, and the treating surgeon must not hesitate to repeat them if the clinical suspicion remains high, even though an earlier test may be negative.

### Blood tests

White cell count and C-reactive protein level are routinely checked, they have limitations in the early postoperative phase when they are elevated due to a systemic inflammatory reaction. White cell count has an 80% sensitivity for the detection of an anastomotic leakage, but only after postoperative day eight. On the other hand, a C-reactive protein level >136 mg/L achieves the same level of accuracy from postoperative day two onward.

### Imaging

A chest radiograph can be performed quickly but it lacks sensitivity and does not provide the topical information of the anastomosis required to direct management. Conversely, CT imaging is a non-invasive, fast, and safe modality to be performed even in the critically ill patient. CT scan has a sensitivity of 80% in identification of an anastomotic leak as well as the ability to assess the severity of a leakage while providing topical visualization of the neck, thorax, and abdomen on a single examination, thus allowing other causes such as pneumonia, empyema, fluid collection, or an abscess to be excluded. When present, CT-guided interventions can be used in the management of complications, including percutaneous drainage of fluid collections. Meanwhile, the Gastrografin swallow study, which was often used as a routine postoperative test, has since fallen out of favor in detecting an anastomotic leak [5]. This is due to the aqueous contrast used which has a low radiographic density with low mucosal adherence, thus limiting the ability to detect small leakages. These studies, however, have some value in providing functional information such as the capacity of conduit and gastric emptying.

### Endoscopy (esophagogastroscopy)

Endoscopy permits not only the assessment of the integrity of the anastomosis but also the viability of the gastric conduit. It can be safely performed by an experienced endoscopist at the bedside and also on patients who are on mechanical ventilators. A recent in-vivo porcine model has demonstrated that disruption of the esophagogastric anastomosis requires an intraluminal pressure >80 cmH$_2$0 while the maximum insufflation of the endoscopy does not exceed 9 cmH$_2$0. In addition to being a diagnostic test, endoscopy also has therapeutic advantages, such as permitting a washout to be done, placement of a decompression tube, clipping the site of the leak, and/or allowing the placement of a stent. Endoscopy has largely replaced the Gastrografin swallow study in the detection of an anastomotic leak. However, endoscopy is still an invasive procedure and may still fail to detect a small anastomotic dehiscence. Furthermore, it confers no extraluminal information limiting its ability to assess local complications, if present.

### The order of investigations

*Clinical features, together with a raised leukocyte and C-reactive protein level in the patient on day three to four after surgery, were suggestive of all complications including anastomotic leakage. Although the neck wound appeared normal and there were no clinical signs of pneumonia. Our initial assessment was focused on ruling out an anastomotic leak (with an intrathoracic manifestation) as this needs early treatment. The first diagnostic test we favor is a CT thorax with oral contrast. Although the sensitivity and specificity may be high, in our patient this appeared to be falsely negative. Hence an endoscopy was performed given the high index of suspicion for a leak. Endoscopy has better specificity and sensitivity compared to contrast swallow in detecting a leak and simultaneously permits assessment for conduit ischemia, which was negative in this patient. Despite that, the patient's clinical condition did not improve and thus a reassessment by CT scan was carried out. This CT scan showed features of mediastinitis (the presence of mediastinal free air and fluid (Figure 7.1).*

## TREATMENT OF AN ANASTOMOTIC LEAK

*The cervical wound was opened for drainage at the patient's bedside and a 16-Fr Foley catheter was placed into the cavity to allow daily flushing. The patient was commenced on broad-spectrum antibiotics and a CT-guided percutaneous drainage of the mediastinal collection was performed (Figure 7.2). Gastric conduit decompression was achieved with a nasogastric tube. The patient was kept nil by mouth and nutrition was supplemented via a feeding jejunostomy which was inserted at the time of esophagectomy. Effluent was seen draining from the neck upon flushing of chest drain, demonstrating a channel between the neck and chest. Daily flushing of the cervical and chest drains were performed in the ward.*

The general principles in the management of an esophageal anastomotic leak include control of sepsis by draining any collections, assessment and management of the gastric conduit/anastomosis, maintenance of adequate nutrition, and finally, rehabilitation of the patient.

### Control of sepsis

Broad-spectrum antimicrobials that provide coverage for aerobes and anaerobes should be administered, such as piperacillin/tazobactam or a carbapenem. In addition, antifungal therapy should be empirically administered as these patients would have been on acid suppression therapy prior to surgery, increasing the risk for fungal infections. The patient should be put on a proton pump inhibitor to reduce gastric secretion and limit contamination of the thorax. Feeding through the oral route must be withheld while simultaneously diverting saliva, and decompression of gastric

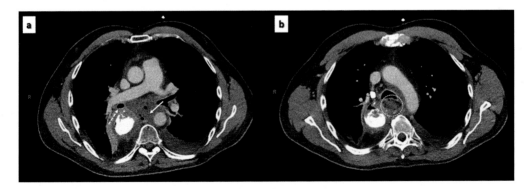

**Figure 7.1** Contrast-enhanced CT scan sections of the thorax. Axial post-contrast CT section showing: (a) Mediastinal air (dashed white line) and fluid (solid white arrow), (b) further mediastinal air and fluid posterior to the trachea (dotted circle).

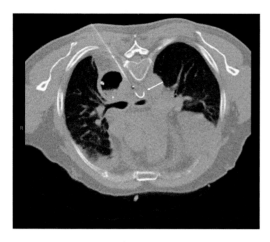

**Figure 7.2** Contrast-enhanced CT scan section of the thorax demonstrating a pigtail drain into the mediastinal collection (white arrow).

conduit should be achieved with nasogastric tube placement to prevent further contamination by bile or gastric content. Meanwhile, all collections and contaminated spaces must be drained adequately. Image-guided percutaneous drainage of collections is preferred but surgical washout should always be considered if inadequate drainage of intrathoracic collections is suspected. Endoscopy is safe when performed cautiously by experienced endoscopists. Endoscopic washout or stent placement may be considered, if necessary.

### Maintenance of nutrition

Nutritional intake must be maintained, especially during the acute phase, to facilitate recovery from sepsis and to ensure healing of the anastomosis. Enteric feeding is the preferable option unless contraindicated. Adequate nutrition can then be supplemented while circumventing the anastomotic site, either by an endoscopically guided nasojejunal feeding tube placement or a feeding jejunostomy placed at the time of the esophagectomy.

### Management of the anastomosis and gastric conduit

The management of the esophagogastric anastomosis is determined by the severity of the leak, clinical condition of the patient, and viability of the gastric conduit. Currently, there is no consensus on the classification for severity of leakage, let alone a standardized treatment of an esophageal anastomotic leakage. At the time of this writing, an international retrospective cohort study on patients with an anastomotic leakage after esophagectomy

(TENTACLE) is being performed to determine the severity of leakage and to provide a standardized guide to treatment options.

Generally, a severe anastomotic leakage with presence of incipient sepsis invariably will require surgical intervention. When the anastomotic dehiscence is small and surrounding tissues are healthy, these can be repaired with absorbable sutures, while larger dehiscence can be controlled with a T-tube insertion and tissues approximated around it. This allows for sepsis to be controlled with the formation of a controlled esophagogastro-cutaneous fistula and with time, when the patient's condition improves, this tube can be removed after four to six weeks. In the rare event of re-exploration during the early postoperative period where only limited necrosis is present, a segmental resection and re-anastomosis can be performed. More commonly, when anastomotic dehiscence is larger than 30% of the circumference with concomitant sepsis, disconnection of the anastomosis is inevitable. Gastric conduit ischemia occurs in approximately 9% of patients and they can vary from limited necrosis to complete loss of conduit. Gastric conduit with only minimal necrosis can be salvaged, and a delayed anastomosis can be performed when the patient's condition improves. However, a total gastrectomy may need to be performed if a large portion of the conduit is ischemic and a cervical esophagostomy needs to be created to allow diversion of saliva and prevent further mediastinal contamination.

In contrast, when the leakage is minimal and well contained without features of sepsis, endoscopic treatment of the anastomosis can be attempted. Endoscopic clipping is a novel technique where the metal clip acts like a surgical suture holding the edges of fistulous opening together occluding the lumen. Another novel technique of endoscopic Vicryl® mesh and fibrin glue application into the fistula opening was reported to achieve an 87% success in sealing a leak up to 3 cm in diameter. Both techniques seem interesting, however, in our experience they have not worked given the inflammatory reaction, stiffness of tissue, and/or presence of necrosis. Nevertheless, it may be that antibiotics alone will suffice for this subset of patients. The application of an endo-vacuum dressing system has also been described recently where a sponge is inserted endoscopically into the leakage cavity and a negative suction pressure is applied to collapse the cavity. All these techniques, however, are still experimental and are yet to undergo large-scale studies comparing them to surgical alternatives.

### Rehabilitation and reconstruction

An esophageal anastomotic leak is a major dilemma in comparison to any other bowel anastomotic leak because these patients must abstain from oral nutrition for a prolonged period of time. Oral feeding should be reintroduced gradually whenever possible while maintaining nutrition supplementation through other routes until the patient is able to tolerate sufficient nutrition intake orally. Once the patient has recovered from the acute stage, reconstruction in patients with a resected conduit can be planned. This surgery usually takes place months later and will require a colonic interposition.

### Isolated cervical anastomosis leakage

Occurrence of an isolated cervical anastomosis leakage is a distinct entity from its intrathoracic counterpart since they usually run a milder clinical course. Isolated cervical anastomosis leakage can be sufficiently managed with opening the neck wound to allow adequate drainage. Severe sepsis occurs less frequently in these patients. Healing occurs within a few weeks. However, luminal stenosis will often develop later which requires endoscopic dilatation.

### Order of treatment and patient progress

*Although this patient had a cervical anastomosis, the leaked contents had tracked into the mediastinum with resultant abscess formation. Endoscopic assessment was unable to visualize any anastomotic dehiscence, while CT scan assessment also did not show a large extravasation of contrast, suggesting that the leak was likely minimal and contained. Additionally, the patient's condition remained stable and did not deteriorate further. However, opening the neck wound is insufficient in attaining control of the sepsis owing to the presence of mediastinal contamination. Therefore, image-guided percutaneous drainage was necessitated. In combination with anti-microbial therapy and enteral nutrition supplementation, the patient successfully recovered from sepsis. The nasogastric tube was removed on postoperative day 20 and the patient was discharged to home with a pigtail drain in the chest. A week following discharge, oral feeding was gradually reintroduced in the outpatient setting. The chest drain was removed on postoperative day 27, after a repeat CT thorax with oral contrast reassessment confirmed complete resolution of the mediastinal collection.*

## KEY MESSAGES

- The incidence of cervical esophageal anastomotic leaks is higher than intrathoracic anastomosis.
- Sepsis control and appropriate drainage of all collections is important in an anastomotic leak.
- A cervical anastomotic leak may present with non-specific clinical features and 50% of patients can have intrathoracic involvement.
- There is a need for a low threshold for focused diagnostic investigations to pursue even subtle clinical manifestations instead of relying on routine control imaging.
- An aggressive approach guided by the patient's condition, viability of the conduit, anastomotic integrity, and local complication is warranted.

## REFERENCES

1. Low DE, Kuppusamy MK, Alderson D et al. Benchmarking complications associated with esophagectomy. *Ann Surg* 2019 Feb;269(2):291–298.
2. Busweiler LAD, Wijnhoven BPL, van Berge Henegouwen MI et al. Early outcomes from the Dutch upper gastrointestinal cancer audit. *Br J Surg* 2016;103(13):1855–1863.
3. Gooszen JAH, Goense L, Gisbertz SS et al. Intrathoracic versus cervical anastomosis and predictors of anastomotic leakage after oesophagectomy for cancer. *Br J Surg* 2018;105(5):552–560.
4. Seesing MFJ, Gisbertz SS, Goense L et al. A propensity score matched analysis of open versus minimally invasive transthoracic esophagectomy in the Netherlands. *Ann Surg* 2017 Nov;266(5):839–846.
5. Nederlof N, de Jonge J, de Vringer T et al. Does routine endoscopy or contrast swallow study after esophagectomy and gastric tube reconstruction change patient management? *J Gastrointest Surg* 2017;21(2):251–258.

# PART 2
# STOMACH

# 8 Obese Patient (BMI 32) with Reflux Disease and Diabetes Mellitus

*Jacob Chisholm and Lilian Kow*

## CONTENTS

## CASE SCENARIO

A 35-year-old woman presented to the bariatric clinic with a body mass index (BMI) of 33 $kg/m^2$ (weight = 85 kg; height = 162 cm). She had gained 15 kg during her second pregnancy three years prior and had struggled to lose weight ever since. During the pregnancy she developed significant symptoms of acid regurgitation which failed to improve after the birth of her daughter. She was commenced on regular proton pump inhibitor medication which inadequately controlled her symptoms. She had been diagnosed with type 2 diabetes mellitus within the last 12 months. Although she was initially able to control her blood sugar level with diet alone, a recent elevation in her serum HbA1c (to 8.1%) had prompted her general practitioner to start her on Metformin. This medication had not resulted in any significant weight loss. She had unsuccessfully tried several nonsurgical strategies to help her lose weight. These included diets, exercise, meal replacement programs, as well as several courses of the appetite suppressant medication, Duromine (Phentermine). The recent deterioration in her diabetes prompted her presentation to the clinic in an attempt to address both her weight and related comorbidities.

## BACKGROUND OF THE PATHOLOGY

The prevalence of obesity has continued to increase worldwide. There is now a better understanding that the etiology is not fully explained by "energy in is greater than energy out." There are complex interactions between energy homeostasis and genetic, behavioral, environmental, or societal factors that ultimately determine our weight. There is now established evidence that bariatric surgery achieves superior and more sustained weight loss compared to diet and lifestyle modification alone. This resulted in 1991 recommendations by the National Institute of Health that surgery be offered to those patients with severe (BMI ≥40) or morbid obesity (BMI ≥35) in the presence of weight related comorbidities. Surgery has since resulted in reduced all-cause mortality as compared to morbidly obese patients who are not offered bariatric surgery [1].

Now, however, mounting evidence suggests a benefit for surgery in patients with class I obesity (BMI between 30–35 $kg/m^2$). Prospective studies indicate that all-cause mortality risk is 30% greater for each 5 $kg/m^2$ gained, and the life span for class I obesity is decreased by three years [2]. The impact on life expectancy by surgery is thought to be due to the amelioration in risk of obesity related comorbidities, especially type 2 diabetes mellitus. The age-adjusted relative risk of developing type 2 diabetes mellitus increases with BMI and is significant for class I obesity. Multiple randomized controlled trials have demonstrated superiority of weight loss surgery over diet and lifestyle intervention alone for the treatment of type 2 diabetes mellitus in the morbidly obese [3]. There would be no reason why this effect wouldn't extend to patients with class I obesity. This has been borne out in randomized, controlled trials dedicated to the low BMI patient [4].

Obesity is also an independent risk factor for gastroesophageal reflux disease. This risk is thought to relate to increased intra-abdominal pressures as well as a higher incidence of hiatal hernias. An appropriately selected bariatric operation can also effectively manage this issue.

## APPROACH TO A PATIENT REQUESTING BARIATRIC SURGERY

The management of an obese patient seeking bariatric surgery should always be multidisciplinary. In addition to the bariatric surgeon, the team should consist of a dietitian, clinical psychologist, bariatric physician, nurse, and specialist anesthetist. Assessment always begins with history and examination.

### History

It is important to explore the development of our patient's obesity. Questions regarding age at which obesity became an issue, subsequent stability of weight, and maximum and minimum weights over their adult life need to be asked. Important also is to clarify our patient's insight into why they have struggled with their weight and what may have led to periods of weight gain. Previous non-surgical methods of weight loss (including medication) and which ones worked, if only temporarily, need to be understood. If non-surgical methods of weight loss were unsuccessful, reasons why need to be asked. The patient then needs to reflect on how surgery will correct their eating patterns. The patient's lifestyle and work routine needs to be discussed and how it impacts on food choices. An understanding of the patient's willingness to change also needs to be determined.

### Medical assessment

It is important to identify all weight-related comorbidities in the patient. One must understand when these diseases were diagnosed and how they are currently treated. The more recent the diagnosis of type 2 diabetes mellitus, the greater the likelihood that surgery will induce remission. Gastroesophageal reflux disease needs to be properly defined, namely how it was diagnosed, previous endoscopic findings, as well as treatments used and their ability to control symptoms.

The presence or absence of other weight-related comorbidities, such as obstructive sleep apnea, hypertension, hypercholesterolemia, and osteoarthritis of weight bearing joints need to be clarified. It is particularly important to understand how obstructive sleep apnea was diagnosed (screening test or sleep study) and, if significant, whether it has been adequately treated with a continuous positive airway pressure mask. This will help plan the postoperative management of the airway. The management of all comorbidities need to be optimized before embarking on any weight loss surgery.

It is important to rule out medical causes of obesity, such as hypothyroidism or Cushing's disease. A complete list of current medications needs to be obtained. Many different medications can contribute to weight gain, including antidepressants. The potential for nonsteroidal anti-inflammatory medication to cause ulceration after bariatric surgery must also be discussed.

It is important to ask the patient if they smoke as this can negatively influence the outcome of bariatric surgery. Smoking is associated with an increased risk of immediate postoperative and even long-term complications. The patient's plans regarding future pregnancy also need to be understood as this should be deferred for at least 12 months after weight loss surgery due to the risk of poor nutritional supply to the growing fetus.

Specific inquiries must be made to determine if the patient has undergone any previous abdominal surgery, as the adhesions from these operations may influence the type of bariatric operation suggested. A sleeve gastrectomy is preferred over a Roux-en-Y gastric bypass if extensive adhesions are suspected.

### Dietary assessment

It is important to appreciate that nearly 50% of patients presenting for bariatric surgery may have macro- and/or micronutrient deficiencies. A complete dietary assessment of the patient must be carried out with the assistance of a dietitian. This would include the content and frequency of meals (including drinks) as well as any snacking or grazing between those meals or after dinner. It is also paramount to tease out the impact of work and daily living on the patient's eating patterns, and how this will need to be altered if it is impacting on the patient's dietary choices. The dietitian will also be able to advise on how to achieve preoperative weight loss through the use of a very low calorie diet. This will help shrink the fatty liver, thereby facilitating surgery.

### Psychological assessment

It is necessary to perform a complete psychological evaluation to exclude any undiagnosed and/or untreated conditions prior to surgery.

Unstable psychiatric illness is considered a contraindication to any weight loss surgery.

## PREOPERATIVE INVESTIGATIONS
### Blood investigations

The various blood tests routinely performed include:

a) Complete blood count

b) Electrolyte profile

c) Iron studies (iron, ferritin) – iron deficiency anemia is commonly detected and needs to be investigated and, if possible, corrected before surgery

d) Vitamin B12 and folate – important to establish a baseline before an operation that may result in a deficiency (such as the Roux-en-Y gastric bypass)

e) Liver function tests

f) Thyroid function tests – to exclude hypothyroidism as a medical cause of obesity

g) 25-OH vitamin D3 – there is evidence that reduced vitamin D and calcium within the first two years of weight loss surgery can lead to an increased risk of reduced bone density

h) Lipids

i) Fasting glucose and HbA1c

As mentioned earlier, it is not uncommon for micronutrient deficiencies to be detected prior to bariatric surgery. These need to be identified and corrected before any surgery.

### Radiological investigations
#### Abdominal ultrasound

The utility of routine abdominal ultrasound prior to bariatric surgery remains controversial, with definitive evidence lacking. The authors continue to perform it routinely to exclude the presence of gallstones prior to weight loss surgery. If symptomatic gallstones are present, it is the authors' preference to perform a laparoscopic cholecystectomy prior to any weight loss surgery. If gallstones are detected on preoperative ultrasound but the patient remains asymptomatic, the authors' preference is to not perform a cholecystectomy, either before or during the weight loss operation. The ultrasound report in our Case Scenario patient was unremarkable.

### Gastroscopy

The routine use of gastroscopy in the preoperative bariatric patient also remains controversial.

The authors believe that in an Roux-en-Y gastric bypass, where the distal stomach will no longer be accessible endoscopically, it seems prudent to exclude any pathology prior to surgery. Additionally, in the setting of long-standing symptoms of gastroesophageal reflux disease, it is important to exclude any associated complications, such as Barrett's esophagus or peptic strictures. Gastroscopy is also useful to preoperatively identify the presence of a hiatal hernia that will need to be repaired at the time of surgery. The patient presented in our Case Scenario had a normal gastroscopy apart from mild reflux esophagitis.

## SELECTION OF THE OPERATION

The four commonly performed bariatric operations around the world are the adjustable gastric band, sleeve gastrectomy, Roux-en-Y gastric bypass, and the one-anastomosis gastric bypass. In recent years, the adjustable gastric band has become less popular due to the increased incidence of late complications and need for subsequent explantation. The sleeve gastrectomy has now surpassed the Roux-en-Y gastric bypass as the most performed weight loss procedure around the world.

Regardless of popularity, the choice of operation needs to be tailored to the patient and their attendant comorbidities. In the only randomized controlled trial powered to assess the difference in remission rates of type 2 diabetes mellitus between sleeve gastrectomy and Roux-en-Y gastric bypass, the Roux-en-Y gastric bypass was found to be superior at 12 months follow-up [5]. Besides, sleeve gastrectomy can lead to worsening symptoms of reflux due to disruption of the lower esophageal sphincter as well as increased intragastric pressure. The presence of preoperative gastroesophageal reflux disease is thus considered to be a relative contraindication to a sleeve gastrectomy by some surgeons. The Roux-en-Y gastric bypass has been demonstrated as having effective control of gastroesophageal reflux disease symptoms even three years post-surgery. The patient presented in our Case Scenario had both type 2 diabetes mellitus and gastroesophageal reflux disease. She was offered a Roux-en-Y gastric bypass as a result.

## SURGICAL MANAGEMENT: ROUX-EN-Y GASTRIC BYPASS

The authors' preference for performing a Roux-en-Y gastric bypass is a five-port technique with one port used for the Nathanson liver retractor (Figure 8.1) [6]. Entry into the abdomen is performed using a 12 mm optical trocar in the left upper quadrant. The abdomen

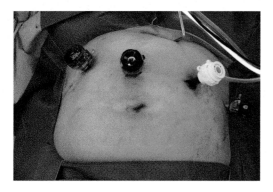

**Figure 8.1** Clinical photograph demonstrating the port placement for a laparoscopic Roux-en-Y gastric bypass.

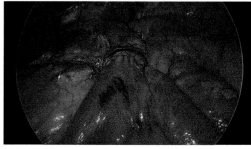

**Figure 8.2** Intraoperative photograph depicting a completed gastrojejunal anastomosis (performed to the gastric pouch).

is insufflated to 15 mmHg and a 45° camera is used for optimum "top down" viewing. The other three ports are from 5–12 mm in size and are placed in a configuration that allows access to both the infra- and supracolic compartments of the abdomen. The two ports in the right upper quadrant will be utilized by the primary surgeon while the two left upper quadrant ports will be used by the assistant. This will include camera operation in the assistant's left hand. The patient is placed in a steep reverse Trendelenburg position.

It is possible to separate the operation into three distinct phases. The first is the creation of a non-distensible lesser curve–based gastric pouch using an endoscopic stapler. This is achieved through dissection at the angle of His, followed by the lesser curve using an energy device, such as the Harmonic Ace. The first staple firing is then performed horizontally no more than 5 cm distal to the gastroesophageal junction. A 36-Fr bougie is then inserted to calibrate the size of the pouch following which further staple firings are performed in a vertical direction toward the angle of His until pouch creation is complete.

The second step is to perform a gastrojejunostomy (Figure 8.2). This begins with the division of the greater omentum down to the transverse colon. This reduces the tension on the small bowel that will be brought up to form the Roux limb. The duodenojejunal flexure needs to be clearly identified by sighting the inferior mesenteric vein. A loop of jejunum 50 to 70 cm from the duodenojejunal flexure is then brought up to the gastric pouch with care taken to maintain the correct orientation of the small bowel. This length of jejunum from the duodenojejunal flexure to the gastrojejunostomy will be the biliary limb. An anchoring suture between the small bowel and gastric

pouch can be used to keep the small bowel in position while the anastomosis is performed. There are three different techniques for performing a gastrojejunostomy, including handsewn, linear stapled, and circular stapled. There is no evidence of superiority of one technique over the other in terms of leak rate, stricture formation, or incidence of marginal ulcers. The authors' preference is a hand-sewn single layer closure using a 2/0 absorbable suture such as 2-0 polydioxanone. A 10 mm transverse gastrotomy is performed anterior to the first horizontal staple line. A small 10 mm enterotomy is then created on the adjacent jejunum. The single layer running suture posteriorly incorporates the staple line. The anterior running suture is completed after the bougie is placed within the small bowel to prevent inadvertent suturing of the posterior wall.

The third step is completion of the enteroenterostomy. This defines the length of the Roux limb. There is no difference in weight loss outcomes between a Roux limb length of 100 cm or 150 cm. It is, however, important that the Roux limb is long enough to prevent any bile reflux.

The authors' preference for the Roux limb is an antecolic antegastric pathway as opposed to retrocolic retrogastric. This eliminates the potential for an internal hernia at the mesocolon. The surgeon, however, should be able to perform a retrocolic and retrogastric approach if there is too much tension on the gastrojejunostomy with an antecolic approach. The enteroenterostomy, or side-to-side jejunojejunostomy, is performed using a single fire of a 60 mm EndoGIA tan stapler. Anchoring sutures are used to align the two lengths of small bowel with the stapler. The remaining enterotomy is closed with a running 2-0 polyglyconate suture. The small bowel is then divided using another EndoGIA 60 mm tan

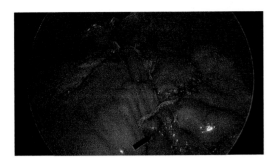

**Figure 8.3** Intraoperative photograph depicting a completed Roux-en-Y gastric bypass (enteroenterostomy marked with a black bold arrow).

stapler separating the Roux limb from the enteroenterostomy (Figure 8.3). Most surgeons would then believe that the jejunal and Petersen's space need to be closed with a 2-0 non-absorbable suture, although evidence for this is still inconclusive.

## POSTOPERATIVE PROGRESS

The patient presented in the Case Scenario made an uneventful recovery. By postoperative day one, she was commenced on a liquid diet and was able to take oral analgesia to manage her pain, which was minimal. Our patient's blood sugar level dropped by day two and her Metformin was not recommended when she was discharged later that day. Paracetamol was the only analgesia required following discharge. She remained on a liquid diet for two weeks followed by a pureed diet for a further two weeks. Normal consistency food was started at the beginning of the fifth week as well as regular multivitamin intake. Postoperative dietary, nursing, and surgical review was performed at week two and week four. Her local doctor also reviewed her with regard to ongoing glycemic control. The first vitamin B12 supplemental injection was administered at three months and continued three monthly thereafter.

Regular review continued three monthly within the bariatric clinic for a further year. At 12 months her excess weight loss was 75% which represented a weight of 65 kg and total weight loss of 16 kg. Her reflux symptoms subjectively had resolved and her proton pump inhibitor medication was no longer required. She remained off her Metformin at 12 months. Repeat blood tests performed 12 months post-surgery revealed an HbA1c of 5.9%. Ongoing lifelong follow-up with appropriate dietary and

psychological support as required was encouraged through the clinic.

## SALIENT POINTS

- The prevalence of obesity continues to increase worldwide along with rates of weight loss surgery.
- The evidence supports offering weight loss surgery to patients with a BMI of between 30 and 35 in the presence of weight-related comorbidities.
- The management of patients presenting for weight loss surgery needs to be multidisciplinary in approach.
- The current surgical options for weight management include the adjustable band gastroplasty, sleeve gastrectomy, Roux-en-Y gastric bypass, and one anastomosis gastric bypass.
- The Roux-en-Y gastric bypass has demonstrated superior outcomes for patients with type 2 diabetes mellitus and gastroesophageal reflux disease.
- Long-term postoperative support is essential.

## REFERENCES

1. Adams TD, Gress RE, Smith SC et al. Long-term mortality after gastric bypass surgery. *N Engl J Med* 2007 Aug 23;357(8):753–761.
2. Whitlock G, Lewington S, Sherliker P et al. Body-mass index and cause-specific mortality in 900 000 adults: Collaborative analyses of 57 prospective studies. *Lancet* 2009 Mar 28;373(9669):1083–1096.
3. Schauer PR, Bhatt DL, Kirwan JP et al. Bariatric surgery versus intensive medical therapy for diabetes –5-year outcomes. *N Engl J Med* 2017 Feb 16;376(7):641–651.
4. Lee WJ, Chong K, Ser KH et al. Gastric bypass vs sleeve gastrectomy for type 2 diabetes mellitus: A randomized controlled trial. *Arch Surg* 2011 Feb;146(2):143–148.
5. Hofso D, Fatima F, Borgeraas H et al. Gastric bypass versus sleeve gastrectomy in patients with type 2 diabetes (Oseberg): A single-centre, triple-blind, randomised controlled trial. *Lancet Diabetes Endocrinol* 2019 Dec;7(12):912–924.
6. Barreto S, Chisholm J, Schloithe A et al. Outcomes following revisional bariatric surgery – the reason for the band explantation matters, *Obes Surg* 2018 Feb;28(2):520–525.

# 9 Locally Advanced Resectable Gastric Cancer

*Savio George Barreto and Shailesh V. Shrikhande*

## CONTENTS

## CASE SCENARIO

A 55-year-old man presented with vague abdominal pain, early satiety, and occasional vomiting after meals. His blood investigations only revealed a hemoglobin at the lower end of normal and so an endoscopy was performed that demonstrated a gastric cancer involving the antrum of the stomach. A contrast-enhanced computed tomography (CT) scan performed demonstrated thickening in the region of the distal body and antrum of the stomach especially along the lesser curvature with perigastric lymphadenopathy. He was referred to us for further management of this likely malignancy.

## BACKGROUND OF THE PATHOLOGY

Gastric cancer is the fifth most commonly diagnosed cancer in the world and is ranked third among the leading causes of cancer-related deaths. The most important risk factors for gastric cancer include *Helicobacter pylori* and Epstein-Barr virus infections, smoking, alcohol, atrophic gastritis, and diets rich in smoked foods and foods containing nitrates and nitrosamines with a paucity of fresh fruits and vegetables. Hereditary cancer syndromes may also contribute to the development of the cancer in a proportion of patients. Over the last few decades, owing to the successful treatment of *Helicobacter pylori* in the west, the location of gastric cancers has migrated from distal stomach to the proximal gastroesophageal region. However, in the developing world, cancers are still seen originating all over the stomach.

Given that symptoms in early gastric cancer are subtle resulting in patients presenting more often in an advanced, and often, incurable stage, it is important for clinicians and general practitioners seeing patients with new-onset dyspepsia, dyspepsia refractory to treatment, or upper gastrointestinal (GI) "sounding" symptoms to consider an early gastroscopy.

Only 10–15% of patients, even in the West, present with early gastric cancer [1]. A significant proportion of patients present with locally advanced, non-metastatic disease. This subset of patients has been the focus of tremendous research in the last two decades. Perioperative chemotherapy, with optimal surgery (gastrectomy and D2 lymphadenectomy) sandwiched in between, is the currently recommended therapeutic strategy for locally advanced, asymptomatic patients with resectable gastric cancer, and will be discussed in this chapter. The other option in symptomatic patients (obstruction and refractory bleeding) is to offer them an upfront surgery and adjuvant chemotherapy.

## APPROACH TO A PATIENT WITH SUSPECTED GASTRIC CANCER

Most patients present with dyspepsia and/or iron deficiency anemia, as was the case in the patient presented. Symptoms such as anorexia, fatigue, and weight loss usually occur much later in the course of the disease. Symptoms of severe reflux followed by dysphagia may be seen in tumors of the cardia and gastro-esophageal junction. Vomiting of undigested food within two to three hours of a meal raises the suspicion of gastric outlet obstruction and warrants further investigation. The passage of black tarry stools (melena) should also alert the treating doctor to the need for a gastroscopy.

Clinically, a patient with locally advanced gastric cancer may have pallor as a result of bleeding. Less commonly, a succession splash from a distally situated obstructing tumor may be auscultated.

The various blood investigations performed are as follows:

a) Complete blood counts: May demonstrate anemia.

b) Liver and renal function tests: It is important to check renal function before undertaking a contrast-enhanced CT scan. These tests are also important prior to commencing chemotherapy.

c) Tumor markers (carcinoembryonic antigen [CEA] and carbohydrate antigen 19-9 [CA 19-9]) – useful in postoperative surveillance if they are elevated prior to surgery and normalize after the operation.

### Gastroscopy

The role of gastroscopy in the diagnosis of gastric cancer cannot be overstated. It not only helps to confirm the presence of the cancer and obtain confirmatory biopsies, but also clarifies the location of the tumor, its proximal and distal extent, rules out synchronous lesions, determines if there is gastric outlet obstruction (in which case, helps place a nasoenteric tube for feeding), and secures hemostasis in the event of a bleeding tumor (using strategies such as adrenaline injections or other hemostatic techniques).

### Endoscopic ultrasound (EUS)

EUS plays an invaluable role in defining the T-stage of the tumor in early gastric cancer. Only patients with T1a disease (involving the mucosa) and favorable histology may be considered for therapeutic endoscopic procedures (endoscopic submucosal dissection [ESMD]) by trained and proficient endoscopists. For tumors with infiltration in the submucosa and beyond, surgery remains the gold standard in view of the risk of lymph node metastases.

### Radiological investigations

In order to appropriately stage the tumor, it is imperative that imaging be carried out and the most important tests include:

a) Triphasic multi-detector computed tomography (MDCT) scan of the chest, abdomen, and pelvis with multi-planar reconstruction:

MDCT scans provides enough information about the T-stage to guide therapy. The presence of peritumor fat stranding is considered suspicious for T3 disease and these patients are offered perioperative chemotherapy. MDCT scans are also useful to define locoregional and nodal spread, as well as distant intra-abdominal disease. It also helps delineate the vascular anatomy which is essential for preoperative surgical planning.

b) Magnetic resonance imaging (MRI) of the abdomen and pelvis:

MRIs may be used as an alternative to MDCT in patients with contrast allergies, or in the absence of facilities for performing, or the expertise needed to report, a CT scan. In these patients, an additional chest X-ray should be performed to rule out lung metastases.

### Complementary investigations

a) PET-CT is not useful in gastric cancer as mucin-containing tumors do not take up fluorodeoxyglucose. Thus, false negative results may be seen.

b) Staging laparoscopy – For patients with locally advanced disease (T3 by radiology with or without perigastric lymphadenopathy) who are being considered for perioperative chemotherapy, the performance of a staging laparoscopy is indicated as this will alter the intent of therapy from curative to palliative should the evidence of peritoneal spread of disease be noted.

### FURTHER MANAGEMENT

A patient who has been fully and adequately worked-up must be discussed in a multidisciplinary team meeting comprising of surgeons, medical and radiation oncologists, pathologists, and radiologists.

The options available for the treatment of locally advanced, non-metastatic gastric cancer, based on the evidence in literature are:

a) Surgery sandwiched between perioperative chemotherapy.

b) Upfront surgery followed by adjuvant chemotherapy/chemoradiotherapy.

Surgery sandwiched between perioperative chemotherapy is the current standard of care for locally advanced, asymptomatic, resectable gastric cancer. The initial impetus to this concept was provided by the Medical Research Council Adjuvant Gastric Infusional

Chemotherapy (MAGIC) trial conducted by the UK Medical Research Council which demonstrated a 13% five-year survival advantage for perioperative chemotherapy versus surgery alone [2]. In India, the authors noted that owing to the toxicity profile of epirubicin, cisplatin, and 5-fluorouracil (ECF), patients were able to tolerate epirubicin, oxaliplatin, and capecitabine (EOX) better (Sirohi B, et al. 2014). The recent success (median survival 50 months vs 35 months, respectively) of the 5-fluorouracil, leucovorin, docetaxel, and oxaliplatin (FLOT-4) regimen compared to ECF/ECX (capecitabine instead of 5-fluorouracil) in a randomized phase 2/3 trial published in the Lancet [3], is likely to see FLOT-4 being increasingly used worldwide. Like the MAGIC trial (45%), only 46% of patients completed the FLOT-4 regimen.

The option of upfront surgery is generally reserved for patients who present with symptoms of gastric outlet obstruction or bleeding refractory to (hemostatic) radiotherapy, or endoscopic attempts at hemostasis. It is supported by evidence from the CLASSIC (D2 gastrectomy followed by capecitabine and oxaliplatin) and ARTIST (D2 gastrectomy followed by capecitabine and cisplatin, with or without radiotherapy) trials from East Asia.

### Surgical management

From a surgical viewpoint, the principles remain the same despite the use of chemotherapy – a complete surgical resection with negative microscopic (R0) margins and a D2 lymphadenectomy (removal of the lymph nodes up to the second echelon). The authors have previously shown that the addition of perioperative chemotherapy may result in complete pathologic response rates in the primary tumor, however, the draining lymph nodes continue to harbor malignancy [4]. Given that locoregional recurrence remains the bane of resectable gastric cancer, performance of a D2 lymphadenectomy should thus be considered standard practice [5] (Figure 9.1).

*Extent of gastric resection (determined by the location of the primary tumor)*

- Total gastrectomy (with a Roux-en-Y esophagojejunostomy with or without a pouch):

    Lesions in the upper third and the upper portion of the middle-third of the stomach, or in linitis plastica lesions involving the entire stomach.

    A total gastrectomy must be considered in all patients in whom a safe oncological proximal margin cannot be achieved when performing a distal subtotal gastrectomy.

- Proximal gastrectomy:

    Lesions in the upper third of the stomach, so long as at least half of the stomach can be preserved.

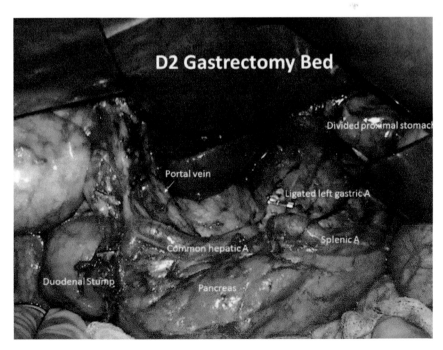

**Figure 9.1** Intraoperative photograph of the gastric bed following a D2 lymphadenectomy.

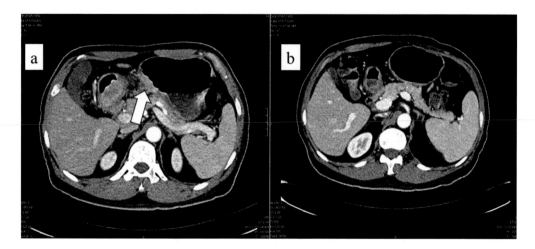

**Figure 9.2** Contrast-enhanced CT scan sections of the abdomen demonstrating: (a) Pre-chemotherapy: Axial post-contrast CT section showing locally advanced gastric cancer along the lesser curvature of the distal body and antrum (*white arrow*). (b) Post-chemotherapy: Axial post-contrast CT section showing complete radiological regression of the tumor.

■ Subtotal (distal) gastrectomy:

Lesions in the lower half of the middle third, or in the distal third of the stomach.

The addition of a bursectomy does not improve survival when compared to a standard omentectomy and D2 lymphadenectomy (JCOG1001).

### Multivisceral resections (including splenectomy)

Multivisceral resections (including organs such as the pancreas, duodenum, and colon) should be considered by experienced surgeons only if they ensure the likelihood of achieving a margin negative (R0) resection. These operations are fraught with the risk of operative morbidity and mortality and thus surgeons must consider the extent of the disease and the performance status of the patient before embarking on these procedures.

The addition of a splenectomy to a gastrectomy must only be considered when performed as part of total gastrectomy for gastric cancers (T2–4) located along the greater curvature with lymph node metastases to station 4sb, and/or in patients in whom a clearance of station 10 lymph nodes would be unable to be satisfactorily performed without the removal of the spleen.

### Role of laparoscopic resections for gastric cancer

Laparoscopic gastric cancer surgery (especially for early stage disease) is feasible. However, randomized controlled data that includes long-term survival outcomes is necessary to establish if laparoscopic surgery is superior to open surgery.

The patient presented in this scenario received epirubicin, cisplatin, 5-fluorouracil (ECF) chemotherapy, and had a good response to preoperative chemotherapy as per the response evaluation criteria in solid tumors (RECIST) criteria (Figure 9.2). He underwent a distal subtotal gastrectomy with D2 lymphadenectomy and made an uneventful recovery. He then went on to complete his postoperative chemotherapy regimen.

### SALIENT POINTS

■ Gastric cancer is a leading cause for cancer-related mortality around the world.

■ Patients with non-metastatic, locally advanced, asymptomatic, resectable gastric cancer should be offered perioperative chemotherapy.

■ Current options for perioperative chemotherapy include FLOT 4, ECF, ECX, or EOX. These protocols should be tailored to the patient tolerability and toxicity profile.

■ Gastrectomy plus D2 lymphadenectomy remains the standard of care despite perioperative chemotherapy.

■ Multivisceral resections must be performed by trained surgeons only in patients in whom the possibility of achieving a margin negative resection is certain.

■ Patient tolerability and extent of disease burden must be considered before embarking on multivisceral resections.

## CONFLICTS OF INTEREST
None to declare.

## REFERENCES

1. Barreto S, Windsor J. Re-defining early gastric cancer. *Surg Endosc* 2016;30:24–37.
2. Cunningham D, Allum WH, Stenning SP et al. Perioperative chemotherapy versus surgery alone for resectable gastroesophageal cancer. *N Engl J Med* 2006 Jul 6;355(1):11–20.
3. Al-Batran SE, Homann N, Pauligk C et al. Perioperative chemotherapy with fluorouracil plus leucovorin, oxaliplatin, and docetaxel versus fluorouracil or capecitabine plus cisplatin and epirubicin for locally advanced, resectable gastric or gastro-oesophageal junction adenocarcinoma (FLOT4): A randomised, phase 2/3 trial. *Lancet* 2019 May 11;393(10184):1948–1957.
4. Shrikhande S, Barreto S, Talole S et al. D2 Lymphadenectomy is not only safe but necessary in the era of neoadjuvant chemotherapy. *World J Surg Oncol* 2013;11:31.
5. Barreto SG, Sirohi B. Why should we perform a D2 lymphadenectomy in gastric cancer? *Future Oncol* 2017 Oct;13(23):2009–2012.

# 10 Locally Advanced, Unresectable Gastric Cancer

*Manish S. Bhandare, Vikram A. Chaudhari, and Shailesh V. Shrikhande*

## CONTENTS

## CASE SCENARIO

A 54-year-old gentleman without any comorbidities or significant past medical history presented with complaints of epigastric pain for a month prior to presentation along with vomiting after food intake for a duration of ten days. These symptoms were associated with weight loss and anorexia. There were no significant findings on clinical examination apart from epigastric fullness. A gastroscopy was performed which demonstrated an ulcerative growth in the pylorus extending into the first part of the duodenum. Biopsy from the growth was performed which was reported to be moderately differentiated adenocarcinoma. A contrast-enhanced computed tomography (CT) scan of the abdomen and pelvis was performed which revealed diffuse thickening of distal body and pyloric region of stomach with extension into the first part of the duodenum, with invasion of the pancreatic head and few enlarged perigastric nodes (Figure 10.1). An endoscopic guided nasojejunal tube was inserted to ensure adequate nutritional supplementation as he was in complete gastric outlet obstruction. Although he had locally advanced unresectable disease to begin with, in view of a good performance status and only one adverse factor, i.e. focal pancreatic head involvement in the absence of significant lymph node involvement, he was discussed at the multidisciplinary team meeting and was planned for initial chemotherapy followed by reassessment for surgery. A staging laparoscopy was performed which confirmed the absence of any peritoneal disease. The patient was commenced on four cycles of 5-fluorouracil, leucovorin, docetaxel, and oxaliplatin (FLOT) [1]. A repeat CT scan to assess treatment response demonstrated a partial response with development of small fistula at the site of pancreatic invasion (Figure

10.2). The patient was subjected to an exploration with an intent for trial of resection. In the absence of peritoneal metastases, the decision was made to proceed with a radical subtotal gastrectomy with pancreatoduodenectomy. R0 resection was achieved. He recovered well and was discharged on the ninth postoperative day. His final pathology report confirmed a moderately differentiated adenocarcinoma of the stomach with involvement of the pancreatic head and peripancreatic soft tissue with 2 out of 34 nodes showing metastasis (pT4N1M0). The patient went on to complete adjuvant chemotherapy and is currently disease free at a follow-up of 16 months.

## BACKGROUND OF THE PATHOLOGY

Gastric cancer is associated with a poor prognosis with a reported overall five-year survival rate of between 20–25% across all stages. Patients diagnosed with earlier stages of gastric cancer have a distinct survival advantage compared to those with more advanced-stage disease. As is the case for many cancers, the epidemiological distribution of gastric cancer demonstrates a marked variation in regional incidence, with as much as a ten-fold difference between the highest- and lowest-risk populations. Countries from South East Asia such as Japan, China, and South Korea, report the highest incidence.

For gastric adenocarcinomas, the most commonly used histological classification schemes are the Lauren classification and the World Health Organization (WHO) scheme. As per the Lauren classification, gastric carcinomas are divided into two main histological types, diffuse and intestinal, with the latter having a significantly better prognosis. The WHO categories are based on the predominant histological patterns of carcinoma, i.e. tubular,

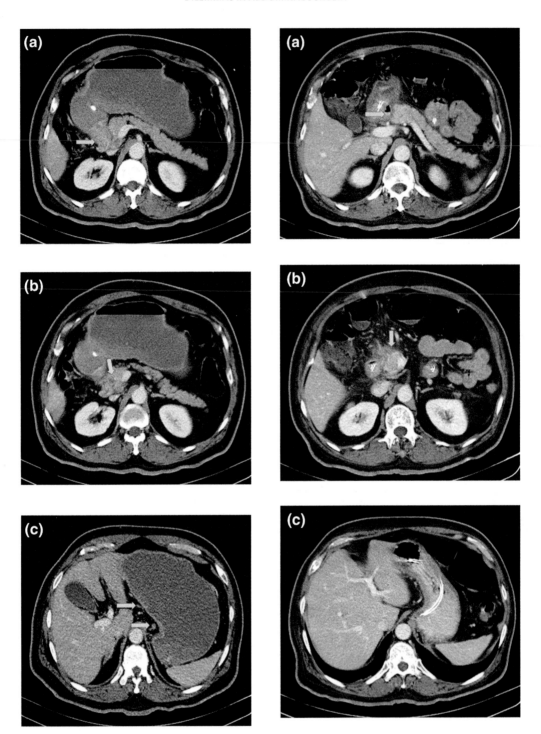

**Figure 10.1** Contrast-enhanced CT scan showing sections of the abdomen. Pre-chemotherapy: Axial CE-CT section showing (a) antropyloric growth (marked by arrow), causing gastric outlet obstruction, (b) growth invading into pancreatic head (marked by arrow), (c) few enlarged perigastric nodes (marked by arrow).

**Figure 10.2** Contrast-enhanced CT scan showing sections of the abdomen. Post-chemotherapy: Axial post-contrast CT section showing partial response, (a) pancreatic invasion with fistulization (marked by arrow), (b) loss of fat planes with pancreatic head, (c) post-chemotherapy regression of perigastric lymphadenopathy.

papillary, mucinous, poorly cohesive, and rare variants. The WHO tubular and papillary carcinomas roughly correspond to the intestinal type described by Lauren, and poorly cohesive carcinomas (encompassing cases constituted partly or totally by signet ring cells) correspond to the Lauren diffuse type.

Gastric cancers are best managed by a multidisciplinary team approach. All patients are staged according to the American Joint Committee on Cancer (AJCC) classification. Patients with stage I–III are treated with "curative" intent, while patients with stage IV disease are considered for "palliative" treatment.

In clinical practice, for investigations and treatment purpose, gastric cancer is divided into the following groups:

**Early gastric cancers** [T1a/T1b N0/N+ M0]: WHO defines early gastric cancer as cancer which is confined to the mucosa and submucosa regardless of lymph node status. However, a more recent evidence-based definition of early gastric cancer takes into account its depth of invasion (mucosa alone), histology, absence of nodal metastasis, and prognosis [2].

**Gastric cancer with locoregional disease** [T1b – T4 N+ M0]:

**Advanced gastric cancers** [unresectable/ metastatic T4 N+ or M1]:

## APPROACH TO MANAGEMENT

### Clinical findings (symptoms and signs)

Common symptoms associated with locally advanced gastric cancer include vomiting and nausea, bleeding (hematemesis and/or melena), abdominal pain, lump in epigastric region, unexplained weight loss, loss of appetite, and early satiety. Patients with tumors at the gastroesophageal junction or proximal stomach might also present with dysphagia. A symptom complex is more suggestive of gastric cancer rather than a single sign or symptom.

### Investigations

a) Endoscopy: Gastroscopy is often the first investigation performed for patients with symptoms of dyspepsia and other upper gastrointestinal symptoms. This enables identification of the primary tumor, its anatomic localization (i.e. disease mapping), as well as the ability to obtain tissue for diagnosis. Any suspicious-appearing gastric ulceration needs to be biopsied.

b) Radiology: A contrast-enhanced CT scan is performed early following the diagnosis of gastric cancer by endoscopy and biopsy (Figures 10.1 and 10.2) for the purpose of accurate staging of the cancer. It provides information regarding the local extent of the tumor, involvement of adjacent structures (left lobe of liver – segments 2/3, pancreatic head, invasion of porta hepatis, etc.), and helps in predicting resectability by detecting distant visceral spread. However, it lacks sensitivity in detecting peritoneal metastases and hematogenous metastases smaller than 5 mm, even with modern CT techniques. The PET-CT scan was not considered useful in primary evaluation of gastric cancers as most diffuse type (signet ring cell tumors) are not fluorodeoxyglucose avid. However, its role in preoperative evaluation is evolving.

c) Staging laparoscopy: Although laparoscopy is more invasive than CT or endoscopic ultrasound, it has the advantage of directly visualizing the liver surface, the peritoneum, and local lymph nodes for assessing metastatic disease. Another advantage of laparoscopy is the ability to perform peritoneal cytology in patients who have no visible evidence of peritoneal spread. Staging laparoscopy upstages the disease which leads to change in the management plan in about 20–30% of patients who have disease that is beyond T1 stage despite having a negative CT scan. Hence, staging laparoscopy is recommended for all patients with gastric cancer who appear to have more than T1 lesion, without any histological confirmation of stage IV disease.

d) Tumor markers: Serum levels of carcinoembryonic antigen and carbohydrate antigen 19-9, may be elevated in patients with gastric cancer. However, due to low sensitivity and specificity, they are not considered as essential or diagnostic of gastric cancer. They can be used in the follow-up evaluation if levels at baseline were elevated.

### Principles of management

The management of GC requires a multidisciplinary approach. All patients are staged according to the AJCC classification.

Surgical resection is the principal therapy for gastric cancer, as it offers the only potential for cure. The aim of surgery is to offer a resection with negative margins and adequate D2 lymph node dissection [3]. Neoadjuvant chemotherapy (perioperative chemotherapy) has an established role in patients with locally advanced resectable disease and is considered as standard of care in most parts of the world.

Postoperative chemotherapy or postoperative chemo radiation are alternative approaches for these tumors.

For advanced unresectable/metastatic gastric cancers, the mainstay of treatment is palliative chemotherapy which improves survival marginally and also improves quality of life. Apart from chemotherapy, palliation of symptoms such as gastric outlet obstruction and management of ascites, pleural effusion, and pain is also essential.

### Treatment options with benefits and risks

The patient presented in the Case Scenario had a locally advanced gastric cancer with duodenal and pancreatic head involvement. Pancreatic head involvement of gastric cancer is considered an advanced, inoperable disease, and the standard treatment for these patients is palliative chemotherapy. Patients presenting with gastric outlet obstruction should be managed with either endoscopic gastroduodenal self-expanding metal stent placement or with a palliative gastrojejunostomy before initiating chemotherapy. The choice between the two options depends on the overall disease burden, predicted life expectancy, and availability of endoscopic expertise. In general, surgical bypass, i.e., gastrojejunostomy, is preferred over gastroduodenal self-expanding metal stent in patients with a life expectancy of more than six months because stents can get blocked over a period of time. Also, stents are associated with a risk of migration and perforation.

Certain patients also present with bleeding from the primary tumor, which can be acute or chronic manifesting as hematemesis or melena. Endoscopic treatment involving the injection of adrenaline or ablative therapy (e.g. argon-plasma coagulation), or angiographic embolization is generally preferred as first-line therapy with palliative emergency gastrectomy reserved when these options fail or are unavailable. Hemostatic radiation therapy has also been attempted with some success. In patients with chronic blood loss, the use of proton pump inhibitors and sucralfate may be considered along with blood transfusions and/or iron infusions.

The chemotherapy regimens used to treat advanced, unresectable tumors generally consist of a 5-fluorouracil and platinum doublet. In some centers, a combination of a third agent, i.e. docetaxel and epirubicin, has been used with some success. Based on the REAL-2 and ML17032 studies, an epirubicin-5-fluorouracil, capecitabine-cisplatin, and oxaliplatin triplet is a regimen of choice in fit patients with a good performance status [4]. A docetaxel, cisplatin, and 5-fluorouracil triplet combination is also associated with good response rates and improvement in median overall survival, although with high rates of grade 3 and grade 4 toxicity. When triplet combination is not feasible, a cisplatin-oxaliplatin doublet – 5-fluorouracil/capecitabine or single agent docetaxel, paclitaxel, and capecitabine have also shown feasibility and can be used as palliative chemotherapy. In this subset of patients, it is important to test for the Her-2 receptor status since the results of the trastuzumab for gastric cancer (ToGA) trial demonstrated a significant survival advantage with the use of trastuzumab, in addition to the doublet chemotherapy, in patients who are Her-2 positive [5]. The use of other targeted agents, such as bevacizumab and ramucirumab, has not shown statistical or clinically significant benefits in combination chemotherapy when used in first-line therapy. The median survival with palliative chemotherapy is reported to be in the range of 12–18 months.

Although the standard treatment is palliative chemotherapy for advanced unresectable gastric cancer, in well selected patients (such as the patient presented in the Case Scenario), there exists a possibility to carry out extended resections with the promise of improved survival. Ideally, such patients who are being considered for multivisceral resection with a likelihood of achieving R0 resection leading to improvement in survival should be evaluated for surgery at high volume centers. The patient presented had a good performance status at presentation, limited disease burden confirmed on contrast-enhanced CT and staging laparoscopy, and had a good response to initial chemotherapy, which convinced us to plan a radical surgery to achieve R0 resection. The testament to appropriate patient selection is evident form the fact that the patient remains disease-free at 16 months of follow-up.

There is some retrospective data to suggest that selected patients with distal gastric cancers with isolated pancreatic head involvement in the absence of peritoneal and gross lymph nodal disease can be offered curative surgery, i.e. radical gastrectomy with pancreaticoduodenectomy, in high volume centers, to achieve R0 resection and this can lead to improvement in survival [6]. Also, unresectable gastric cancer patients initially exhibiting only one non-curative factor (like the case in discussion with pancreatic head involvement alone as an incurable factor), who receive a conversion surgery after good response to chemotherapy and undergo R0 resection, have been shown to enjoy a significant improvement on overall survival [7].

However, such extended and multivisceral resections for locally advanced gastric cancer should only be offered to well-selected patients at high volume centers, so as to get the desired benefit in improving their long-term survival while keeping the operative morbidity and mortality to a minimum.

## KEY MESSAGES

- The standard treatment for locally advanced unresectable gastric cancer is palliative chemotherapy with surgery reserved for palliation of symptoms like obstruction and/or bleeding.
- Well-selected patients with locally advanced unresectable disease should be evaluated for a radical surgery at high volume centers, with or without multivisceral resection after initial chemotherapy with good response, when there is high likelihood of achieving R0 resection, which can lead to improvement in survival.

## REFERENCES

1. Al-Batran S-E, Homann N, Schmalenberg H et al. Perioperative chemotherapy with docetaxel, oxaliplatin, and fluorouracil/leucovorin (FLOT) versus epirubicin, cisplatin, and fluorouracil or capecitabine (ECF/ECX) for resectable gastric or gastroesophageal junction (GEJ) adenocarcinoma (FLOT4-AIO): A multicenter, randomized phase 3 trial. *J Clin Oncol* 2017 May 20;35:4004.

2. Barreto SG, Windsor JA. Redefining early gastric cancer. *Surg Endosc* 2016;30(1):24–37.

3. Shrikhande SV, Barreto SG, Talole SD et al. D2 lymphadenectomy is not only safe but necessary in the era of neoadjuvant chemotherapy. *World J Surg Oncol* 2013;11:31.

4. Okines AFC, Norman AR, McCloud P et al. Meta-analysis of the REAL-2 and ML17032 trials: Evaluating capecitabine-based combination chemotherapy and infused 5-fluorouracil-based combination chemotherapy for the treatment of advanced oesophago-gastric cancer. *Ann Oncol* 2009 Sep 1;20(9):1529–1534.

5. Bang Y-J, Van Cutsem E, Feyereislova A et al. Trastuzumab in combination with chemotherapy versus chemotherapy alone for treatment of HER2-positive advanced gastric or gastro-oesophageal junction cancer (ToGA): A phase 3, open-label, randomised controlled trial. *Lancet* 2010 Aug;376(9742):687–697.

6. Roberts P, Seevaratnam R, Cardoso R et al. Systematic review of pancreaticoduodenectomy for locally advanced gastric cancer. *Gastric Cancer* 2012 Sep 1;15(1):108–115.

7. Fukuchi M, Ishiguro T, Ogata K et al. Prognostic role of conversion surgery for unresectable gastric cancer. *Ann Surg Oncol* 2015 Oct 1;22(11):3618–3624.

# 11 Post Total Gastrectomy Complications: Duodenal Stump Leak

*Kailash Kurdia and Rajneesh Kumar Singh*

## CONTENTS

## CASE SCENARIO

A 70-year-old man presented with complaints of dyspepsia, anorexia, and weight loss over three months. Upper gastrointestinal endoscopy showed a large ulcerated growth in the antropyloric region of the stomach and the biopsy was reported as an adenocarcinoma. Blood investigations confirmed anemia. A contrast-enhanced computed tomography (CT) scan of the abdomen and pelvis staged the tumor as cT3N1M0. After a discussion by the multidisciplinary tumor board, the patient was taken up for planned neoadjuvant chemotherapy as part of a perioperative chemotherapy regime. Following a re-staging CT scan four weeks after chemotherapy that confirmed absence of disease progression, the patient underwent a staging laparoscopy. The operative findings revealed a small circumferential tumor involving the gastric antrum and a few perigastric lymph nodes for which the patient underwent a distal subtotal gastrectomy, D2 lymphadenectomy with a Roux-en-Y gastrojejunostomy and feeding jejunostomy. The duodenal stump was divided with a stapler and sewn over with interrupted 3-0 polypropylene sutures. Two intra-abdominal drains were placed, one in the region of the duodenal stump and the other in the left retrogastric area. While the early postoperative course appeared uneventful, by the fourth postoperative day, the patient developed abdominal distension and intolerance to feeding. He was in pain, febrile with tachycardia, and had developed mild tachypnea by postoperative day five. The wound examination showed some tenderness and minimal discharge. The drain adjacent to the duodenal stump was draining about 100 ml of serous fluid daily. He had an elevated white cell count (16,000/cmm) with a chest X-ray suggestive of basal consolidation on the right side with a pleural effusion. An ultrasound examination of the abdomen provided inadequate evaluation due to abdominal distension and excessive bowel gas. The drain fluid amylase was found to be normal. Microbiologic assessment of the drain fluid showed *Escherichia coli* on culture.

## BACKGROUND OF THE PATHOLOGY

The risk factors for duodenal stump leaks can be broadly classified into modifiable factors and non-modifiable factors. The modifiable (or partially modifiable) factors include patient factors like poor nutrition and poorly controlled comorbid conditions; surgical factors like inadvertent devascularization of duodenal stump due to excessive dissection and diathermy use, inadequate surgical closure of duodenal stump, local hematoma or incorrect abdominal drain placement; and other factors like neoadjuvant therapy, neoplastic involvement of duodenal resection margin (R1–R2 resections) or postoperative distension of duodenum due to distal obstruction. Non-modifiable factors include advanced age and an advanced stage of cancer. The method of closing the duodenal stump has been a subject of much scrutiny in this regard. However, no single method (stapled or hand sewn) has been convincingly shown to be superior to the other. A recent comparative study did show that purse-string suture closure may have a lower leak rate than stapled or inter-rupted suture closure. Several surgeons use reinforcement of the duodenal staple or suture line to try to prevent duodenal stump leak. However, there is no universal agreement on the superiority of any one technique (including the use of fibrin glue, oversewing suture line, or omental buttress) over the other. Oversewing with barbed suture has been shown to have lower leak rates in one study of laparoscopic gastrectomy. At least one study reported a novel naso-gastro-duodenal tube to keep the duodenum decompressed in the postoperative period and help in reducing leak rates.

### Clinical presentation

Duodenal stump leaks usually present at the end of the first postoperative week (fifth to tenth day). The most common presentation is in the form of abdominal pain and fever. These may be accompanied by tachycardia, vomiting, ileus, distension, and in severe cases, perito-nitis; and in unrecognized cases, progress to multiorgan failure.

While fever in the immediate postoperative period after gastrectomy may be due to non-infective causes, such as surgical trauma and/or basal atelectasis within the first 48 hours, postoperative fever beyond 48 hours is usu-ally due to an infective focus. The search for such an infective focus may be divided into causes directly related to the surgical field (e.g. anastomotic leaks, collections, abscesses, etc.) or related to other nonsurgical causes (e.g. central venous lines, urinary catheters, hospi-tal acquired pneumonia, etc.). An experienced surgical team learns to keep a high index of suspicion for an intra-abdominal complication in these scenarios.

In this patient, the surgical wound was sug-gestive of superficial surgical site infection. The wound was laid partially open at the bedside, and purulent fluid removed with open dressing of the wound. The incidence of wound infec-tion following open gastrectomy can be as high as 20%. Some of the contributory factors may be anemia, hypoalbuminemia, preoperative chemotherapy, and gastric outlet obstruction. However, surgical complications often tend to occur in clusters. Hence, a severe wound infec-tion may be associated with an intra-abdominal complication like an anastomotic leak or duo-denal stump blowout. In this case, the patient continued to have fever and tachycardia even after drainage of the surgical wound. Hence a suspicion of an intra-abdominal complication was raised. Further, this patient underwent a contrast-enhanced CT scan of the abdomen and pelvis that revealed a 5x5 cm collection

in the right subhepatic region with few small pockets of entrapped air. The drain adjacent to the duodenum was noted to be anterior to the pancreatic head and away from this collection. The duodenum was seen to be collapsed and the duodenal stump could be identified by the radio-opaque staple line on the CT scan. In addition, there was a small pleural effusion on the right side with basal lung consolidation.

### Investigations

The initial investigations in case of suspected duodenal stump leak include blood investiga-tions, ultrasound, and X-ray examination of the chest. Further workup is dependent on the index of suspicion.

a) *Blood investigations*: Blood workup should include complete blood counts; renal func-tion parameters, like blood urea nitrogen, serum creatinine, and electrolytes; and liver function tests including serum total proteins and albumin. Ancillary blood tests that may be needed in florid sepsis include blood sugar monitoring, blood gas parameters, and inflammatory markers like C-reactive protein. Further, these may need to be repeated depending on the severity of the sepsis and progress of the patient. Patients needing interventions or surgery will also need a basic coagulation workup including platelet counts and international normalized ratio. Cultures of blood, urine, and drain fluids should be sent routinely as these may help in directing antibiotics therapy and should be repeated as needed.

b) *Imaging*

i) *Chest X-ray*: A chest X-ray is useful in diagnosis and follow-up of chest complica-tions like pleural effusions or pneumonitis that are usually secondary to intra-abdomi-nal sepsis.

ii) *Ultrasound*: An ultrasound examina-tion is often the first abdominal imaging advised in case of a suspected leak. The usual findings are intra-abdominal collec-tions/abscesses, free fluid in the abdomen, and distended bowel loops. However, the sensitivity of ultrasound is lowered in the presence of distended bowel loops and an inexperienced operator. Since most intra-abdominal interventions are done with ultrasound guidance, it is a useful start-ing point for investigating patients with suspected intra-abdominal complications.

iii) *Contrast-enhanced CT scan of the abdo-men and pelvis (with or without oral contrast)*: If the suspicion of a duodenal stump remains high (clinical or radiology), a contrast-enhanced CT scan of the abdomen and pelvis is the investigation of choice. The usual findings are intra-abdominal collections/abscesses, free fluid, and distended bowel loops (Figure 11.1). The

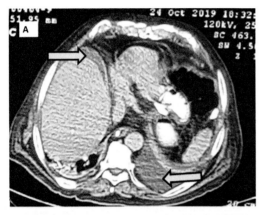

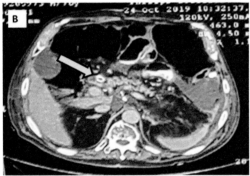

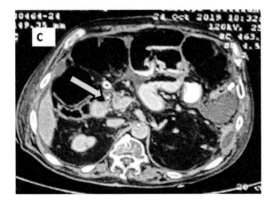

**Figure 11.1** Axial sections of a contrast-enhanced CT scan of the abdomen demonstrating: (A) Perihepatic fluid collection and left sided pleural effusion (yellow arrows), (B) the tip of right flank drain anterior to the head of pancreas (yellow arrow), (C) duodenal stump with the radio-opaque staple line visible (yellow arrow).

interpretation of the CT scan performed for a suspected duodenal stump blowout is fraught with several pitfalls. Identification of the duodenal stump may be facilitated by the fact that the radio-opaque staple line is easily visualized on the CT scan. It must be remembered that in this form of postgastrectomy reconstruction, the duodenum is excluded from the food stream. Hence, ordinarily orally ingested water-soluble contrast would not fill up the duodenum and there is no contrast leak to look for. However, sometimes the oral contrast may travel retrograde to fill up the duodenal stump in case of distal bowel obstruction, edema, or ileus. In such instances, the duodenal loop may be seen to be distended with contrast. Milder forms of duodenal stump leak will only present with collections in relation to the duodenal stump. These collections may be seen in the Morison's pouch or anterior to the pancreatic head or occasionally tracking into the right paracolic gutter, and often may have pockets of air to indicate bowel communication. It must be remembered that not all collections or abscesses in the right upper abdomen are related to duodenal stump leakage, but the suspicion remains high.

### Role of surgical drains in detecting postoperative complications

While surgical drains are usually placed for draining any serous fluid exuding due to surgical dissection, it is also hoped that drains would provide the first indicators of a surgical complication such as an anastomotic leak. Postgastrectomy, the presence of bilious fluid in the right abdominal drain, or a high drain fluid amylase is highly suggestive of a duodenal stump leak. However, it is well appreciated that surgical drains may not function the way they were intended to due to reasons such as clogging off secondary to coagulum, displacement from the surgical field, etc. Studies on postgastrectomy analysis of drain fluid amylase for detecting complications have provided inconsistent results. Drain fluid amylase sometimes may not rise, even in patients with clinical leaks. Even in those with high drain fluid amylase, this rise may not antedate the symptoms of leak, thereby being of questionable utility in clinical practice.

### Management

The management of duodenal stump leak depends, to a certain extent, on the clinical presentation of the patient. On one end of the spectrum is a patient like in the present case, with a minor leak and collection in the right upper abdomen. At the other extreme, a major leak would lead to severe spillage of infected contents all over the peritoneal cavity with consequent peritonitis, necessitating immediate surgical re-exploration. In the latter, the generalized peritonitis is often accompanied by organ dysfunction, including respiratory distress or acute renal failure.

Measures used to manage duodenal stump leak can be considered in the following subheadings.

### Control of sepsis

a) *Intravenous antibiotics*: Broad-spectrum antibiotics to cover gram-negative, gram-positive, and anaerobic bacteria should be started empirically if needed, and thereafter changed based on culture-sensitivity results as available.

b) *Drainage of collections*: Intra-abdominal collections/abscesses are preferably drained by placement of percutaneous ultrasound guided drains. Occasionally, a difficult access may prompt a CT-guided approach for the placement of a drain. In a few cases with widespread spillage of the duodenal contents in the peritoneal cavity, surgical lavage and the placement of drains may be needed.

### Ancillary/supportive measures

a) *Nil per oral and nutritional supplementation*: In most patients (with minor leaks), the inflammation is confined to the upper abdomen, and the rest of the bowel function is usually preserved. Hence, small bowel feeding through a feeding jejunostomy tube or a nasojejunal tube is often well tolerated and an effective way of delivering enteral nutrition. Keeping the patient nil by mouth is initially recommended in view of upper abdominal inflammation. The patient may then be gradually started on an oral diet as the inflammation resolves during treatment, even without waiting for the duodenal fistula to close completely. This is possible as the duodenal stump is blind after surgery and not part of the food passage (except in case of gastroduodenal anastomosis). Occasionally, total parenteral nutrition is needed (often initially) when enteral nutrition is not well tolerated due to inflammation and ileus.

b) *Physiotherapy and supportive measures*: Often, these patients develop secondary complications such as pneumonitis in the presence of intra-abdominal sepsis. Hence mobilization and physiotherapy plays a major role in early recovery and prevention, and management of these secondary complications, including deep vein thrombosis.

### Management of high-output duodenal fistula

a) *Fluid and electrolyte management*: The loss of fluid and electrolytes from the duodenal fistula should be factored in the daily requirements of the patient and should be adequately replaced. Re-feeding of the duodenal fistula contents into the enteral tube feeding is often practiced in resource-constrained situations as a low cost solution to reduce the impact of duodenal fistula loss. However, this can only be done once the patient is free of sepsis and has a persistent high-output fistula.

b) *Measures to reduce the high-output duodenal fistula*: Temporary withholding of enteral intake may be needed in case of a high-output duodenal fistula as this may be due to retrograde reflux of the enteral feed. Latert, enteral feeding can be reintroduced in gradual increments. Somatostatin and its analogs are useful in reducing duodenal, pancreatic, and biliary secretion and hence reducing duodenal fistula output. However, this must be weighed against the increased cost of treatment and the fact that the fistula closure duration are not much improved with these drugs.

c) *Investigations*: A persistently high-output fistula should lead to investigation for downstream obstruction at the level of the gastrojejunostomy, jejunojejunostomy, or feeding jejunostomy. In such a case, a CT scan of the abdomen will show a dilated duodenum, often filled with retrograde reflux of oral contrast agent from the gastro-jejunostomy. Such an obstruction may need surgical correction.

d) *Surgery*: If adequately managed, most duodenal fistulae would close with non-surgical treatment. The indications of surgical treatment include a persistent high-output duodenal fistula, secondary complications such as associated bowel fistulae or bleeding, extensive contamination of the peritoneal cavity, and down-stream obstruction leading to a high-output duodenal fistula.

### Management of a minor duodenal stump leak

"Minor leakage" refers to localized spill of duodenal contents without major sepsis

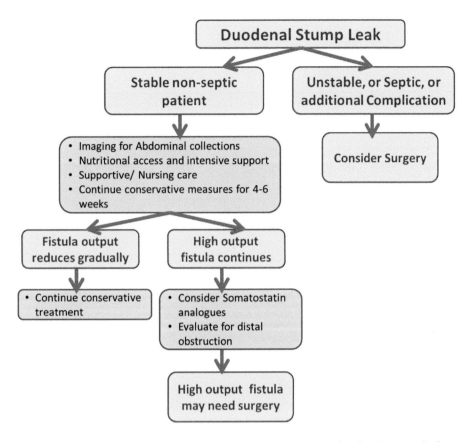

**Figure 11.2** Flowchart for the management of a postgastrectomy duodenal stump leak.

and may be managed non-surgically with percutaneous drainage of any collections/abscesses along with appropriate antibiotics and supportive care (Figure 11.2). The aim of intervention is to convert the leak into a controlled duodenal fistula. An important part of the supportive care is good nutritional intake. The non-surgical measures listed above would be successful in most cases to manage a small duodenal leak. With the conservative approach, the mean reported fistula closure time is 39 days (22–68) [1].

*Management of a major duodenal stump leak*
"Major duodenal leaks" refers to severe peritoneal spill, general peritoneal signs, and sepsis. It is usually managed with surgery (Figure 11.2). The mandatory steps at surgery are a thorough peritoneal lavage, wide drainage, and placement of a feeding tube jejunostomy (if not already performed). If the duodenal stump is of reasonable health, a suture closure may be attempted and reinforced with omentum or falciform ligament. Otherwise, a tube duodenostomy with a soft drainage tube through the duodenal leak site

may be done. We have successfully used a latex T-tube (no. 16 or 18) or a Foley's catheter (latex, size 16–18) that are brought out through the flank, alongside a paraduodenal drain. In some cases of severe peritonitis, it may not be possible to primarily close the midline fascia and a planned laparostomy may be undertaken. A meta-analysis of the existing data on the management of duodenal stump leaks determined that while all patients underwent peritoneal lavage, additional surgical procedures performed included: repair of duodenal stump (53%), tube duodenostomy (36%), biliary procedures (11%), and laparostomy (2%) [2]. A large multicenter study from Italy showed that 37% of the patients underwent surgical treatment, 12% needed surgery twice, and 6% needed to undergo three surgical procedures [3]. Multivariate analysis of factors predicting delayed healing were multiple surgeries, abdominal abscesses, colonic fistula, and central line sepsis.

Duodenal fistula following a major duodenal stump leak may be associated with other complications, such as secondary hemorrhage, pneumonitis, acute renal failure, etc. These will need to be managed simultaneously with the duodenal leak for optimal recovery of the patient. A multicenter study found associated complications such as abdominal abscesses (38%), wound infection (28%), sepsis (26%), central line infection (15%), pneumonia (13%), acute renal failure (10%), colonic fistula (7%), etc. [4,5].

Endoscopic treatment of duodenal stump blowout has been rarely employed. Published literature consists of only a few case reports and therefore it is not a standard modality of management of these patients.

### Case scenario (continued)

The patient was commenced on broad spectrum intravenous antibiotics. These were initially empiric but were then guided by the drain fluid culture. An ultrasound-guided percutaneous drain was placed by the intervention radiologist into the subhepatic collection. It drained 100 ml of bilious fluid immediately. The fever and tachycardia responded in 48 hours and the abdominal distension decreased. The total leucocyte count reduced to 11,000/cmm within 48 hours of drainage. The patient was gradually started on oral and tube feeding. Output from the drainage tube gradually reduced and it was removed after a week. Thereafter, the patient was progressively weaned off tube feeding and was able to fulfill his nutritional requirements solely through oral feeding.

### KEY MESSAGES

■ Meticulous surgical technique should be adhered to in order to prevent a duodenal stump blowout.

■ Abdominal pain, fever, and tachycardia in the late first postoperative week should be viewed with a high index of suspicion and investigated.

■ Adequate drainage of collections/abscesses, appropriate antibiotics, and good nutrition are the cornerstones of treatment.

■ Major leaks need surgery, and may have severe associated complications and a high mortality.

### REFERENCES

1. Cornejo Mde L, Priego P, Ramos D et al. Duodenal fistula after gastrectomy: Retrospective study of 13 new cases. *Rev Esp Enferm Dig* 2016 Jan;108(1):20–26.
2. Zizzo M, Ugoletti L, Manzini L et al. Management of duodenal stump fistula after gastrectomy for malignant disease: A systematic review of the literature. *BMC Surg* 2019 May 28;19(1):55.
3. Cozzaglio L, Giovenzana M, Biffi R et al. Surgical management of duodenal stump fistula after elective gastrectomy for malignancy: An Italian retrospective multicenter study. *Gastric Cancer* 2016 Jan;19(1):273–279.
4. Cozzaglio L, Coladonato M, Biffi R et al. Duodenal fistula after elective gastrectomy for malignant disease: An Italian retrospective multicenter study. *J Gastrointest Surg* 2010 May;14(5):805–811.
5. Aurello P, Sirimarco D, Magistri P et al. Management of duodenal stump fistula after gastrectomy for gastric cancer: Systematic review. *World J Gastroenterol* 2015 Jun 28;21(24):7571–7576.

# 12 Post Total Gastrectomy Complications

## *Esophagojejunal Anastomosis Leak*

*Kailash Kurdia and Rajneesh Kumar Singh*

## CONTENTS

## CASE SCENARIO

A 30-year-old man presented with complaints of dyspepsia followed by progressive dysphagia over a period of three months. Upper gastrointestinal endoscopy revealed an ulceroproliferative mass extending from the gastroesophageal junction into the proximal body of stomach with a biopsy confirmatory for an adenocarcinoma. A staging contrast-enhanced computed tomography (CT) scan of the abdomen and pelvis demonstrated a mass involving the proximal stomach staged as cT3N+M0. The patient's findings were discussed in the multidisciplinary tumor board and planned for neoadjuvant chemoradiotherapy (45 Gy external beam radiotherapy and two cycles of chemotherapy – cisplatin, and capecitabine based). Following a re-staging computed tomography (CT) scan four weeks after therapy that confirmed absence of disease progression, the patient underwent a staging laparoscopy. The operative findings confirmed thickening of the proximal stomach extending up to the gastroesophageal junction with small perigastric nodes. In the absence of peritoneal metastases, he went on to have a total gastrectomy with a Roux-en-Y esophagojejunostomy, D2 lymphadenectomy, splenectomy, and feeding jejunostomy. The duodenum was divided with a stapler and oversewn with interrupted polypropylene sutures. The esophagojejunal anastomosis was performed in an end-to-side fashion employing a 25 mm circular stapler, with a 50 cm Roux limb of the jejunum. Drains were placed in the regions of the esophagojejunostomy and the duodenal stump. The final histopathologic tumor stage was ypT0N0M0 (no residual tumor). In the early postoperative period, the patient appeared well and could be gradually started on feeding through the jejunostomy. The intraoperatively placed transanastomotic nasogastric tube continued to drain 300–400 ml bilious fluid per day. On the sixth postoperative day, the patient complained of left shoulder pain. This was accompanied with the clinical signs of tachycardia and a raised total white cell count (25,000/cmm) on routine investigation. A day later, the drain near the esophagojejunostomy anastomosis started draining bilious output.

## BACKGROUND OF THE PATHOLOGY

The esophagojejunostomy anastomosis is the Achilles heel of a total gastrectomy. esophagojejunostomy anastomotic leak is a serious and potentially fatal complication that may result in delayed oral feeding, a prolonged hospital stay, increased costs, and the long-term risk of an anastomotic stricture.

The risk factors for an esophagojejunostomy leak include advanced age, pulmonary comorbidities, high HbA1c, multiple organ resections, increased operative time, significant blood loss, the need for intraoperative blood transfusions, macroscopic esophageal invasion of the cancer, extent of lymph node dissection, and an elevated postoperative creatinine level [1]. The contribution of chemoradiotherapy to the development of an esophagojejunostomy leak cannot be underestimated. An intraoperative air leak test and endoscopic examination can detect technical failure of the anastomosis during surgery and the placement of additional, buttressing sutures may prevent a leak [2,3].

Meticulous surgical techniques, experience with anastomotic devices, and a thorough understanding of various risk factors and the institution of preventive measures are essential to mitigate the risk of an esophagojejunostomy leak.

## CLINICAL PRESENTATION

Early diagnosis of esophagojejunostomy leak plays an important part in successful management with a good outcome. Unfortunately, the initial clinical signs of an esophagojejunostomy leak may be nonspecific. A clinical leak is defined by the presence of pyrexia, increased abdominal pain, systemic sepsis, or gastrointestinal content within the abdominal drain. Suspicious appearance (turbid, purulent, bilious, or enteric) of the effluent from the juxta-anastomotic surgical drain may be an early warning sign. These findings generally prompt further evaluation to confirm or rule out an esophagojejunostomy leak.

## INVESTIGATIONS

The initial investigations include blood investigations, ultrasound, and X-ray examination of the chest and abdomen. Further workup is dependent on the index of suspicion.

a) *Blood investigations*: Blood workup should include complete blood counts; a renal function test, such as blood urea nitrogen, serum creatinine and electrolytes; and liver function tests, including serum total proteins and albumin. Ancillary blood tests that may be needed in florid sepsis include blood sugar monitoring, blood gas parameters, and inflammatory markers like C-reactive protein. Further, these may need to be repeated depending on the severity of the sepsis and progress of the patient. Patients needing interventions or surgery will also need a basic coagulation workup including platelet counts and international normalized ratio. Cultures of blood, urine, and drain fluids should be sent routinely as these may help in directing antibiotics therapy and should be repeated as needed.

b) *Imaging*

i) *Oral contrast radiography*: An anastomotic leakage is confirmed by the extravasation of orally ingested water-soluble contrast during the radiological examination or as a full-thickness defect visualized at flexible video endoscopy. The leak is considered subclinical if detected during routine oral contrast examination in an asymptomatic patient. It must be remembered that poor mucosal coating property is an important pitfall of water soluble contrast agents. This may result in a false negative study even in the presence of a clinical leak. On the flip side, over-interpretation of mucosal folds may be diagnosed as a leak on the contrast study. Hence, such contrast studies should not be interpreted in isolation but with the clinical context in mind. Barium is not the preferred contrast agent in this study because of its property of retention around the leaking anastomosis. The retained barium can induce further inflammation and fibrosis, in addition to interfering with subsequent imaging like a CT scan by inducing radio-opaque artefacts.

ii) *Upper gastrointestinal endoscopy*: Oral contrast radiography may at times give a false negative or even a false positive result. It should be correlated with clinical evidence of a leak and sometimes a careful upper gastrointestinal endoscopy can detect a leak in case of doubt. Even though an endoscopy is considered to be safe and effective in such a scenario, we have not resorted to doing endoscopy in such patients and prefer to manage the patient using clinical signs and other investigations.

iii) *CECT scan*: Patients with evidence of sepsis in the form of fever, raised total leukocyte count or C-reactive protein would need to be investigated with a CECT scan (with oral and intravenous water-soluble contrast) of the thorax, abdomen, and pelvis. Thoracic CT scan is useful in demonstrating associated pulmonary complications like pleural effusion, basal consolidation, pneumonitis, etc. An abdominal CT scan may show active contrast extravasation from the anastomotic leak, subdiaphragmatic collections/abscesses, free fluid in the abdomen, dilated bowel loops, and any potential site of bowel obstruction that may have contributed to the leak. Though it suffers from the same pitfalls in demonstrating active contrast leak as the oral contrast study in the previous section, but it is a useful investigation to guide drainage of any residual collections and diagnosis of bowel obstruction, if any.

## TREATMENT OPTIONS

Once diagnosed, the management of an esophagojejunostomy leak depends on the patient's clinical condition, location of anastomosis, time point of diagnosis of leakage, extent of anastomotic disruption, perfusion/ischemia/ necrosis of conduit, involvement of surrounding organs, whether or not the leakage is contained, and tumor resection margin status. Treatment options include conservative treatment, endoscopic therapy, or surgery. Early and aggressive treatment is vital in order to prevent a further deterioration in the patient's clinical condition. Based on recent improvements and developments in conservative and endoscopic treatment options, not all esophagojejunostomy leaks warrant surgical reintervention.

### Conservative treatment

Conservative treatment is an option for clinically stable patients with small leakage. Severity of the leak also strongly influences clinical symptoms and appropriate treatment. In the presence of mild clinical symptoms and laboratory signs (fever, leucocytosis, and abnormal C-reactive protein), low output fistulas from the drains, and small radiologic leaks, conservative therapy is the treatment of choice, especially if adequate nutrition can be maintained. This would include nil by mouth, parenteral or enteral nutrition (jejunostomy tube), and culture-based antibiotics. Percutaneous radiologic-guided drainage of undrained intra-abdominal fluid collections is mandatory. The role of somatostatin or its analogs is questionable. We have tended not to use somatostatin or related drugs and have achieved good results with good nutrition, appropriate drainage, and supportive care.

### Endoscopic treatment

This is one field in which technologic advances have made a major headway in terms of the management of esophagojejunostomy leaks. Broadly, the endoscopic options can be classified into a) non-stent endoscopic therapy (such as endoscopic clips, over the scope clips, biologic sealants, etc.), and b) self-expanding metal stents [4]. According to published studies, the option choice exercised seems to depend on the size of the anastomotic insufficiency and margins status. An appropriate scenario for endoscopic treatment is a leakage up to 50% of the circumference and preserved vascularity (absence of conduit necrosis). Biological sealants or clip placement can be considered for smaller defects (<30% of the circumference) but sealants have limited success. Clip placement is a safe and effective method in the treatment of digestive fistulas. Multiple clips can be placed beginning at either edge of a defect and making one's way toward the

center of the defect. However, limitations may be represented by the inability to adequately grasp the damaged tissue and the partial success in full-thickness perforations. The new over-the-scope-clip system has shown fewer drawbacks with improved results for early leaks (<1 week) without fibrosis. In patients with larger defects (30–50% of the circumference) without necrosis, partially or fully covered plastic or self-expanding metal stents seem to be more effective. However, the associated problem is a high stent migration rate (reported to be up to 61%) that may need additional procedures to recover the stent. There is emerging evidence for the use of endoscopically placed vacuum sponge-assisted therapy in the management of anastomotic leakages with associated undrained collections in the perianastomotic region.

One must be aware about the paucity of robust evidence for the use of endoscopic modalities in esophagojejunostomy leaks. Most series are retrospective and without an adequate comparison with conservative or surgical treatment.

### Surgical treatment

Early surgical management is warranted in patients who are in sepsis with diffuse peritonitis, or in those in whom adequate drainage through a radiological or endoscopic approach has not been achieved or in the case of jejunal limb necrosis [5]. Resurgery is fraught with the risk of high morbidity and even mortality and hence should only be considered when conservative management is unsuccessful or in the case of uncontrolled sepsis. If surgery is carried out following esophagojejunostomy leak, a few basic principles would need to be adhered to. First, exploration of the anastomotic site to fully assess the extent of leakage and potential ischemia/necrosis is essential to guide further treatment. Second, a thorough lavage of the surgical site with warm saline, decortication of the thoracic cavity from necrotic and fibrotic tissue (if necessitated), and abscess debridement are crucial for sepsis control. Third, adequate internal and external drainage of the leakage has to be established by using large drains and nasogastric tubes. A T-tube drain can be placed directly into the defect to enable a controlled drainage of the leak. Surgical options include direct repair of the anastomosis, redo of the anastomosis, or take-down of anastomosis with abdominal jejunostomy and closure of the esophagus combined with endoluminal drainage. Early leakage (<72 hours after initial operation) is usually due to a technical error. Surgical reintervention is recommended with the aim to potentially redo the anastomosis, or to directly close the site of leakage. The latter must only be attempted if the leakage is small and the anastomosis is without (or with only minimal) signs of ischemia/necrosis, and if

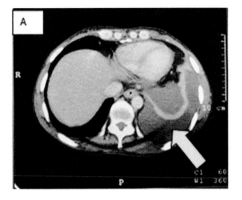

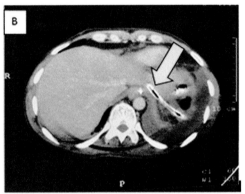

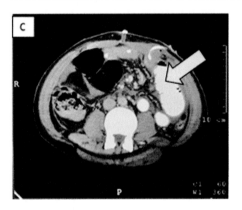

**Figure 12.1** Axial sections of a contrast-enhanced CT scan of the abdomen demonstrating: (A) Left pleural effusion with underlying collapsed lung (yellow arrow), (B) intraoperatively placed drain lying adjacent to the anastomosis without evidence of contrast leak (yellow arrow), (C) dilated jejunal loop next to the feeding jejunostomy site – probable cause of obstruction (yellow arrow).

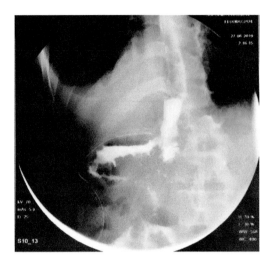

**Figure 12.2** Oral contrast study showing no extravasation of contrast on postoperative day eight after successful management of the patient.

the patient is not septic. In case of major leakage with severe mediastinitis/peritonitis, takedown of the anastomosis and establishment of a controlled fistula must be performed. The role of maintaining nutrition and correction of micronutrient deficiencies (with the help of a dietitian) is vital.

## CASE SCENARIO (CONTINUED)

With a suspicion of an anastomotic leak the patient was investigated with a CECT scan of the abdomen (Figure 12.1). This revealed a left subdiaphragmatic collection and a mild left pleural effusion. The Roux limb of the jejunum was found to be dilated and the dilatation could be traced to the feeding jejunostomy site, although the orally administered contrast demonstrated passage distally. In this patient, the surgically placed drain was adequately functioning lying well within the subdiaphragmatic collection. Besides, the CT scan ruled out the presence of undrained collections. The leak seemed to be related to the proximal distension due to obstruction at the feeding jejunostomy site (as seen in the CT scan). While surgical correction of the etiology was considered, the obstruction resolved. The patient was initially managed with antibiotics (based on culture results) and enteral feeding through the jejunostomy tube. Since it appeared on the CT scan that the feeding jejunostomy site was the site of jejunal obstruction, a relaparotomy was contemplated after this initial treatment. However, the bilious output from the began to reduce, all the while the patient's nutrition being well maintained through the jejunostomy. The drain output changed to a serious nature, and a repeat fluoroscopic study with oral water-soluble contrast failed to demonstrate a leak after eight days (Figure 12.2). The patient was commenced on oral nutrition and discharged ten days after surgery.

### KEY MESSAGES:

- Early diagnosis of an esophagojejunostomy leak is the important for successful management.
- Clinical signs, contrast imaging studies, and endoscopy all need to be used judiciously to contribute to the diagnosis and the clinician should aware of their shortcomings.
- Conservative measures work well for a small controlled leak, while surgery is needed for major leaks with uncontrolled sepsis.
- Endoscopic modalities are gaining in popularity in the management of esophagojejunostomy leak, but high-quality studies are lacking for their indications in the clinical scenario.

- Establishment of an enteral feeding access is vital for the successful management of esophagojejunostomy leak.

### REFERENCES

1. Deguchi Y, Fukagawa T, Morita S et al. Identification of risk factors for esophagojejunal anastomotic leakage after gastric surgery. *World J Surg* 2012;36(7):1617–1622.
2. Kanaji S, Ohyama M, Yasuda T et al. Can the intraoperative leak test prevent postoperative leakage of esophagojejunal anastomosis after total gastrectomy? *Surg Today* 2016 Jul;46(7):815–820.
3. Lamb PJ, Griffin SM, Chandrashekar MV et al. Prospective study of routine contrast radiology after total gastrectomy. *Br J Surg* 2004 Aug;91(8):1015–1019.
4. Shim CN, Kim HI, Hyung WJ et al. Self-expanding metal stents or nonstent endoscopic therapy: Which is better for anastomotic leaks after total gastrectomy? *Surg Endosc* 2014 Mar;28(3):833–840.
5. Hummel R, Bausch D. Anastomotic leakage after upper gastrointestinal surgery: Surgical treatment. *Visc Med* 2017 Jun;33(3):207–211.

# 13 Metastatic Gastrointestinal Stromal Tumor with Bleeding

*Inian Samarasam and K. Senthilnathan*

## CONTENTS

## CASE SCENARIOS

### Patient 1

A 45-year-old man, with a prior history of anemia, presented to the emergency department after two episodes of bright red hematemesis. In addition to reporting fatigue and tiredness, he did not have any other significant symptoms. He denied any change in bowel habits and was otherwise in good health. He was not on regular medications, occasionally had a glass of alcohol, did not smoke, and was not on any regular medications. On examination, he was stable, with a blood pressure of 128/78 mmHg, pulse rate of 98/minute, and respiratory rate of 23/minute. Abdominal examination revealed a vague epigastric mass. His hemoglobin value was reported as 6 gm% and the coagulation profile including platelet count were normal.

After initial stabilization and blood transfusion, he underwent a gastroscopy which showed a large polypoidal growth in the stomach. The biopsy from the growth confirmed a gastrointestinal stromal tumor. A staging computed tomography (CT) scan revealed a large gastrointestinal stromal tumor tumor arising from the stomach, with multiple liver metastasis involving both lobes of the liver (Figure 13.1).

### Patient 2

An 80-year-old man presented to the surgical outpatient clinic with a prior history of melena. He had been investigated at another center and was referred to us with a diagnosis of a metastatic gastrointestinal stromal tumor. The CT scan revealed a large tumor of the stomach, infiltrating the pancreas, crura of the diaphragm, and the vessels of the coeliac axis, with metastatic deposits in the liver (Figure 13.2). Based on the locallyadvanced nature of the primary tumor on CT scan, even a palliative resection was deemed not feasible. In addition, the patient had multiple medical comorbidities, and was unfit for any operative intervention. He was admitted to the hospital and on the second day of admission had multiple episodes of large volume hematemesis with significant drop in hemoglobin.

## BACKGROUND OF THE PATHOLOGY

Gastrointestinal stromal tumors are the most common mesenchymal neoplasms of the gastrointestinal tract. They can occur anywhere in the gastrointestinal tract though most commonly in the stomach (60%) followed by the small intestine (30%) [1]. First described in the year 1983, these tumors originate from interstitial cells of Cajal (pacemaker cells), located within the myenteric plexus. The tumor cells express a tyrosine kinase receptor encoded by the oncogene KIT2. Immunohistochemical marker CD117 (c-kit) codes for the KIT protein and has been helpful in distinguishing gastrointestinal stromal tumors from other mesenchymal tumors. Discovered on GIST1 (DOG1) was shown by gene expression profiling to be highly expressed in gastrointestinal stromal tumors. Several recent studies have demonstrated the higher sensitivity of antibodies that recognize DOG1 in the diagnosis of a gastrointestinal stromal tumor compared with KIT.

The majority of patients with gastrointestinal stromal tumors benefit from tyrosine kinase inhibitor therapy (Imatinib and Sunitinib).

## CLINICAL FINDINGS

Gastrointestinal stromal tumors are more common in males and are encountered in the fourth or fifth decades of life. These tumors

Acute presentations such as gastrointestinal bleeding, perforation, and obstruction generally warrant surgical management. Acute gastrointestinal bleeding is not an uncommon presentation of a gastrointestinal stromal tumor. In the setting of a surgically resectable gastrointestinal stromal tumor, an emergency surgical resection may be performed. However, management of a patient with a locally advanced or a metastatic gastrointestinal stromal tumor, when associated with acute gastrointestinal bleeding, may pose a treatment dilemma since surgical resection of the primary tumor may be difficult or unlikley. This chapter deals with two such case scenarios – the first patient with a bleeding metastatic gastrointestinal stromal tumor and a potentially resectable primary, and the second one with a bleeding, non-resectable metastatic gastrointestinal stromal tumor.

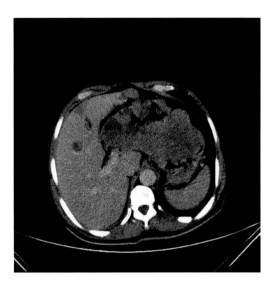

**Figure 13.1** CECT scan section of the abdomen. Axial post-contrast section showing metastatic GIST, but primary potentially resectable (Patient 1).

## INVESTIGATIONS
### Diagnosis and staging

- Gastroduodenoscopy with six to eight biopsies from the tumor for confirmation of the diagnosis (c-kit/DOG1 testing on immunohistochemistry). The biopsies may be non-representative if the mucosa is intact and if the tumor is predominantly exophytic with no mucosal involvement.

- A percutaneous biopsy is best avoided (due to risk of bleeding and percutaneous seeding). However, it may be necessary in large tumors when neoadjuvant therapy is being considered or in patients with metastates, especially if the endoscopic biopsies are non-diagnostic.

- Triple phase CT scan (multi-detector or helical) of the abdomen and pelvis is useful for staging of the disease and in preoperative planning. If the patient is allergic to contrast media, then a magnetic resonance imaging (MRI) of the abdomen may be performed.

The Indian Council of Medical Research (ICMR) consensus guidelines give an excellent overview of the evidence pertaining to the investigation and management of gastrointestinal stromal tumors [3].

## APPROACH TO MANAGEMENT

- **General guidelines for management of gastrointestinal stromal tumors**

    The general guidelines for management of gastrointestinal stromal tumors are as

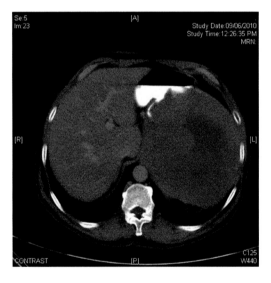

**Figure 13.2** CECT scan section of the abdomen. Axial post-contrast section showing a large, locally advanced, potentially unresectable gastrointestinal stromal tumor (Patient 2).

are commonly asymptomatic but clinical presentation of these gastrointestinal stromal tumors may range from indolent vague abdominal pain, chronic anemia, palpable abdominal masses, and dysphagia. Abdominal pain and intestinal bleeding are the most common clinical presentations in symptomatic patients [2].

follows. A non-metastatic gastrointestinal stromal tumor ≥2 cm should be offered a complete surgical resection (R0) without breach of the pseudocapsule. Laparoscopic excision may be offered, depending on the size of the tumor and technical feasibility and expertise. Lymphadenectomy is not indicated as part of surgery for gastrointestinal stromal tumors as they seldom metastasize to lymph nodes. However, enlarged lymph nodes that appear suspicious may be sampled at the time of surgery. For locally advanced but resectable gastrointestinal stromal tumors, downstaging of the tumor with the use of neoadjuvant therapy (tyrosine kinase inhibitor and Imatinib), followed by surgery, is the preferred option. Upfront surgery may be considered in these cases, only if complications due to the tumo\r are present such as major bleeding or gastric outlet obstruction.

Optimal management of patients diagnosed with a gastrointestinal stromal tumor is multidisciplinary, and requires input from experts from different fields, including surgery, medical gastroenterology, radiology, medical oncology, radiotherapy, and interventional radiology.

- **Investigations and management plan for a bleeding gastrointestinal stromal tumor**

The initial management (as in any acute gastrointestinal bleed) would include stabilization of the patient, adequate resuscitation taking care of the airway, breathing, and circulation. Routine blood investigations, including a coagulation profile, are performed to rule out systemic causes of bleeding. Patients on anticoagulants and antiplatelet medications may need to be adequately reversed, based on the clinical setting. The next step would involve a gastroscopy under general anesthesia and cross-sectional imaging, such as a CT scan. The treatment would then depend on the stage of the disease, the general condition of the patient, and the expected treatment goals.

- **Treatment option for an acutely bleeding, metastaticgastrointestinal stromal tumor (primary lesion in the stomach potentially resectable) – Patient 1**

The first patient had a bleeding metastatic gastrointestinal stromal tumor, but the primary tumor in the stomach was potentially resectable. In addition, the patient was

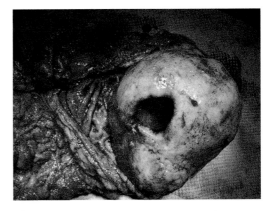

**Figure 13.3** Photograph of the total gastrectomy resection specimen (Patient 1).

also fit for surgical intervention. In such a scenario, palliative or debulking resections may be undertaken in patients who have acute bleeding, provided they are medically fit with a reasonable anticipated life expectancy.

This patient therefore underwent an emergency total gastrectomy (Figure 13.3) and made an uneventful recovery. He was started on adjuvant Imatinib postoperatively.

In cases of small volume peritoneal metastasis, debulking surgery along with resection of the bleeding primary tumor may be offered.

- **Treatment options for acutely bleeding, metastatic gastrointestinal stromal tumor (primary lesion in the stomach unresectable) – Patient 2**

Not uncommonly, one might encounter a more difficult situation wherein the bleeding primary gastrointestinal stromal tumor is unresectable. The causes for unresectability include locally advanced tumors, an unfavorable location, or the patient being unfit for major resectional surgery. In such circumstances, endoscopic measures (clipping, electrocoagulation, or adrenaline injection) may be attempted. If not feasible in view of a large bleeding tumor or bleeding from areas of necrosis, then as a next option, transarterial chemo-embolization may be undertaken, as was carried out in the second patient of our Case Scenario. As part of this, the first step is to perform a CT angiography to localize the bleed. This is then followed by embolization of one or two of the major vessels of the stomach (Figures 13.4A & B).

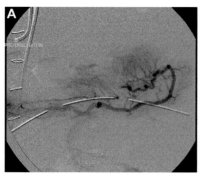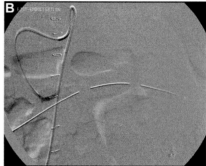

**Figure 13.4** Digital subtraction angiography images of patient showing: (A) right gastroepiploic vessel with bleeding, (B) post-therapeutic embolization of the right gastroepiploic artery absence of arterial blush.

The various embolic materials that have been tested include N-butyl cyanoacrylate (NBCA) mixed with iodized oil micro coils (Cook and Inc), polyvinyl alcohol particles, and gelatin sponge. A recent study addressed the efficacy and safety of transarterial chemoembolization in acutely bleeding gastrointestinal stromal tumors, and concluded that it is an effective option in patients where endoscopic or surgical options are not feasible [4].

There have been reports of advanced endoscopic techniques, such as endoscopic ultrasonographyguided angiotherapy, for large bleeding gastrointestinal stromal tumors [4]. In this report, a curved linear array echoendoscope was used to identify a bleeding vessel right under a large gastrointestinal stromal tumor. Under direct echoendoscopic vision, the vascular anatomy was delineated and needle puncture of the target artery was performed. Subsequent to this, targeted embolization therapy was done using 2 ml of N-butyl- 2-cyanoacrylate. Furthermore, immediate assessment of efficacy of the embolization was performed using a color Doppler. endoscopic ultrasonography-guided angiotherapy appears safe, effective, and technically feasible for the management of select suitable cases of bleeding gastrointestinal stromal tumors. An additional point to note is that its application is not limited by the lesion's size. Future clinical indications for its use may include patients with bleeding gastrointestinal stromal tumors requiring a bridging therapy prior to surgery and those not suitable for surgical resection [4].

Historically, gastrointestinal stromal tumors have been considered radiation-resistant, but there may be a role for radiotherapy in the palliative management of patients with gastrointestinal stromal tumors. It has been predominantly used in palliation of bone metastasis. It is also now being realized that gastrointestinal stromal tumors are not universally radioresistant to radiotherapy, and if combined with molecularly targeted therapy, can improve the outcomes for patients diagnosed with gastrointestinal stromal tumor. In the setting of acute bleeding in a non-resectable gastrointestinal stromal tumor, radiotherapy may be considered as a palliative option [5]. The efficacy achieved could result possibly from the combined effects of radiotherapy and tyrosine kinase inhibitors, and might possibly be less with radiation alone. But more studies are warranted to standardize the role of radiotherapy in acute bleeds. The effective dosage and the irradiation techniques also need to be standardized [6].

**KEY MESSAGES**

- Management of a patient with a bleeding metastatic gastrointestinal stromal tumor of the stomach may be a challenge (Figure 13.5).
- Therapeutic endoscopic measures may not be an option in large tumors.
- Surgical resection of the primary tumor, when feasible, is the treatment of choice.
- In cases where this may not be possible, non-surgical methods such as embolization, endosocopic ultrasonography-guided therapy, and radiation therapy may be attempted based on the tumor status, patient condition, and availability of resources.

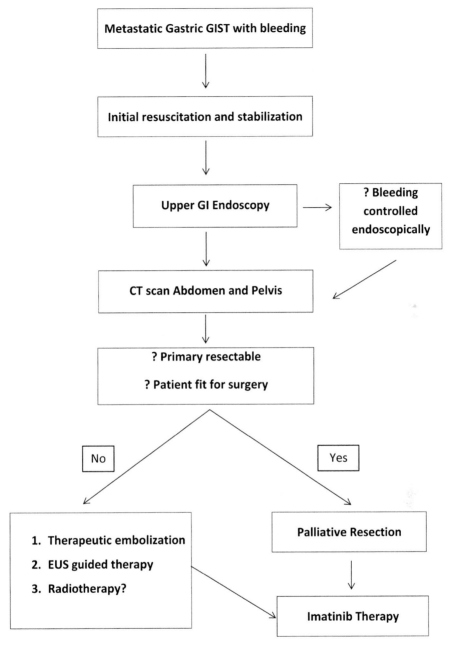

**Figure 13.5** Algorithm for approach to a patient with a bleeding gastrointestinal stromal tumor of the stomach that is metastatic. (*Abbreviations:* GI – gastrointestinal; CT – computed tomography; EUS – endoscopic ultrasonography.)

## REFERENCES

1. Roggin KK, Posner MC. Modern treatment of gastric gastrointestinal stromal tumors. *World J Gastroenterol* 2012;18(46):6720–6728.
2. Yacob M, Inian S, Sudhakar CB. Gastrointestinal stromal tumours: Review of 150 cases from a single centre. *Indian J Surg* 2015;77:S505–S510.
3. Shrikhande SV, Sirohi B, Barreto SG et al. Indian Council of Medical Research consensus document for the management of gastrointestinal stromal tumors. *Indian J Med Paediatr Oncol* 2014;35(4):244–248.

4. Koo HJ, Shin JH, Shin S et al. Efficacy and clinical outcomes of transcatheter arterial embolization for gastrointestinal bleeding from gastrointestinal stromal tumor. *J Vasc Interv Radiol* 2015;26(9):1297–1304.

5. Kumbhari V, Gondal B, Okolo PI et al. Endoscopic ultrasound-guided angiotherapy of a large bleeding gastrointestinal stromal tumor. *Endoscopy* 2013;45:E326–E327.

6. Gatto L, Nannini M, Saponara M et al. Radiotherapy in the management of GIST: State of the art and new potential scenarios. *Clin Sarcoma Res* 2017;7:1.

# PART 3
# DUODENUM

# 14 Two Centimeter D1–2 Anterior Perforation Presenting 24 Hours Later

*Peush Sahni and Rajesh Panwar*

## CONTENTS

## CASE SCENARIO

A 60-year-old man presented to the emergency services with severe pain in the abdomen that started suddenly, around 24 hours prior. The pain began in the upper abdomen but soon became generalized. There was no history of vomiting, diarrhea, or gastrointestinal bleeding. He had not passed flatus or stools after the onset of pain and had passed urine only once, about 12 hours earlier. The patient was a known diabetic who also suffered from hypertension and coronary artery disease. He had been having pain in his joints for the past two months for which he had been prescribed nonsteroidal anti-inflammatory drugs.

At presentation, he was conscious but disoriented and was lying still in bed. He had tachycardia with a feeble radial pulse. Abdominal examination revealed distension with generalized tenderness, guarding, and rigidity. There was obliteration of liver dullness and the bowel sounds were absent.

A diagnosis of a hollow viscus perforation causing peritonitis was made. The perforation was likely due to a peptic ulcer.

## BACKGROUND OF THE PATHOLOGY

*Helicobacter pylori* infection or chronic use of nonsteroidal anti-inflammatory drugs are the most common risk factors for complications of peptic ulcer disease, including perforation. Peptic ulcer perforation may occur in patients with a history of prolonged dyspeptic symptoms. However, in some patients, perforation may be the first presentation of a peptic ulcer. The first part of the duodenum is the most common site for peptic ulcer perforation, followed by the antrum and body of the stomach.

Sudden onset of abdominal pain, tachycardia, and abdominal rigidity constitute the classic triad of a perforated peptic ulcer. The clinical manifestations evolve over three phases [1]. The first phase lasts for around two hours from the onset of perforation. The entry of acid into the peritoneal cavity results in chemical peritonitis which is initially localized to the upper abdomen. Thus, the pain starts in the epigastrium but soon becomes generalized. The release of vasoactive mediators due to peritoneal reaction results in tachycardia and cold extremities. The second phase begins around two hours from the onset and lasts till around 12 hours. Pain may become less severe initially as the acid gets diluted by the fluid released due to peritoneal reaction. However, pain is more generalized and becomes worse on any movement. The signs of peritonitis (tenderness, guarding, and rigidity) also become apparent. The third phase usually begins after 12 hours as the peritoneal inflammation progresses further. There is increasing abdominal distension as paralytic ileus sets in and fluid accumulates in the peritoneal cavity. The patient becomes febrile and third space loss of fluid in peritoneal cavity and sepsis result in hypotension and circulatory collapse. The patient may also develop electrolyte imbalance and renal failure.

Early diagnosis and treatment, especially within six hours, results in an excellent outcome. Delay in treatment (>12 hours), advanced age, shock at presentation, renal failure, and presence of comorbid conditions, such as diabetes, are associated with poor prognosis.

A number of scoring systems (Boey, Peptic Ulcer Perforation Score, American Society of Anesthesiologists, and Mannheim peritonitis index) have been used for predicting mortality and morbidity of peptic ulcer perforation [2].

## APPROACH TO MANAGEMENT
### Initial assessment
The initial management begins as soon as the patient arrives in the emergency department. The airway (A), breathing (B), and circulation (C) must be assessed. Patients with perforative peritonitis generally have tachycardia (heart rate of > 120/minute), a feeble pulse with cold clammy hands, and hypotension (blood pressure of <90/60 mmHg).

The patient should be started on high flow oxygen and fluid resuscitation should be commenced with normal saline using wide bore intravenous cannula. Blood samples need to be drawn just prior to this for an urgent hemoglobin, hematocrit, total leucocyte count, blood glucose levels, serum electrolytes, blood urea, and serum creatinine.

A nasogastric tube must be inserted and left on free drainage. The patient must be catheterized to monitor urine output, and a central venous catheter must be placed in order to monitor resuscitation.

A detailed history must be taken, and a complete physical examination done after the initial resuscitation. Presence of multiple comorbid conditions especially diabetes mellitus and delayed presentation (>24 hours) are important with regard to the outcome. In the patient presented in our Case Scenario, all the above were done. Additionally, the history of sudden onset upper abdominal pain and recent nonsteroidal anti-inflammatory drug use were important pointers for the diagnosis.

A general physical examination will likely confirm evidence of shock and dehydration while an abdominal examination will reveal signs of generalized peritonitis (including tenderness with voluntary guard, with or without rigidity).

An intravenous proton pump inhibitor and a combination of intravenous antibiotics (third generation cephalosporin and metronidazole) must be started.

A plain chest radiograph in the erect position must be performed to include both domes of the diaphragm. In the patient presented in our Case Scenario, this revealed free gas under the diaphragm, thereby confirming the diagnosis of a hollow viscus perforation. A lateral decubitus film may be obtained if the patient is unable to maintain an erect posture. A computed tomography (CT) with oral contrast, which is more sensitive, may be obtained if the plain radiograph does not show any free air, but the clinical suspicion for a perforation is strong.

Once the diagnosis is confirmed, the patient must be taken up for an emergency exploratory laparotomy after obtaining informed consent. Surgery is the standard treatment for peptic ulcer perforation and should be done as early as possible. The morbidity and mortality rates increase with delayed treatment.

### Surgery vs non-operative management
Although most patients with peptic ulcer perforation are candidates for surgical treatment, non-operative management may be an option in some of them [3]. Non-operative management consists of keeping the patient nil per oral, with nasogastric drainage, intravenous antibiotics, and proton pump inhibitors or histamine (H2) receptor antagonists. Non-operative management may be considered in patients with a presumed sealed perforation. These patients are clinically stable, have less severe symptoms, and do not have clinical signs of generalized peritonitis. A CT with oral contrast also does not show any extravasation of contrast. These patients may be managed conservatively, and surgery offered only if there is clinical deterioration. Non-operative management has also been used with some success in patients with minor leaks. Another subset of patients who are managed non-operatively are those with severe comorbid conditions that preclude any surgical intervention. These patients are managed non-operatively with percutaneous drainage. Endoscopic placement of over the scope clips and covered stents are some novel methods that may be used for patients who are not candidates for surgery.

### Open vs laparoscopic surgery
Laparoscopic surgery has been found to be feasible for duodenal ulcer perforation. Meta-analysis of randomized trials has not shown any difference in overall morbidity and mortality, however, laparoscopic approach had lower rate of surgical site infection, shorter nasogastric tube duration, and less postoperative pain than an open approach [4]. Thus, laparoscopic approach may be preferred if technical expertise is available. However, laparoscopic approach is considered safe only in younger patients (<70 years), who present early (<24 hours), do not have shock at presentation, and do not have significant comorbid illnesses. Thus, only patients with Boey score 0 and 1 (Table 14.1) are suitable candidates for laparoscopic surgery. As our patient had presented

## Table 14.1 Boey Score for Peptic Ulcer Perforation

**Boey score**

1 point for each of the following factors
- Duration of perforation >24 hours
- Preoperative shock
- Severe medical comorbid illness

Score range 0–3

after 24 hours, had significant comorbid illnesses, and had shock at presentation, we chose the open surgical approach.

## CASE SCENARIO (CONTINUED)

### Operative findings and details

The patient was found to have 1.5 L of bilio-purulent fluid in the peritoneal cavity and the bowel was covered with fibrin exudates. There was a 2 cm perforation on the anterior wall of the junction of the first and second part of the duodenum. The margins of the perforation were unhealthy but the surrounding tissues were supple with minimal scarring. The margins were freshened and the perforation was repaired with an omental patch (Graham patch repair). Interrupted 3-0 atraumatic silk sutures were used for the repair (alternatively, Polydioxanone can also be used). The first suture was placed at the proximal margin of the ulcer with each bite around 5 mm from the ulcer edge. Both ends of the suture were held separately using artery clips which allowed the placement of subsequent sutures under direct vision, thereby avoiding the risk of incorporation of the posterior wall of the mucosa in the sutures. Subsequent sutures were placed 5 mm apart. A vascularized omental pedicle was placed over the defect in the duodenal wall and the sutures were gently tied over the omental pedicle. The sutures were neither too tight nor too loose.

No definitive acid-reducing procedure was attempted. A feeding jejunostomy was done using a 12-Fr Malecot catheter (alternatively, a nasogastric tube of the same size can also be used) and fashioned by the Witzel technique. The peritoneal cavity was irrigated with warm saline. A drain was placed in Morison's pouch and the abdomen was closed.

**Rationale for choice of the procedure:** Simple omental patch closure is a quick procedure ideally suited for patients with significant comorbid illnesses and those who present late with features of shock. The availability of potent anti-secretory agents and antibiotic therapy for *Helicobacter pylori* have made acid-reducing procedures less preferred. Nonsteroidal anti-inflammatory drug related perforations (as in our patient) usually do not require acid-reducing procedures as the drug can be stopped or substituted in most instances. The location of perforation also determines the surgical approach. A perforation located in the first part of duodenum just beyond the pylorus may be easily incorporated in a pyloroplasty, and hence may be treated with a pyloroplasty. In such situations, a truncal vagotomy can be added. A distally located perforation (as in our case) cannot be included in a pyloroplasty, and thus would require a separate drainage procedure if truncal vagotomy is added. Although, a highly selective vagotomy without a drainage procedure is possible, but it is time consuming and may not be suitable for such sick patients.

A feeding jejunostomy is not done routinely but may be considered in cases of large perforations, delayed presentation, unhealthy surrounding duodenal wall that may not hold sutures, and debilitated and malnourished patients.

Thus, simple omental patch closure is the preferred surgical procedure for most patients with a perforated duodenal ulcer [5]. If the closure has a high risk of leakage owing to large size of perforation or significant surrounding inflammation or scarring, a pyloric exclusion with gastrojejunostomy may be added to protect the suture line. Another option is to do a triple tube ostomy which includes a gastrostomy, retrograde tube duodenostomy, and a feeding jejunostomy. Rarely, large perforations may not be amenable to simple patch closure. These may be treated with truncal vagotomy, antrectomy, closure of the duodenal stump, and gastrojejunostomy. This may not be possible if the ulcer extends to the second part of duodenum beyond the ampulla. In that case, jejunal serosal patch, jejunal graft, pyloric exclusion, or wide bore drainage alone may be chosen on a case-to-case basis. Figure 14.1 describes the algorithmic approach to the management of a perforated duodenal ulcer.

**Peritoneal lavage:** Thorough peritoneal lavage (5–10 L of saline) is commonly practiced during surgery for perforation causing peritonitis in order to decrease the risk of infection despite the lack of evidence to support its use. We usually irrigate the peritoneal cavity to get rid of the solid debris and remove gross contamination.

**Drains:** Drain or no drain is again a matter of individual choice as there is no clear evidence to suggest any significant benefit. We prefer to

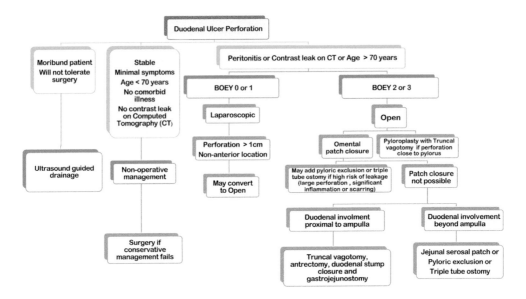

**Figure 14.1**    Approach to the management of a perforated duodenal ulcer.

place a 32-Fr soft abdominal drain in Morison's pouch after repair of a duodenal perforation.

## POSTOPERATIVE CARE

Intravenous fluid resuscitation and antibiotics are continued in the postoperative period. Antibiotics are stopped once the patient remains afebrile for 48 hours and has a normal leucocyte count. The nasogastric tube is kept on free drainage. It is removed only when the daily output decreases to <200 ml which may take some days due to the postoperative ileus. The drain is removed when the daily output decreases to <100 ml. We perform a contrast study selectively for patients who have symptoms and signs suggestive of a leak. Oral feeding is resumed once the nasogastric tube has been removed and patient has passed flatus. The patient is started on oral sips initially and gradually progressed to liquid and semisolid diet. *Helicobacter pylori* eradication therapy is offered to all patients of perforated duodenal ulcer once they resume oral diet. Another reasonable approach is to perform an endoscopy to determine the *Helicobacter pylori* status and offer eradication therapy to only those who test positive.

## GASTRIC ULCER PERFORATION

The surgical management of a perforated gastric ulcer is similar, except for the following deviations:

a) The ulcer should either be excised or multiple biopsies should be taken from its edges to rule out a malignancy.

b) A follow-up endoscopy should be done to document healing of the ulcer and to biopsy any suspicious areas.

### KEY MESSAGES

- Peptic ulcer perforation occurs in 2–10% of patients with peptic ulcer disease, and the duodenum accounts for 60% of such perforations.
- Typical clinical presentation and demonstration of free gas under the diaphragm are sufficient for diagnosis.
- Management involves prompt resuscitation and early surgery.
- Non-operative management may be offered to stable patients with sealed perforation (no contrast leak on imaging) or those in a poor general condition that precludes surgery.
- Laparoscopic surgery may be offered to younger and stable patients who have presented early.
- Simple omental patch closure is the preferred surgical technique for a majority of patients.
- A small subset of patients with a large perforation or significant inflammation or scarring may require more extensive procedures.

### CONFLICTS OF INTEREST

None to declare.

## REFERENCES

1. Chung KT, Shelat VG. Perforated peptic ulcer – An update. *World J Gastrointest Surg* 2017;9(1):1–12.
2. Thorsen K, Søreide JA, Søreide K. Scoring systems for outcome prediction in patients with perforated peptic ulcer. *Scand J Trauma Resusc Emerg Med* 2013 Apr 10;21:25.
3. Crofts TJ, Park KG, Steele RJ et al. A randomized trial of nonoperative treatment for perforated peptic ulcer. *N Engl J Med* 1989;320(15):970–973.
4. Tan S, Wu G, Zhuang Q et al. Laparoscopic versus open repair for perforated peptic ulcer: A meta analysis of randomized controlled trials. *Int J Surg* 2016;33 Pt A:124–132.
5. Chan KS, Wang YL, Chan XW et al. Outcomes of omental patch repair in large or giant perforated peptic ulcer are comparable to gastrectomy. *Eur J Trauma Emerg Surg* 2019 Oct 14. [Epub ahead of print]. doi:10.1007/s00068-019-01237-8.

# 15 Biliary Leak after Pancreatoduodenectomy for Duodenal Neuroendocrine Tumors

*Gayatri Balachandran and Sadiq S. Sikora*

## CONTENTS

## CASE SCENARIO

A 58-year-old man presented with a lesion in the second part of the duodenum, incidentally detected during a routine screening esophago-gastroduodenoscopy. Triple-phase computed tomography (CT) scan of the abdomen showed an enhancing 2 × 2 cm lesion in the medial wall of the duodenum with features suggestive of a neuroendocrine tumor (Figure 15.1). After pre-operative optimization, he underwent a classi-cal pancreatoduodenectomy. Intraoperatively, the bile duct was 4 mm in size and an end-to-side hepaticojejunostomy was performed in Blumgart-Kelly fashion (interrupted sutures with 5–0 polydiaxone sodium). End-to-side dunking pancreaticojejunostomy and end-to-side loop gastrojejunostomy were performed to complete the reconstruction. A nasojejunal tube was placed across the gastrojejunal anastomo-sis to permit early enteral feeding. A 22-Fr por-tex drain was placed in the subhepatic space.

The patient developed early intraluminal postpancreatectomy hemorrhage, as evidenced by blood in the nasogastric aspirate. He showed no features of hemodynamic compromise and was therefore managed conservatively along with transfusion of a bag of packed red cells. The bleeding subsequently subsided. The abdominal drain amylase level on postopera-tive day three was diagnostic of a postopera-tive pancreatic fistula. The levels, however, normalized by postoperative day five. As there was no clinically relevant manifestation of the pancreatic leak, it was labeled a grade A

postoperative pancreatic fistula. Nasojejunal feeds were initiated from the second postopera-tive day and gradually stepped up. On the sixth postoperative day, the drain effluent was noted to be bilious. Ultrasonogram of the abdomen showed no intraperitoneal collections and no intrahepatic biliary radicle dilatation. Liver function tests were normal.

## BACKGROUND OF THE PATHOLOGY

With advances in operative techniques and perioperative patient care, mortality rates associated with pancreatoduodenectomy have drastically reduced from initial reports of 27% to less than 5%. The overall perioperative morbidity for pancreatoduodenectomy ranges from 33–67%. The most common complications are delayed gastric emptying, postpancreatec-tomy hemorrhage, postoperative pancreatic fistula, and intra-abdominal abscess formation. Less frequent complications include surgical site infection, biliary leak (from the hepatico-jejunostomy), and other complications such as urinary tract infection, pneumonia, deep vein thrombosis, and pulmonary thromboembolism.

### Bile leak after pancreatoduodenectomy

Hepaticojejunostomy leaks are less frequent, with rates of 3–8% [1–4]. Surgical literature on hepaticojejunostomy leak after pancreatoduo-denectomy is sparse to the extent that a univer-sal definition of post-pancreatoduodenectomy bile leak and biliary fistula is lacking. Most surgeons employ the definition proposed by

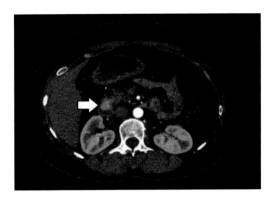

**Figure 15.1** Axial section of a contrast-enhanced CT scan of the abdomen in the arterial phase demonstrating an enhancing lesion in the anteromedial wall of the second part of the duodenum (marked by a white arrow) suggestive of neuroendocrine tumor.

the International Study Group of Liver Surgery (ISGLS). As per the ISGLS, bile leak after hepatobiliary and pancreatic surgery is defined as drain fluid bilirubin concentration more than thrice the serum levels at or after the first postoperative day, or presence of any biliary collections or peritonitis requiring either radiological or surgical intervention.

In 2012, a single center study from Japan first described hepaticojejunostomy leaks after pancreatoduodenectomy occurring in about 8% of patients (9/107 pancreatoduodenectomy) [1]. Combined hepaticojejunostomy and pancreaticojejunostomy leaks are also described, occurring in about 3%.

## APPROACH TO A PATIENT WITH A SUSPECTED BILIARY LEAK (FROM A HEPATICOJEJUNOSTOMY)

### Presentation

Most biliary leaks are suspected by the visualization of a biliary effluent from the intraoperatively placed drains, or from percutaneous drainage tubes placed postoperatively under radiological guidance. Most instances of hepaticojejunostomy leak manifest within the first postoperative week. Fever, abdominal pain, and leucocytosis are non-specific presenting signs. Bile leak after surgery resulting in an intraperitoneal bile collection is typically not contaminated by bacteria and usually does not result in the classical symptoms of biliary peritonitis. The fistula output may vary depending upon the extent of disruption of the anastomosis and therefore the volume of output may directly correlate with size of disruption and also the outcome. Most observational studies reporting hepaticojejunostomy leaks after

pancreatoduodenectomy have defined high-output fistulae as those with daily drain output greater than 250 mL/day [2].

### Imaging

- *CT or magnetic resonance imaging (MRI):* Cross-sectional imaging of the abdomen and pelvis remains the investigation of choice to evaluate the morphology of intra-abdominal collections that require drainage. CT scan provides excellent spatial resolution and is readily available. MR cholangiogram has the added advantage of demonstrating communication between the high-intensity intra-abdominal collection and the anastomotic site, involvement of any aberrant ducts (if any), and may provide a reasonable appreciation of the size of anastomotic dehiscence.

- *Sinograms:* Biliary leak may be confirmed by imaging with a contrast study through the abdominal drain, which demonstrates the fistulous communication with the hepaticojejunostomy site as well as the presence of any residual intra-abdominal collections. Sinograms are also useful to rule out bilious drainage secondary to pancreaticojejunostomy dehiscence, in which the hepaticojejunostomy is clearly visualized to be intact.

- *Hepatobiliary scintigraphy (Hepatoiminodiacetic acid/HIDA) scan:* This may provide functional information demonstrating the presence of an active leak, but spatial resolution is poor and identification of the leak site can be challenging. In up to 80% of patients, hepatobiliary scintigraphy does not identify the site of leak, thereby limiting its feasibility in deciding whether to use endoscopic, percutaneous, or a surgical treatment approach.

## DETERMINING THE APPROACH TO THE MANAGING THE LEAK: A PLACE FOR "CLASSIFICATION"

Once a bile leak has been diagnosed, the next step is to decide which patients require intervention, and what would be the appropriate approach. To aid in this process, there are a few classification systems. Surgeons must decide which of these best suits their practice. Bile leaks may be classified, and management strategies assigned based on the site and severity of leak. There are three classification systems for biliary leak, namely, one proposed by the ISGLS, another by Burkhart et al. [2], and, finally, the Modified Accordion Severity Grading System described by Porembka and colleagues [5].

*ISGLS classification*: ISGLS classification stratifies patients based on clinical impact of the bile leak, i.e. requiring little or no change in clinical management (grade A), requiring additional diagnostic or interventional procedure (without relaparotomy), or bile leak lasting longer than a week (grade B), and bile leaks requiring relaparotomy (grade C).

*Burkhart classification*: Burkhart et al. [2] proposed a grading system inspired by that of International Study Group for Pancreatic Surgery (ISGPS) for postoperative pancreatic fistula that categorizes patients into three grades of biliary leaks (below).

1) Grade A bile leaks are diagnosed by the presence of bile in surgically placed drains but are not associated with any change in clinical condition or infection.

2) Grade B leaks are associated with mild signs of infection, such as a leukocytosis and fever. A sinogram may be performed to define the leak, and a CT scan is generally necessary to evaluate for undrained collections.

3) Grade C leaks are associated with significant physiologic derangements or sepsis requiring an increased level of care (e.g. transfer to the intensive care unit or step-down unit). A sinogram often demonstrates a substantial and uncontrolled leak, and early drain outputs are high.

Treatment may be recommended as per the category: conservative management of the controlled external fistula for Group A, antibiotics and optimization along with peritoneal drainage for Group B, and biliary drainage / laparotomy, as indicated, for Group C.

*Modified accordion classification*: The classification can be modified to grade patients with bile leak. Patients are assigned to a grade from zero to six based on the severity of biliary leak and the implication of the resultant complications (Table 15.1).

The clinical utility of these systems has been studied and all three systems have been shown to be reliable in categorizing biliary fistulae according to clinical outcomes and financial impact. But none of these classifications take into consideration the incidence, or implication, of concomitant postoperative pancreatic fistula. The coexistence of the two complications contributes to significant morbidity and is associated with highest risk of postpancreatic hemorrhage, relaparotomy, and death. Therefore, it is worthwhile to consider the presence of a postoperative pancreatic fistula while categorizing the severity and management strategies of a biliary leak.

## MANAGEMENT OF BILE LEAK AFTER A PANCREATODUODENECTOMY

The management of biliary leak after pancreatoduodenectomy is determined by the following factors:

- Timing of presentation: Early (<48 hrs) vs late (>48 hrs)

- Volume of bile leak (high volume >250 ml/day)

- Associated features of sepsis

- Associated complications such as postpancreatectomy hemorrhage or postoperative pancreatic fistula

- Underlying biliary anatomy, site of leak, and nature of defect

## CONSERVATIVE MANAGEMENT

Low-volume fistulae with no features of peritonitis may be managed conservatively with continued abdominal drainage. Imaging is crucial in this group of patients to rule out any undrained

## Table 15.1 The Modified Accordion Classification as Applied to Bile Leak

| Grade | Modified Accordion Classification |
|---|---|
| 0 | No complication |
| 1 | Mild complication: Discharge with original surgical drain or treatment of fistula by nil per os alone |
| 2 | Moderate complication: Pharmacological treatment, such as use of therapeutic octreotide, antibiotic, and parenteral nutrition |
| 3 | Severe complication: Intervention without general anesthesia, such as percutaneous drain placement, interventional procedures, and complex wound management |
| 4 | Severe complication: Reoperation under general anesthesia, OR single organ failure secondary to the leak |
| 5 | Severe complication: Reoperation under general anesthesia with single organ failure secondary to the leak, OR multisystem (two or more) organ failure secondary to the leak |
| 6 | Postoperative death secondary to the leak |

intra-abdominal collections; these need to be addressed with percutaneous drainage or drain repositioning/upsizing. Periprocedural antibiotics are administered, but there is usually no indication for long-term antibiotics. Spontaneous closure of biliary fistula occurs in around 50% of cases with expectant management over a variable period ranging from 2–12 weeks. Correction of electrolyte disturbances and nutritional optimization are important in these patients.

## INTERVENTIONAL PROCEDURES

Uncontrolled, high volume leaks (through the drain and/or through the laparotomy wound) that present with/without superadded infection warrant some form of intervention. The goal of treatment in these cases is to ensure adequate abdominal drainage and establish a controlled biliary fistula. Percutaneous catheter drainage of intra-abdominal collections should be done, and appropriate antibiotics are to be initiated. Due attention must be paid to the electrolyte disturbances (hypokalemia, etc.) that ensue as well as on maintaining adequate macro- and micro-nutrient intake.

Percutaneous transhepatic biliary drainage is the only endoluminal treatment option for biliary leakage post-pancreatoduodenectomy. It provides an opportunity to create a low-pressure system along the biliary tract, redirecting the bile flow from the defect into the bile ducts permitting time for the leak to heal. Percutaneous transhepatic biliary drainage therefore may avoid further surgery or serve as a bridging therapy while stabilizing the patient's condition prior to surgery. Transhepatic biliary drainage should be considered in prolonged high-output fistulae associated with fluid and electrolyte derangements, especially with a significant anastomotic disruption. In the clinical scenario of non-dilated biliary ducts, percutaneous transhepatic biliary drainage can be challenging, but several reports have demonstrated feasibility of the procedure with good technical success, and rates comparable to percutaneous transhepatic biliary drainage in patients with dilated bile ducts. The average time from percutaneous transhepatic biliary drainage placement to resolution of bile leak varies from 9–150 days.

### Resurgery

The most common indication for early reoperation is a poorly controlled/unmanageable bile leak with either biliary peritonitis or bile leaking through the abdominal wound. Operative strategy is essentially to achieve a thorough abdominal lavage and source control. In the presence of sepsis, no attempts should be made to do a redo/revision hepaticojejunostomy. Simple lavage and placement of large bore drains around the hepaticojejunostomy leak site are the best options in the presence of sepsis warranting early reexploration. Placement of a T-tube exiting through the anastomotic defect is an option for biliary diversion. Occasionally, bile leaks detected early (<48 hours) without sepsis may be amenable to suture closure. In patients with >50% circumferential disruption, or biliary fistula with associated stricture, revision of the hepaticojejunostomyshould be performed. Redo hepaticojejunostomy should be performed by experienced hepatobiliary surgeons after control of sepsis and preferably after an interval of four to six weeks for local inflammation to subside to ensure a durable hepaticojejunostomy. Transanastomotic stents may be used for revision hepaticojejunostomy.

Surgical intervention may also be indicated for complications such as catastrophic post-pancreatectomy hemorrhage or postoperative pancreatic fistula grade C. In these situations, hemorrhage control obviously takes precedence, and damage control principles are to be followed to quickly stabilize the patient. Lavage and drain placement are typically carried out in these situations.

Leakage from aberrant ducts, though rare, has also been described after pancreatoduodenectomy. Because the transected duct is small and decompressed, achieving good results with surgical reconstruction is difficult, even in experienced hands. Although anecdotal reports have been published describing percutaneous and endoscopic rendezvous approach to managed accessory bile leak after pancreatoduodenectomy, the most established form of management is bilioenteric anastomosis to the same Roux loop after adequate control of sepsis and at the appropriate time.

In all patients with bile leak, there is a need to obtain the help of a nurse wound manager as bile is damaging to the skin. The use of zinc-based barrier creams, as well as stoma bags to minimize contact of bile with the skin, should be pursued. Total/peripheral parenteral nutrition must be considered in patients in whom enteral nutrition cannot be sustained. Macro- and micro-nutrient, as well as electrolyte deficiencies, must be treated aggressively.

A proposed algorithm of management is detailed below (Figure 15.2).

### Prevention of an hepaticojejunostomy leak

Hepaticojejunostomy leaks may be prevented by adhering to principles of sound surgical technique and ensuring good vascularity at the level of anastomosis.

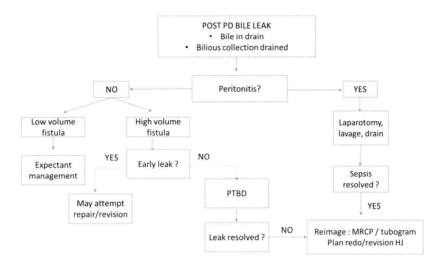

**Figure 15.2** Management algorithim for post-pancreatoduodenectomy bile leak. (*Abbreviations:* PD – pancreatoduodenectomy; HJ – hepaticojejunostomy; MRCP – magnetic resonance cholangiopancreatography; PTBD – percutaneous transhepatic biliary drainage.)

■ Tension-free vascularized anastomosis: Ensure adequate mobilisation of the transected bile duct, as well as adequate length of the jejunal Roux limb.

■ Ensure that the anastomosed mucosal edges are healthy with no inflammation or ischemia.

■ Use a standardized technique of single-layer, end-to-side hepaticojejunostomy with fine monofilament absorbable sutures.

■ While performing a hepaticojejunostomy with "skinny ducts" (<5 mm):

• The ropeway method can be used to stabilize the bile duct and jejunal limb as it allows precise mucosa-to-mucosa anastomosis.

• A transanastomotic transjejunal stent may be placed.

### Case scenario (continued)

The patient was clinically stable, with no features of sepsis. He was managed conservatively as an external biliary fistula with prolonged abdominal drainage. By the second postoperative week, the drain output had ceased. An abdominal ultrasound showed no residual collections or intrahepatic biliary dilatation. The drain was removed.

Two weeks later, he developed mild abdominal pain. Liver function tests were deranged, with grossly elevated serum alkaline phosphatase. An abdominal CT scan was done, which showed a large subdiaphragmatic and gallbladder fossa collection. A percutaneous catheter was placed and the biloma drained. A subsequent magnetic resonance cholangiopancreatography demonstrated a leak from an aberrant right posterior sectoral duct, draining into the subdiaphragmatic collection (Figure 15.3). On serial imaging, the collection resolved and the drainage tube was subsequently removed. The patient is planned for a review and possible definitive surgical reconstruction after an interval of six to eight weeks.

### KEY MESSAGES

■ Bile leak is an infrequent complication following pancreatoduodenectomy.

■ An anastomosis involving a small-diameter (<5 mm) common hepatic duct is one of the established risk factors for a leak.

■ Sound surgical technique to ensure a well-vascularized tension-free anastomosis is critical while performing a hepaticojejunostomy

■ Once diagnosed, stratification of severity of bile leaks helps in the appropriate choice of therapy.

■ The need for, and means of intervention, may be dictated by the volume of leak, biliary anatomy, and clinical manifestations of sepsis and/or local complications.

■ The majority of bile leaks post-pancreatoduodenectomy are self-limiting and may be managed expectantly.

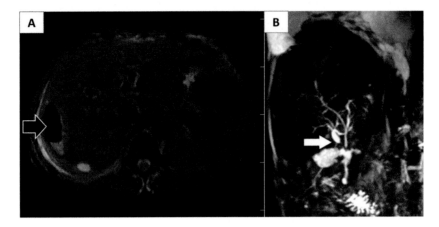

**Figure 15.3**   Postoperative MRCP demonstrating: (A) Axial section and (B) coronal section depicting a subdiaphragmatic collection (solid black arrow), and a dilated aberrant right posterior sectoral duct (solid white arrow).

## REFERENCES

1. Suzuki Y, Fujino Y, Tanioka Y et al. Factors influencing hepaticojejunostomy leak following pancreaticoduodenal resection; importance of anastomotic leak test. *Hepatogastroenterology* 2003;50(49):254–257.
2. Burkhart RA, Relles D, Pineda DM et al. Defining treatment and outcomes of hepaticojejunostomy failure following pancreaticoduodenectomy. *J Gastrointest Surg* 2013;17(3):451–460.
3. Andrianello S, Marchegiani G, Malleo G et al. Biliary fistula after pancreaticoduodenectomy: Data from 1618 consecutive pancreaticoduodenectomies. *HPB* 2017;19(3):264–269.
4. Jester AL, Chung CW, Becerra DC et al. The impact of hepaticojejunostomy leaks After pancreatoduodenectomy: A devastating source of morbidity and mortality. *J Gastrointest Surg* 2017;21(6):1017–1024.
5. Porembka ML, Hall BL, Hirbe M et al. Quantitative weighting of postoperative complications based on the accordion severity grading system: Demonstration of potential impact using the American college of surgeons national surgical quality improvement program. *J Am Coll Surg* 2010;210(3):286–298.

# 16 Duodenal Neuroendocrine Tumors

## A Discrete 1 cm Lesion on D2 – Antipancreatic Surface vs Pancreatic Surface

*Valentina Andreasi, Stefano Partelli, Francesca Muffatti, and Massimo Falconi*

## CONTENTS

## CASE SCENARIO

A 76-year-old man with a past medical history of atrial fibrillation, hypertension, and obesity presented with dyspepsia and was submitted to upper gastrointestinal endoscopy. During this procedure, a 12 mm polypoidal submucosal lesion arising from the antipancreatic surface of duodenum, at the junction between the first and the second part, was observed. A deep biopsy of the lesion was then performed and the pathology report showed a G1 duodenal neuroendocrine tumor with a Ki-67 proliferative index <2%. The diagnostic workup was completed with a [68]Gallium positron emission tomography (PET) scan showing an intense duodenal radiotracer uptake. The duodenal neuroendocrine tumor was clearly discernible on an abdominal computed tomography (CT) scan with contrast medium. The patient was then submitted to an endoscopic ultrasound showing an 8 mm duodenal neuroendocrine tumor, finally treated with endoscopic submucosal dissection. The final histopathology confirmed the presence of a 7 mm duodenal neuroendocrine tumor G1 confined to the submucosal layer (pT1b) and extended to the deep resection margin (R1). Endoscopic follow-up at one year was negative for disease recurrence.

## BACKGROUND OF THE PATHOLOGY

Duodenal neuroendocrine neoplasms are heterogeneous tumors representing approximately 1–3% of all primary duodenal neoplastic lesions and about 3% of all gastrointestinal neuroendocrine tumors, with an overall incidence of 0.19/100,000 in the United States. These neoplasms are nowadays discovered more frequently, as it has been estimated that their incidence has increased by 400% over the last 27 years [1].

The vast majority of duodenal neuroendocrine neoplasms (90%) are non-functioning. Therefore, most of these tumors are incidentally detected during upper gastrointestinal endoscopy. A functional clinical syndrome can be observed when hormonal hypersecretion is present. Symptoms related to Zollinger-Ellison syndrome are present in about 10% of cases, whereas carcinoid syndrome occurs rarely (3%) [1]. Duodenal neuroendocrine neoplasms may be sporadic or genetically determined, when associated with multiple endocrine neoplasia type 1 [2].

Duodenal neuroendocrine neoplasms are usually small (75% less than 2 cm in size), solitary, and restricted to the mucosal or submucosal layer of duodenum. However, nodal involvement is reported in 40–60% of cases, whereas liver metastases occur in <10% of patients [1,3]. The presence of multiple duodenal neuroendocrine neoplasms (9–13%) should arise the suspicion of an underlying genetic disease. Most duodenal neuroendocrine neoplasms (>90%) are located in the first-second part of duodenum, with 20% of them occurring in the ampullary/periampullary region. Ampullary/periampullary neuroendocrine neoplasms are often differentiated from other duodenal neuroendocrine neoplasms, as they differ clinically, histologically, and in their biological behavior [1,2,3]. Lesions are less frequently found in the distal duodenum [1].

Tumor grade is classified according to the World Health Organization (WHO) grading system, into: neuroendocrine tumor (NET)-G1 with Ki-67 index <3%, and NET-G2 with Ki-67 index between 3–20%. Neuroendocrine neoplasms (NEN)-G3 are further divided in NET-G3 when the Ki-67 index is >20% with well-differentiated morphology and neuroendocrine carcinoma (NEC)-G3 with Ki-67 index

>20% and poorly differentiated morphology. The majority (50–70%) of these neoplasms are low-grade and well-differentiated, whereas only a few cases display high-grade and/or poorly differentiated morphology. The estimated five-year survival rate among patients with localized G1-G2 duodenal neuroendocrine neoplasms ranges between 80%–90%, whereas it decreases to 72% in patients with well-differentiated duodenal NET-G3. In contrast, in the presence of a poorly differentiated NEC-G3, the median survival is only ten months [1,2,4].

## APPROACH TO MANAGEMENT
### Clinical findings
The patient described in the Case Scenario is a 76-year-old male with an incidental diagnosis of duodenal neuroendocrine neoplasm. This kind of presentation is consistent with data reported in literature, as the mean age of duodenal neuroendocrine neoplasms appearance is in the sixth decade, although with a wide range from 15 to 91 years. Moreover, a slight male predominance is reported in many series [1]. Duodenal neuroendocrine neoplasms are usually diagnosed at an early stage, despite being asymptomatic, owing to their incidental discovery on high-resolution examinations performed for other symptoms [3,5]. The patient presented in the Case Scenario underwent an upper gastrointestinal endoscopy because of dyspepsia, which is described as the most common non-specific symptom leading to the gastroscopies. In a smaller fraction of cases, patients complain of one or more symptoms, with abdominal pain being the most frequent. Other possible presentations include nausea/vomiting, jaundice, gastrointestinal bleeding, weight loss, and pancreatitis [3,4,5]. The tumor described in the case summary was located on the antipancreatic surface of duodenum, therefore it is unlikely that it could provoke jaundice or pancreatitis. In contrast, patients with ampullary/periampullary duodenal neuroendocrine neoplasms, which are located on the pancreatic surface of duodenum, experience jaundice, and/or pancreatitis more frequently. Finally, this case falls within the 90% of non-functioning duodenal neuroendocrine neoplasms.

### Diagnostic workup
The patient presented in this scenario underwent upper gastrointestinal endoscopy with the finding of a 12 mm submucosal lesion on the antipancreatic surface of duodenum, at the junction between first and second part. **Upper gastrointestinal endoscopy** represents the gold standard in the diagnosis of duodenal neuroendocrine neoplasms, as it is the most sensitive modality to detect primary tumors located in the upper gastrointestinal tract [2]. As recommended by guidelines, the lesion was biopsied and it was assessed as a duodenal NET-G1. It is important to perform a direct tissue **biopsy** in order to histologically confirm duodenal neuroendocrine neoplasm diagnosis and to rule out differential diagnoses such as Brunner's gland hyperplasia, adenomas, and adenocarcinomas [1,2]. Moreover, biopsy permits determination of Ki-67 value. It has been reported that the presence of a duodenal neuroendocrine neoplasm with Ki-67 ≥3% represents a strong predictor of tumor aggressiveness [3,5]. Therefore, the determination of Ki-67 index may influence the subsequent management between surgical or endoscopic resection [1,2].

The patient was then submitted to **endoscopic ultrasound**, which has a crucial role in the locoregional staging, for evaluation of tumor size and depth of invasion (Figure 16.1) [2]. In this case, endoscopic ultrasound described the known duodenal lesion as lying within the

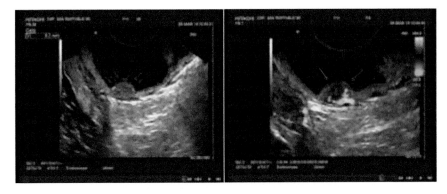

**Figure 16.1**  Endoscopic ultrasound of the patient affected by an 8 mm G1 duodenal neuroendocrine neoplasm (indicated by red arrows) located on the antipancreatic surface of duodenum, at the junction between the first and the second part.

submucosa, close to, but not infiltrating the muscular layer. Moreover, endoscopic ultrasound reported a smaller size of the tumor compared to upper gastrointestinal endoscopy (8 mm vs 12 mm) and was able to rule out the presence of nodal metastases, whose evidence would have represented a clear indication for surgery [2].

In the absence of features of aggressive disease (nodal involvement, invasion beyond submucosal layer, tumor size >2 cm, and tumor grade G2-G3) at both upper gastrointestinal endoscopy and endoscopic ultrasound, the performance of an abdominal CT scan and [68]Gallium-PET is not strictly indicated. In contrast, when at least one feature of aggressiveness is present, both CT scan and [68]Gallium-PET are recommended [1,2]. In the present case, despite the absence of aggressiveness features, CT scan and [68]Gallium-PET were performed in order to obtain a complete total-body disease staging and to rule out the presence of nodal metastases. At **CT scan** with contrast medium, the primary tumor was visible despite its small dimension and there was no evidence of nodal or distant metastases. CT and magnetic resonance imaging (MRI) are usually poorly accurate in detecting duodenal neuroendocrine neoplasms, with false negative rate around 80% [2]. Therefore, the routine use of CT scan in small localized duodenal neuroendocrine neoplasms is questionable, although CT and/or MRI with contrast medium are always indicated for patients with advanced disease [1,2]. Finally, the patient was submitted to [68]**Gallium-PET,** which showed an intense duodenal radiotracer uptake, confirming the neuroendocrine nature of the lesion and excluding the presence of metastases (Figure 16.2). [68]Gallium-PET is indicated for disease staging,

although it has as well a low sensitivity for the identification of small primary duodenal neuroendocrine neoplasms [1,2].

## Management

Small and incidentally detected duodenal neuroendocrine neoplasms often pose a therapeutic dilemma. The management of these small neoplasms is still controversial and needs to be clarified [2,4,5]. In fact, natural history, ideal extent of resection, and prognostic factors for duodenal neuroendocrine neoplasms have been poorly investigated. However, it is well known that tumor size and depth of invasion are the most important predictors of malignancy [3,5]. In particular, tumor size seems to be highly predictive of nodal involvement [3]: the risk of nodal metastases is <5% for patients with duodenal neuroendocrine neoplasms <1 cm, whereas positive lymph nodes are found in approximately 80% of cases when tumor diameter is >2 cm. The patient had a stage I disease, consistent with the majority (66%) of patients affected by duodenal neuroendocrine neoplasms. His tumor was very small (<1 cm) and it was described at endoscopic ultrasound as located in the submucosal layer, close to, but not infiltrating the muscular layer of duodenum. According to the guidelines proposed by the European Neuroendocrine Tumor Society (ENETS), treatment of localized duodenal neuroendocrine neoplasms ranges from active surveillance to endoscopic excision up to surgical resection [2]. Therefore, the adequate management of these lesions should be generally based on patient and tumor characteristics.

First of all, the presence of aggressiveness features has to be ruled out. **Surgical resection** is mandatory if the neoplasm is >2 cm in size and/or the tumor extends beyond the submucosal layer and/or tumor grade is G2-G3 and/or if the lesion has an ampullary/periampullary location associated to jaundice, alteration of liver enzymes, or pancreatitis [1,2]. Ampullary and periampullary tumors have typically a more aggressive course, with the development of early metastatic disease even when they are small in size [1,4]. Therefore, pancreatoduodenectomy is the treatment of choice for ampullary/periampullary duodenal neuroendocrine neoplasms and, generally, for tumors located on the pancreatic surface of duodenum [1,5]. In contrast, for lesions located on the antipancreatic surface, as the one presented in this scenario, also a local surgical excision can be performed. Although local excision is a more conservative surgical procedure compared to pancreatoduodenectomy, it is associated with the potential risks of postoperative

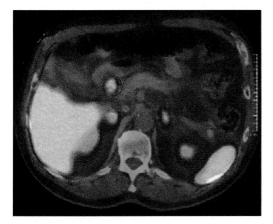

**Figure 16.2** Axial section of a [68]Gallium-PET scan of the patient affected by an 8 mm G1 duodenal neuroendocrine tumor (indicated by the red circle).

complications, mainly related to the presence of a duodenal suture. Based on the tumor size, the low Ki-67, and the absence of features of aggressive disease (as determined by upper gastrointestinal endoscopy and biopsy, endoscopic ultrasound, CT scan, and ⁶⁸Gallium-PET), in our patient, the multidisciplinary team advised the performance of a less invasive curative treatment (endoscopic submucosal dissection), thereby avoiding all the postoperative complications and the long-term functional outcomes possibly associated to surgery, especially in a frail patient. The decision against active surveillance was based on the fact that the tumor invaded the submucosal layer of duodenum.

Several types of endoscopic resection, such as endoscopic mucosal resection, endoscopic mucosal resection with ligation device, and endoscopic submucosal dissection can be performed. However, duodenal neuroendocrine neoplasms removed by endoscopic mucosal resection, and endoscopic mucosal resection with ligation device are more likely to have positive deep resection margins as they frequently arise and involve the submucosal layer. In contrast, endoscopic submucosal dissection is able to allow the removal of deeper lesions, guaranteeing a high rate of oncological radicality, even in the presence of submucosal invasion [1]. This is the reason why endoscopic submucosal dissection was chosen over endoscopic mucosal resection in the present case: tumor size was <1 cm, but submucosal involvement had been clearly described by endoscopic ultrasound. Of note, endoscopic submucosal dissection is also associated with a higher rate of complications, such as bleeding and perforation [1], but in this specific case the post-procedural course was uneventful.

In the current case, the final histopathology report after endoscopic submucosal dissection confirmed the presence of a 7 mm duodenal NET-G1 infiltrating the submucosal layer (T1b) and focally extended to the deep resection margin (R1). Therefore, despite endoscopic submucosal dissection being performed, the complete oncological radicality (R0) was not reached, as a R1-resection was described at the final pathological report. Nowadays, no consensus exists regarding the treatment approach for incompletely resected lesions, although guidelines suggest that surgical resection should be performed [4]. Nevertheless, current guidelines are based on small series with short follow-up. In this case, the decision on how to manage the patient after the histological finding was carefully discussed in a dedicated multidisciplinary tumor board. The possible

indication for a surgical resection was weighted with the risk of severe complications and with tumor characteristics. In the current scenario, the patient was 76 years of age and had several comorbidities, such as hypertension, atrial fibrillation, and obesity. Furthermore, pancreatic gland had radiological risk criteria for pancreatic fistula such as a "soft" texture and no dilated main pancreatic duct. A pancreato-duodenectomy would have been associated with a high risk of complications and mortality. Regarding tumor characteristics, in the present case no risk factors for nodal and distant metastases were present at the final pathological examination. Therefore, given the significant surgical risk related to performing a pancreatoduodenectomy balanced against the low oncological aggressiveness, a strict endoscopic surveillance seemed safe. The follow-up schedule included an endoscopic ultrasound every six months for the first two years and yearly thereafter for at least five years. The patient is currently alive and disease-free at one year from endoscopic resection.

In the absence of features of aggressiveness, tumor dimension has to be considered: when tumor size is <1 cm, both **endoscopic resection** and **active surveillance** are feasible, whereas when tumor diameter is between 1–2 cm, endoscopic resection is recommended.

## KEY MESSAGES

- Duodenal neuroendocrine neoplasms are rare tumors that are often incidentally discovered.
- Upper gastrointestinal endoscopy with biopsy represents the gold standard for their diagnosis.
- Patients with G1 tumors <1 cm, limited to the submucosal layer and without nodal metastases, can be submitted to endoscopic resection or, sometimes, to active surveillance.
- When features of aggressive disease are present, surgery is recommended.
- If the tumor is located on the pancreatic surface of duodenum, pancreato-duodenectomy has to be performed, whereas if the tumor is on the antipancreatic surface, a local surgical excision can be considered as well.
- Various types of endoscopic resection are available: endoscopic submucosal dissection seems to guarantee the higher rate of oncological radicality, even if with a higher rate of complications compared to endoscopic mucosal resection.

- In the case of an incompletely resected lesion (R1), the best approach between additional surgery or regular endoscopic follow-up must be decided on a case-by-case basis, considering the tumor and patient characteristics.

## ACKNOWLEDGMENTS

Dr. Valentina Andreasi, PhD studentship and Dr. Francesca Muffatti research fellowship were supported by Ms. Gioja Bianca Costanza legacy donation.

## REFERENCES

1. Sato Y, Hashimoto S, Mizuno K et al. Management of gastric and duodenal neuroendocrine tumors. *World J Gastroenterol* 2016;22(30):6817–6828.

2. Delle Fave G, O'Toole D, Sundin A et al. ENETS consensus guidelines for the management of patients with gastroduodenal neoplasms. *Neuroendocrinology* 2016;103(2):119–121.

3. Park SG, Lee BE, Kim GH et al. Risk factors for lymph node metastasis in duodenal neuroendocrine tumors: A Retrospective, single-center study. *Medicine* 2019;98:23(e15885).

4. Lee SW, Sung JK, Cho YS et al. Comparisons of therapeutic outcomes in patients with non-ampullary duodenal neuroendocrine tumors (NADNETs) A multicenter retrospective study. *Medicine* 2019;98:26(e16154).

5. Margonis GA, Samaha M, Kim Y et al. A multi-institutional analysis of duodenal neuroendocrine tumors: Tumor biology rather than extent of resection dictates prognosis. *J Gastrointest Surg* 2016;20(6):1098–1105.

# PART 4

# SMALL AND LARGE INTESTINES

# 17 Crohn's Disease

## Multiple Diffuse Strictures with Three Episodes of Subacute Intestinal Obstruction in One Year on Monoclonal Antibodies

*Lohith Umapathi, Divya Manikandan, and Govind Nandakumar*

## CONTENTS

## CASE SCENARIO

A 32-year-old man presented with intermittent pain in the abdomen, and symptoms suggestive of subacute intestinal obstruction. The patient underwent a contrast-enhanced computed tomography (CT) scan of the abdomen that revealed two discrete areas of thickening in the ileum. He responded well to conservative measures that included bowel rest and intravenous fluids. To investigate the regions of ileal thickening noted on the CT scan, a colonoscopy was performed a few weeks later. This revealed a normal colon and rectum but showed the presence of a few aphthous ulcers in the terminal ileum. Biopsies taken confirmed Crohn's disease. The patient was started on oral steroids and azathioprine.

## INTRODUCTION

Crohn's disease is a transmural illness that can involve any portion of the gastrointestinal tract from the mouth to the anal verge. The risk factors implicated in Crohn's disease are multifactorial, including smoking, low-fiber and high-carbohydrate diet, changes in the gut microflora, and nonsteroidal anti-inflammatory drugs [1]. Genetic factors are also known to play a role. A variant of the gene in inflammatory bowel disease protein 1 (IBD1) at locus 16q12, which was named *NOD2* on discovery and later altered to CARD15, is associated with ileal Crohn's disease. Crohn's disease is

characterized by segmental involvement often described as skip lesions owing to normal areas of bowel between diseased segments. Isolated colon involvement is noted in 25% of patients, with an additional 25% involving the ileum, and 50% affecting both. Crohn's disease is subclassified by the Montreal Classification based on: age at diagnosis (<16yrs, 17–40yrs, >40yrs), disease location (ileal, colonic, or ileocolonic), and disease behavior (non-stricturing/non-penetrating or stricturing, penetrating) [2].

## APPROACH TO THE PATIENT

### Clinical features

Abdominal pain is the most common presenting complaint in Crohn's disease (60–70%), with other frequent symptoms including diarrhea (50–60%), weight loss (25–30%), fever, and fatigue. Twenty percent of patients may present with bleeding as an initial symptom. Perianal disease is seen in about 10% of patients.

Extraintestinal manifestations in Crohn's disease are present in 6–40% of patients, the most common being iritis/uveitis (0–6.4%), primary sclerosing cholangitis (0.4–1.2%), ankylosing spondylitis (excluding asymptomatic sacroiliitis, 1.2–8%), peripheral arthritis (12.8–23%), pyoderma gangrenosum (0.6–1.2%), and erythema nodosum (1.9–7.2%). Pauciarticular arthropathy, erythema nodosum, and episcleritis are directly associated disease severity in Crohn's disease.

## BLOOD INVESTIGATIONS

The diagnosis of Crohn's disease is based on clinical, endoscopic, radiological, and histopathological features. Quantifiable markers of immune regulation are used to assess inflammatory status, and the most commonly employed studies include erythrocyte sedimentation rate and C-reactive protein. These studies lack specificity but can be used to monitor disease severity.

Certain antibodies are associated with inflammatory bowel disease. The most studied thus far being perinuclear anti-neutrophil cytoplasmic antibodies, more commonly elevated in ulcerative colitis (48–82% of patients) and less frequently in Crohn's disease (5–20% of patients), and anti-saccharomyces cerevisiae antibodies, elevated in 48–69% of patients with Crohn's disease (c.f. 5–5% in ulcerative colitis). There is evidence that panels of these tests rather than a single one may improve specificity. The specificity and sensitivity for diagnosing Crohn's disease and ulcerative colitis in adults when perinuclear anti-neutrophil cytoplasmic antibodies and anti-saccharomyces cerevisiae antibodies are combined are in the order of 95% and 50%, respectively.

## RADIOLOGICAL WORKUP

In the later stages of Crohn's disease affecting the bowel, patients can develop clinical symptoms of intestinal obstruction. Patients with Crohn's disease may also present with fistula, strictures, abscess, or a malignancy and a good radiological workup is essential to plan care. Barium small bowel follow-through was used frequently in the past. It is a dynamic and functional study and still has value in selected cases.

### The role of CT and magnetic resonance imaging (MRI) scanning

CT and MRI scans have emerged as important modalities to study Crohn's disease. False-positive results may be seen due to under-distention of the bowel or normal bowel peristaltic contractions. Presently, the use of a neutral oral contrast (e.g. Peglec) has minimized these effects, yet the definition of a "stricture" in most studies remains non-uniform, varying from bowel thickening to simple bowel narrowing with pre-stenotic dilatation.

Computed tomographic enterography is superior to the conventional CT in detecting strictures and other associated small bowel pathologies. In the presence of a single stricture, its sensitivity is about 85–93%, with a specificity approaching 100%. The overall accuracy of detecting multiple strictures is around 83% [3]. Computed tomographic enterography tends to over or underestimate the extent of disease in about 31% of complicated disease, and the scan results have been found to alter clinical management plans in approximately 50% of cases [3]. Computed tomographic enterography is also useful in differentiating between inflammatory and fibrostenotic lesions (accuracy of 77% and 79%, respectively) [4].

MRIs have high sensitivity to detect stenosis ranging from 75–100%, with a specificity of 91–100%. A comparison of magnetic resonance enterography and enteroclysis revealed superior bowel distension with the latter, but a comparable sensitivity and specificity for the identification of stenosis. A direct comparison of CT and MRI for diagnosis of this narrowing showed generally similar sensitivity (85% vs 92%) and specificity (100% vs 90%) [4].

Computed tomographic enterography or magnetic resonance enterography may also be used for surveillance of patients following surgery. However, in this indication they run the risk of being unable to differentiate active disease from scarring. Although neither of the scans specifically detects fibrosis, MRIs with a special sequence called *magnetization transfer* may help measure fibrosis semi-quantitatively. It is important to know if the stricture is inflammatory or fibrotic, as fibrotic strictures are best managed surgically.

Fibrosis on a CT or MRI is depicted by a thickened segment of bowel without the mucosal enhancement of increased vascularity (Figure 17.1). In the future, therapeutic approaches may be guided by special MR sequences or a combined ultrasound elastography technique to differentiate fibrosis from inflammatory strictures. In our center we use Computed tomographic enterograph or magnetic resonance enterography for evaluation of Crohn's disease. We prefer CT as the initial study and in follow-up, to decrease the radiation exposure, we use magnetic resonance enterography.

## MEDICAL THERAPY

Medical therapy is the cornerstone of managing Crohn's disease, as the goal is to avoid resectional surgery thereby preserving bowel. Corticosteroids have been traditionally used to induce remission in patients with Crohn's disease, and drugs like prednisolone have proven effective in mild or moderate disease. Steroids have significant side effects and are not preferred in the long term. Aminosalicylates, including 5-aminosalicylic acid (mesalamine

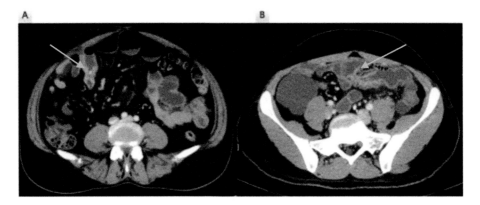

**Figure 17.1**  Contrast-enhanced CT scan sections of the abdomen demonstrating: (A) Axial post-contrast computed tomographic enterographysection showing an ileal stricture which needed resection. (B) Axial post-contrast computed tomographic enterographysection demonstrating an inflammatory stricture, which was managed medically.

and the controlled-release forms asacol and pentasa) and Sulfasalazine (a sulfonamide antibiotic, sulfapyridine, linked to mesalamine) can be used selectively to induce remission. Drugs like azathioprine (prodrug of 6-mercaptopurine), Methotrexate (both oral and injectable forms), and monoclonal antibodies like infliximab (anti TNF-alpha) are being commonly employed as well.

As maintenance therapy, oral azathioprine is recommended daily, with close monitoring for drug-related complications like bone marrow suppression, pancreatitis, and liver enzyme derangements. Another alternative involves weekly injectable methotrexate. However, this requires surveillance for liver toxicity, and should be avoided in women who may want to conceive.

Biological therapies such as infliximab administered every eight weeks have been shown to be effective in maintaining remission among those responsive to the primary round of therapy. Patients may form antibodies to infliximab, leading to acute and delayed hypersensitivity reactions and loss of responsiveness in those who may have responded previously. Other biologicals such as adalimumab, certolizumab, natalizumab, ustekinumab, and vedolizumab are also available as second-line drugs. Detail discussion of these second-line biologicals is beyond the scope of this chapter.

The patient discussed in the Case Scenario presented six months later with a similar history of subacute intestinal obstruction, successfully treated again with bowel rest and intravenous fluids. After the failure of first-line immune suppressor therapy (oral steroids, 5-aminosalicylic acid, and azathioprine), he was started on the monoclonal antibody infliximab at a dose of 5 mg/kg on zero, two, and six weeks, and thereafter an eight-week interval for a year. Infliximab was administered for one year, after which there was disease relapse, this time with acute intestinal obstruction.

## ENDOSCOPIC THERAPY

Endoscopic dilation is controversial but has demonstrated some promise in dilating strictures. It is principally used for short and isolated strictures, which are accessible by regular colonoscopies. Since many of these strictures are located in the terminal ileum or ileocecal region, a balloon with pneumatic dilation can be used. The availability of double balloon enteroscopy makes it possible to dilate stenosis involving the proximal small bowel, however, there is insufficient evidence to support endoscopic dilation. The highest number of endoscopic dilations are performed on anastomotic strictures and the method is best indicated for short (<4 cm) strictures with no ulcers. We do not use endoscopic dilation at our center.

## SURGERY

The patient presented in the Case Scenario had a CT scan with contrast when he presented with obstruction and was found to have multiple areas of thickening in the terminal ileum. He underwent a diagnostic laparoscopy and then subjected to a mini laparotomy during which the bowel assessed for occult strictures or fistulae. One stricture was resected with primary anastomosis and two other strictures were repaired in a Heineke-Mikulicz fashion.

The association between anti-tumor necrosis factor (TNFα) agents and complications in patients with Crohn's disease remains controversial. The pharmacokinetics of monoclonal antibodies, such as infliximab, permit persistent therapeutic concentrations for at least eight weeks post-infusion. Although it is controversial, we prefer to wait at least four weeks after the last dose was administered [5]. Urgent or emergent procedures can be performed while on infliximab.

High dose steroids (prednisolone >20 mg per day for >six weeks) may increase the risk of infectious complications, especially when combined with anti-TNF agents [5]. Timing of surgery and the decision to create stoma should be tailored to the clinical situation at hand.

Several surgical techniques can be utilized to surgically manage the complications of Crohn's disease.

## RESECTION

Patients who have failed medical management or who have had complications will need surgery. There is evidence to suggest that the presence of inflammation at the resection margin and the type of anastomosis does not affect recurrence. A limited resection of the diseased segment is recommended. At our center, we use a combination of gross examination and manual palpation of thickened bowel to assess disease. The Foley balloon technique (Figure 17.2) is helpful to detect occult strictures. In this technique we inflate a Foley catheter balloon with 10 ml of normal saline. This catheter is inserted through enterotomy at the most proximal stricture, which is determined by manual examination. By telescoping maneuver, partial strictures are detected. The decision to resect versus repair bowel should be tailored to the clinical situation.

## STRICTUREPLASTY

Strictureplasty can be used to preserve bowel for the future. Commonly performed techniques can be grouped into three categories: the Heineke–Mikulicz-like technique (commonly used for strictures <10 cm), the intermediate procedures, e.g. Finney procedure (for strictures >10 cm and <25 cm) or enteroenterostomies, e.g. isoperistaltic side-to-side strictureplasty by Michelassi (for strictures >25 cm) (Figure 17.3).

The need for a strictureplasty may arise in the presence of multiple strictures over a lengthy piece of bowel, a previous >100 cm small bowel resection, short bowel syndrome, duodenal stricture, or a recurrent stricture at an anastomotic site (Figure 17.4). Contraindications to strictureplasty include presence of a phlegmon or abscess, perforation with diffuse peritonitis, suspicion of malignancy at the stricture, or the weak nutritional condition of a patient. A strictureplasty can be performed relatively safely in the presence of active disease. Single layered seromuscular stitches are preferable, should make sure that there is no localized abscess or distal obstruction. Overall complication rate of the procedure is reported between 0–57% (avg. 13%), and a 6% incidence of major complications, including anastomotic leakage, formation of an abscess or fistula, and sepsis [3].

## SUMMARY OF THE PATIENT IN THE CASE SCENARIO

In the case of the patient presented, six months postoperatively, the patient is off monoclonal antibodies and steroids. The disease is well controlled with azathioprine and mesalamine.

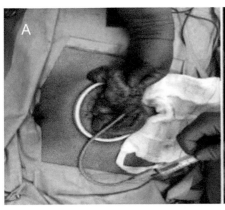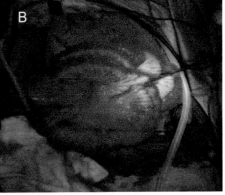

**Figure 17.2**   The Foley balloon technique used intraoperatively to detect strictures. Note in picture B, multiple strictureplasties have been done.

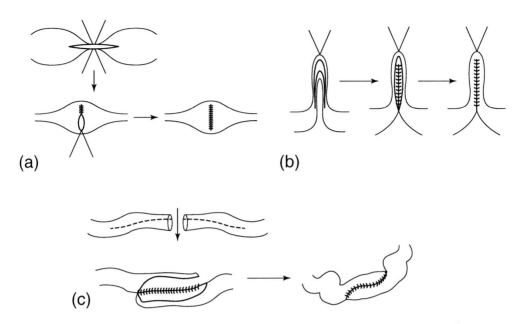

**Figure 17.3** Operative techniques for strictureplasty. (a) Heineke Mikulicz procedure, (b) Finney procedure, (c) isoperistaltic side-to-side strictureplasty by Michelassi [6].

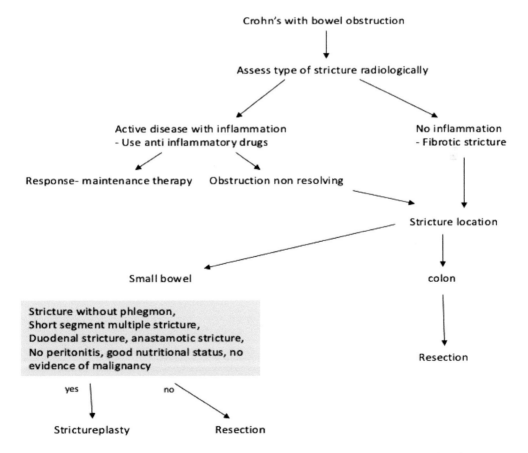

**Figure 17.4** General schemata for management of Crohn's disease strictures with indications for strictureplasty and resection.

## KEY MESSAGES

- There has been significant progress in our understanding of fibrosis and the ability to detect strictures in Crohn's disease.
- Radiologically, CT and magnetic resonance enterography help differentiate fibrotic and inflammatory stenoses.
- The future of Crohn's disease care lies in harnessing new medical therapies and novel biomarkers to predict clinical outcomes, and to utilize medical and surgical therapies more effectively.
- Bowel preservation by way of strictureplasties, limited and selective resection are important principles in the surgical management of Crohn's disease.

## REFERENCES

1. Michelassi F, Nandakumar G, Katdare MV et al. *Fischer's Mastery of Surgery: Surgical Treatment of Crohn's Disease.* 6th ed. Wolters Kluwer India Pvt. Ltd.

2. Nandakumar G, Michelassi F. Crohn disease: General considerations, medical management, and surgical treatment of small intestinal disease. Shackleford's surgery of the alimentary canal. 7th Elsevier Saunders; Chapter 17. Crohn's disease: General considerations, medical management, and surgical treatment of small intestinal disease.

3. Rieder F, Zimmermann EM, Remzi FH et al. Crohn's disease complicated by 3 strictures: A systematic review. *Gut* 2013. U.S. National Library of Medicine.

4. Govind N, Trencheva K, Michelassi F et al. Accuracy of CT enterography and magnetic resonance enterography imaging to detect lesions preoperatively in patients undergoing surgery for Crohn's disease. *Diseases Colon Rectum* 2014 Dec;57(12):1364–1370.

5. Strong S, Steele SR, Boutrous M et al. 2015. *Clinical Practice Guidelines for the Surgical Management of Crohn's Disease.* American Society of Colon and Rectal Surgeons.

6. Michelassi F. Side-to-side isoperistaltic strictureplasty for multiple Crohn's strictures. *Diseases Colon Rectum* 1996;39(3): 345–349

# 18 An Acute Embolic Event Affecting the Superior Mesenteric Artery

*Edward Travers, Alain Nguyen, and Savio George Barreto*

## CONTENTS

## CASE SCENARIO

A 75-year-old obese man with a prior history of paroxysmal atrial fibrillation on Apixaban® and chronic obstructive airway disease presented to the emergency department with sudden onset of severe generalized abdominal pain six hours prior. He was unable to open his bowels. The patient reported ceasing his Apixaban for five days a couple of weeks prior as he had to undergo an excision of a skin lesion on his face. On clinical examination, the patient was dehydrated, with tachycardia and episodes of hypotension transiently responsive to fluid resuscitation. On abdominal examination, his symptoms were out of proportion to the clinical signs. His blood investigations revealed an elevated white cell count of $17 \times 10^9$/L, with renal functions in keeping with the early development of acute kidney injury. His serum lactate was normal. Given the clinical suspicion of mesenteric ischemia, a computed tomography angiography scan of the abdomen and pelvis was performed which revealed an abrupt cutoff of contrast opacification in the superior mesenteric artery with features concerning for small intestinal ischemia (Figure 18.1). Along with the fluid resuscitation and analgesia, the patient was commenced on a heparin infusion and an anesthetic review was urgently sought. A detailed conversation about the diagnosis and need for emergency surgery along with its attendant risks was carried out with the patient and the family by the general and vascular surgeons, and after obtaining informed consent, the patient was shifted to the operating theatre for a laparotomy.

## BACKGROUND OF THE PATHOLOGY

The superior mesenteric artery is the second unpaired branch of the abdominal aorta arising from its ventral surface 1 cm below the origin of the celiac artery. It provides arterial blood supply to the bowel extending from the distal duodenum to the middle of the transverse colon through its branches, namely, the inferior pancreaticoduodenal artery, the jejunal and ileal arteries, the ileocolic, right colic and middle colic arteries. All these branches possess collateral vessels between them, including the marginal artery of Drummond that is the collateral vessel between the branches supplying the colon. The arc of Buhler is the collateral vessel between the celiac artery and superior mesenteric artery.

Acute mesenteric ischemia is a rare condition but is associated with high morbidity and a 30-day mortality rate up to 80%. Thromboembolism of the superior mesenteric artery is the most common cause for mesenteric ischemia accounting for 67% of cases with superior mesenteric venous thrombosis and non-occlusive mesenteric ischemia accounting for the rest [1]. Most patients present in their seventh or eighth decade of life. Embolic events (40–50%) are generally acute in onset presenting with catastrophic symptoms and occur secondary to either pre-existing arrythmias (especially atrial fibrillation) or arrythmias arising in the setting of a recent myocardial infarction with a resultant thrombus in the heart serving as the source of emboli. Less frequent causes include cardiomyopathy, left ventricular aneurysms, rheumatic valvular disease, or recent vascular interventional procedures. The

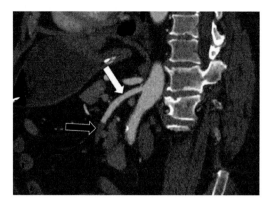

**Figure 18.1** Reformatted curved reconstruction of the computed tomography angiography of the abdomen of the patient performed at the time of admission demonstrating the origin of the superior mesenteric artery/superior mesenteric artery (white arrow) with an abrupt cut-off of the contrast in the vessel down-stream by an embolus (black arrow).

arterial occlusion in embolic disease is usually seen distal to the jejunal branches often involving the ileocolic vessels. The acute angulation of the origins of the middle colic vessels often result in a characteristic pattern of sparing of the transverse colon. Ischemia secondary to thrombosis of the superior mesenteric artery (30%) [2], on the other hand, even when acute in nature, tends to be insidious in progression and most patients report prior symptoms consistent with chronic mesenteric ischemia (characterized by recurrent abdominal pain after meals leading to the fear of eating). The most common underlying cause is atherosclerosis. Less common causes include a hypercoagulable state or prolonged hypotension. Thrombosis is more common in patients with a prior history of a cerebrovascular accident or disseminated cancer [1]. In thrombotic disease, the occlusion commences at the origin of the superior mesenteric artery and extends down contiguously resulting in the involvement of the proximal jejunal vessels, unlike the case of embolism.

## CLINICAL SYMPTOMS

Acute occlusion of the superior mesenteric artery by emboli leads to reduced perfusion to the affected segment with consequent hypoxia and anerobic metabolism. This causes regional acidosis and the production of lactates. These changes result in intense hyperperistalsis that is clinically manifested in the form of sudden onset of nausea and vomiting with severe cramping abdominal pain that is vague and non-localized in distribution owing

to visceral neural stimulation and appears "out of proportion to the physical signs" on abdominal examination. Some patients may have diarrhea. On abdominal examination, the patient may have a mildly distended abdomen with reduced bowel sounds. Poor oral intake coupled with vomiting result in dehydration and reduced urine output which, if untreated, can progress to acute kidney injury. Nearly half the patients report palpitations consistent with an ongoing arrythmia as the underlying cause. However, even in the absence of an arrythmia, these patients tend to have tachycardia unless they are on beta blockers. A prior history of embolism may be reported by in one-third of the patients. The development of localizing clinical signs and/or peritonitis in mesenteric ischemia heralds the development of gangrene of the bowel with or without a perforation. These patients tend be febrile and hypotensive.

It is paramount that the clinician be aware of the signs and symptoms of acute mesenteric ischemia to make a timely diagnosis when vascular intervention and bowel salvage are feasible. The clinician must also attempt to identify underlying risk factors that warrant attention. In 20% of patients, a concomitant embolus within another organ such as the spleen or kidney may occur [3]. A medication history that includes the use of antiplatelets and/or anticoagulation is vital prior to any surgical intervention to ascertain if a reversal of the agent is warranted.

## APPROACH TO MANAGEMENT
### Blood investigations

Every patient presenting to an emergency department with acute abdominal pain must have a complete set of blood investigations that include the following:

a) **Complete blood count:** May be non-specific in the early phases of the disease. However, significant elevation in the white cell count often prompts a search for an underlying cause.

b) **Renal function tests:** Elevation in blood urea is a sign of dehydration. It is important to know a patient's serum creatinine and estimated glomerular filtration rate when planning a computed tomography angiography.

c) **Liver function tests:** Help to rule out other causes of acute abdominal pain, especially biliary problems.

d) **Serum amylase and lipase:** If significantly elevated may help to identify acute pancreatitis although elevations are also noted in acute mesenteric ischemia, as well.

e) **Serum lactate:** Not a sensitive test in early ischemia, especially in patients with a good hepatic function. By the time it is elevated in acute mesenteric ischemia, the bowel is usually beyond salvage. It may be elevated in non-surgical causes, such as renal failure.

f) **Arterial blood gas:** An invaluable test in an acutely unwell patient, especially in elderly patients with respiratory issues. Provides a quick estimation of the metabolic status (acidosis or alkalosis), anion gap, hemoglobin, and lactate levels.

g) **Coagulation profile:** As a minimum, the patient must have their prothrombin time, activated partial thromboplastin time, and international normalized ratio determined. If indicated, an extended coagulation profile including rotation thromboelastometry may be performed. Blood for these tests should be collected before administering heparin to avoid confounding the interpretation of the results.

h) **Blood group and crossmatch:** All patients with acute mesenteric ischemia must have this done. The number of units of packed red cells crossmatched would be dependent on the planned surgical intervention. The choice of other blood products would be dependent on the patient's coagulation status.

### Radiological investigations

a) **Erect chest and abdominal X-rays:** These basic investigations that are universally available are invaluable in the initial assessment of a patient with an acute abdomen. An erect chest X-ray with both domes of diaphragm on view helps to rule out free gas and a bowel perforation as well as pneumonia as a cause or associated pathology. The abdominal X-ray findings may vary from small and/or large bowel dilatation, with bowel wall thickening due to edema. Although non-specific, these findings serve to alert the clinician to a possible abdominal problem prompting further investigation using cross-sectional imaging.

b) **Computed tomography angiography:** This is widely regarded as the investigation of choice in a patient with suspected acute mesenteric ischemia in the absence of established peritonitis. It not only permits a thorough assessment of the abdominal aorta and all its branches, but also an evaluation of the bowel and other organs to confirm the diagnosis and rule out other clinical conditions that may mimic acute mesenteric ischemia (including a bowel perforation, bowel obstruction, acute pancreatitis, acute cholecystitis, etc). The vascular findings in an embolic superior mesenteric artery occlusion include patent superior mesenteric artery origin with an abrupt cut-off of intravascular contrast at the site of the embolus. This helps to differentiate from an underlying thrombosis of the superior mesenteric artery – thereby facilitating appropriate planning of the vascular intervention. Computed tomography angiography helps to determine the number of involved vessels and the site of occlusion. The small and large bowel appear dilated with thickened, edematous walls. Hypoperfusion or lack of perfusion confirms the suspicion of underlying ischemia. Other supportive findings include stranding of mesenteric fat and free fluid. The presence of free gas suggests a bowel perforation. Computed tomography angiography also helps to rule out embolic occluding the vasculature of other organs.

c) **Magnetic resonance angiography:** Although considered a useful alternative to computed tomography angiography in other clinical conditions by virtue of avoiding exposure to ionizing radiation, in the case of acute mesenteric ischemia, its limited availability, longer acquisition times, and poor spatial resolution and artefacts that may arise from the prior placement of stents, rendering magnetic resonance angiography a less useful option.

d) **Echocardiogram:** A transesophageal echocardiogram is the ideal investigation to rule out an atrial thrombus in a patient with an embolic occlusion of the branches of the superior mesenteric artery. If unavailable, a transthoracic echocardiogram is a useful alternative. This test need not be performed immediately but preferably in the intensive care unit (ICU) once the patient has undergone emergency surgery. The presence of an atrial appendage thrombus necessitates therapeutic anticoagulation to avoid further episodes of embolization.

e) **Mesenteric Angiography:** Prior to the availability of computed tomography angiography, mesenteric angiography served as a "one-stop shop" investigation for suspected mesenteric ischemia as a diagnostic and therapeutic tool. However, the rise of computed tomography angiography in terms of its ease of availability, its capability to provide information about the intra-abdominal organs, and the fact that it seldom delays surgery or the initiation of anticoagulation (heparin) has resulted in the diminished use of mesenteric angiography [4]. Its current use is restricted to patients with known vasculopathies with extensive calcification of their vessels, or with stents in situ. As a therapeutic modality, it retains its importance in centers where endovascular procedures are performed, including angioplasty, thrombolysis, and stenting.

f) **Duplex ultrasonography:** This modality does not have a role in acute mesenteric ischemia as bowel gas within the dilated bowel loops as well as mesenteric edema, coupled with patient discomfort, preclude any valuable information being gleaned from it.

## MANAGEMENT

The principles of managing a patient with acute mesenteric ischemia are summarized in the three Rs, namely resuscitation, rapid diagnosis, and early revascularisation [5]. The initial management of a patient with suspected acute mesenteric ischemia due to embolism (as with all other causes) revolves around the cardinal principles of resuscitation that include:

a) Securing the airway, especially in the elderly who may vomit and are at risk of aspiration.

b) Providing high flow (supplementary) oxygen using a mask or nasal prongs.

c) Establishing vascular access with two large bore cannulas and resuscitate the patient with isotonic crystalloids (to counteract the third space losses) after obtaining blood for the investigations listed above. Blood products must be used when indicated especially in an anemic patient. If the patient is hypotensive needing inotropes, vasopressors that result in splanchnic vasoconstriction must be avoided and the preferential use of drugs such as dobutamine, milrinone, and low dose dopamine must be considered [5]. Patients in atrial fibrillation should be rate-controlled after seeking an opinion from the cardiology team.

d) Inserting a nasogastric tube and in-dwelling urinary catheter.

e) Promptly correcting electrolyte disturbances.

f) Commencing the patient on analgesia and broad-spectrum antibiotics (owing to the risk of bacterial translocation from bowel with compromised vascularity).

g) As soon as the diagnosis is confirmed, commencing the patient on a heparin infusion (unless contraindicated) to maintain the activated partial thromboplastin time from 60–80 seconds.

If the resuscitation is happening in the ICU, the intensivists may consider inserting an arterial line and central venous catheter. If not, then these need to be inserted by the anesthetist.

The management of acute mesenteric ischemia due to embolism is multidisciplinary including the vascular and general surgeons, anesthetists, intensivists, cardiologists, and hematologists.

### Surgery

Patients with suspected acute mesenteric ischemia secondary to embolism (especially with signs of peritonism) should undergo a prompt laparotomy with open embolectomy and examination of the bowel [5]. In the absence of bowel ischemia, and if the necessary expertise and resources are available, endovascular techniques can be attempted. However, it is very difficult to identify full-thickness patches of gangrene on computed tomography angiography of the abdomen and hence the authors prefer a thorough assessment of the bowel that is best achieved by a laparotomy.

If on laparotomy and the entire visible bowel (small and large) has full-thickness gangrene, the patient is deemed unsalvageable and must be offered palliative care only.

### *Principles of open embolectomy*

■ Warm saline packs covering the bowel to help with retraction.

■ Infrapancreatic incision at the root of mesentery.

■ Achieve secure control over the main trunk of superior mesenteric artery and its main branches.

■ Transverse arteriotomy on the superior mesenteric artery trunk.

■ Embolectomy carefully performed (without forcing the catheter) with a 3–4 mm Fogarty catheter trolled proximally and distally to ensure free bleeding from both directions.

■ Flush proximally and distally with heparinised saline (10 units / mL).

■ Tension-free, closure of arteriotomy with interrupted polypropylene 6/0 sutures between proximal and distally situated vascular clamps.

- Examination of bowel.

### Principles of bowel surgery

- Assessment of the bowel is based on its gross appearance – color, the lustre of the serosa, visible peristalsis, pulsations in the mesentery, and bleeding of cut ends [5].

- All visible full-thickness gangrenous bowel must be resected and the ends left stapled in situ.

- Less commonly observed tiny <1 cm patches of gangrene may be overrun in one or two layers with polydioxanone 3/0 suture and re-examined at the time of the relook laparotomy.

- Preferably, no attempt at anastomosis must be made at the first laparotomy and the patient must be left with a laparostomy since the intent is damage control surgery [3]. The author's preference of laparostomy dressing is the vacuum-assisted closure ABThera abdominal wound management system (KCI, Australia). However, in the authors' experience, in resource-limited situations, a "Bogota bag" fashioned out of a sterile cut open drainage bag dipped in betadine may be used. In this situation, the bag is sutured to the skin and covered with copious sterile absorbent dressing with Hypafix over the top. The only caveat is that the dressing needs to be replaced within 48 hours after surgery.

The patient is then transferred to the ICU for further resuscitation and care. The heparin infusion is continued. The patient must be commenced on total parenteral nutrition and no enteral feeding must be provided.

### Principles of relook laparotomy

- The timing of the relook laparotomy is guided by the clinical condition of the patient.

- The authors' preference is to relook at 48 hours (planned) to allow the vascularity to declare itself. In which case, the ICU team is informed to cease the heparin infusion 4–6 hours prior to the planned resurgery.

- The indications for relook prior to 48 hours (on-demand) include – worsening hemodynamic instability (increase in the dose or number of inotropes), accompanied by a rising serum lactate in serial arterial blood

gas, and/or evidence of intra-abdominal bleeding.

- At the relook laparotomy, any further gangrenous bowel is resected and the decision is made whether to close the abdomen or persist with a laparostomy (which would be done if the extent of bowel gangrene is unexpected in location and extent).

- If the patient's condition necessitated a resection of the right colon with sufficient amount of small bowel (>100 cm), then an ileostomy may be fashioned. Other considerations favoring the creation of a stoma include ongoing inotrope requirements, and severely edematous bowel that the surgeon deems unsafe to anastomose.

- An anastomosis must only be created if the surgeon deems it safe beyond reasonable doubt – no inotropes or multiorgan failure, need for resection of a limited segment of proximal jejunum (which would result in a high-output stoma), and healthy bowel available for anastomosis. The value of an anastomosis must be strongly considered in patients who undergo an extensive bowel resection to improve functional results. However, this must not be at the cost of an insecure anastomosis as a leak will likely result in a fatal outcome in such patients who are already compromised.

- The authors' preference is a side-to-side hand-sewn anastomosis in two layers with polydioxanone 3/0.

- Abdominal wall closure is preferentially achieved by nylon sutures (with or without interrupted stitches of the same material). The skin may be closed with a continuous subcuticular poliglecaprone 3/0 suture or interrupted staples. The authors' preference is to apply a PREVENA ® incision management system over the skin wound for the first 7–14 days.

- One must be aware of the risk of intra-abdominal hypertension following primary fascial closure. The ICU team needs to be aware of this to anticipate a transient elevation in inotrope requirement in the initial hours after surgery that gradually improves. They need to ensure the patient has adequate renal perfusion during this period. Serial measurements of intra-abdominal pressures via the in-dwelling urinary catheter helps to guide the clinicians in the event of evolving intra-abdominal hypertension/abdominal compartment syndrome.

- If the closure of the rectus sheath is not feasible, then a bridging mesh may be used. Ideally, a biological mesh is best suited for this indication. However, if the option of a biological mesh is not available, then a composite mesh can be used with an attempt to lay the omentum immediately under the mesh.

- Patients who are left with less than 60 cm of small intestine after resection are at high-risk of short bowel syndrome and even lifelong total parenteral nutrition. The value of such endeavors must take into account the resultant morbidity, mortality, and quality of life especially in elderly, moribund patients.

All patients with an embolic cause for the acute mesenteric ischemia must be put on lifelong anticoagulation, unless contraindicated.

The patient presented in the Case Scenario underwent a laparotomy with open embolectomy. The bowel appeared dusky but viable, and so the patient was subjected to a laparostomy with the vacuum-assisted closure ABThera abdominal wound management system (KCI, Australia). He underwent a relook laparotomy within 24 hours due to hemodynamic instability (Figure 18.2), during which 30 cm of the terminal ileum, as well as the cecum and ascending colon, were resected and the stapled ends left in situ. He was subjected to a laparostomy. At the final relook laparotomy in 48 hours, 15 cm of jejunum situated 25 cm from

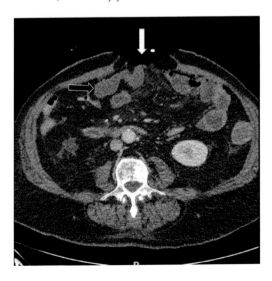

**Figure 18.2** Contrast-enhanced axial CT image of the patient's abdomen performed prior to the first relook laparotomy demonstrating the laparostomy (white arrow) and small bowel with hypoattenuating walls suspicious for ischemia (black arrow).

the duodenojejunal flexure was resected and anastomosed, an end ileostomy was fashioned, and the abdomen closed primarily. He had a slow recovery owing to his underlying chronic obstructive airway disease necessitating a tracheostomy. However, he was discharged home after spending a few weeks at a rehabilitation facility after receiving education on managing his ileostomy.

### SALIENT POINTS

- Embolism from atrial fibrillation is the leading cause for acute mesenteric ischemia.
- A high degree of suspicion is essential to avoid delays in initiating management in these patients.
- Pain disproportionate to clinical abdominal signs is a characteristic presentation of acute mesenteric ischemia.
- In the absence of a sensitive blood test, early computed tomography angiography is essential to investigate these patients.
- Once the diagnosis is confirmed, systemic heparinization and prompt surgical exploration with open embolectomy and damage control surgery is key to success.
- Performing a laparostomy with a planned relook is recommended with resection of all visible gangrenous bowel.
- The decision to perform a stoma versus anastomosing bowel should be guided by the experience of the surgeon and the clinical condition of the patient.
- All patients with an embolic acute mesenteric ischemia should be put on lifelong anticoagulation.

### REFERENCES

1. Acosta S. Epidemiology of mesenteric vascular disease: Clinical implications. *Semin Vasc Surg* 2010 Mar;23(1):4–8.
2. Mansour MA. Management of acute mesenteric ischemia. *Arch Surg* 1999 Mar;134(3):328–330; discussion 31.
3. Bala M, Kashuk J, Moore EE et al. Acute mesenteric ischemia: Guidelines of the World Society of Emergency Surgery. *World J Emerg Surg* 2017;12:38.
4. Ryer EJ, Kalra M, Oderich GS et al. Revascularization for acute mesenteric ischemia. *J Vasc Surg* 2012 Jun;55(6):1682–1689.
5. Tilsed JV, Casamassima A, Kurihara H et al. ESTES guidelines: Acute mesenteric ischaemia. *Eur J Trauma Emerg Surg* 2016 Apr;42(2):253–270.

# 19 Post-Colonic Anastomotic Leak

*Anu Behari*

## CONTENTS

## CASE SCENARIO

A 51-year-old woman with hypertension underwent surgery for cecal cancer. Intraoperatively, she had a hard mass in the cecum along with large nodes along the ileocolic vessels. A right hemicolectomy and a hand-sewn ileocolic anastomosis was done in a single-layer, interrupted fashion. The immediate postoperative recovery was uneventful. On the fifth postoperative day, the patient developed tachycardia, fever, and abdominal tenderness on clinical examination. After initial resuscitation, a contrast-enhanced computed tomography (CT) scan of the abdomen was performed which revealed a small collection adjacent to the site of anastomosis. Based on these findings, the decision was made to manage the patient conservatively with bowel rest and intravenous antibiotics. However, she continued to deteriorate clinically over the next two days and so a repeat contrast-enhanced computed tomography scan was performed. This scan demonstrated significant free intraperitoneal air and fluid in the abdomen. The patient was explained the findings of the scan and after informed consent, she was taken up for an emergency exploratory laparotomy. At laparotomy multiple pus pockets were encountered along with an anastomotic disruption of about one-fourth of its circumference. The anastomosis was taken down and an ileostomy and mucus fistula were fashioned. Thereafter, the patient recovered uneventfully. She was reoperated after six weeks and a successful continuity of the bowel was restored.

## BACKGROUND OF THE PATHOLOGY

Colonic anastomotic leak arises from partial or complete disruption at suture/staple lines. It leads to a leakage of variable quantities of air, fluid, and/or gastrointestinal contents from the site of a colonic anastomosis (ileocolic, colocolic, or colorectal) with often devastating consequences.

Though the overall rates of colonic anastomotic leak are low (colorectal or coloanal: 1–19%; colocolic: 0–2%; ileocolic: 0.02–4%), colonic anastomotic leak is a serious complication that is associated not only with an increase in the morbidity, hospital stay, need for reintervention and cost of treatment, but also mortality. There is also evidence to link colonic anastomotic leak with increased rates of local recurrence and worse long-term prognosis in patients with cancer [1]. Healing with fibrosis leading to stricture formation has also been shown to lead to a significant reduction in the long-term quality of life.

Though we do not completely understand why anastomoses leak, several factors have been implicated in increasing the risk of colonic anastomotic leak [2]. These may be related to the surgical technique, patient characteristics, preoperative therapy (chemo- and/or radiation therapy) as well as intraoperative and postoperative events. Table 19.1 provides a summary of these factors. An understanding of these underlying factors is important as in addition to the basic tenets of doing a technically sound anastomosis, namely ensure good vascularity and absence of tension, the surgeon needs to appreciate the risk factors and modify or tailor operative decisions for an individual patient. Some practices that can help mitigate the risk of a colonic anastomotic leak include encouraging preoperative cessation of alcohol consumption and smoking, nutritional optimisation in malnourished patients, tapering steroids (when feasible) in patients with Crohn's disease, and delaying surgery for six to eight weeks before elective colorectal resections after ceasing

## Table 19.1 Risk Factors for Development of Colonic Anastomotic Leak

| Patient-related factors | Factors related to surgical technique | Intraoperative factors | Postoperative factors |
|---|---|---|---|
| Increasing age<br>Sex (higher risk in males)<br>Obesity<br>High ASA score<br>Malnutrition<br>Smoking<br>Chronic alcohol consumption<br>Diabetes mellitus and Hyperglycemia<br>Chronic steroid use<br>Immunosuppression<br>Preoperative radiotherapy | Tension at the anastomotic site<br>Impaired vascularity of bowel ends<br>Multiple intersecting staple lines<br>Site of anastomosis (colorectal at higher risk than ileocolic) | Emergency surgery<br>Excessive blood loss<br>Prolonged operating time<br>Intraoperative hypotension and contamination<br>Use of inotropes<br>Blood transfusion | Use of NSAIDs and Cox-2 inhibitors |

**Abbreviations:** CAL – colonic anastomotic leak, NSAIDs – nonsteroidal anti-inflammatory drugs, ASA – American Society of Anesthesiologists.

bevacizumab and to delay initiation of therapy for at least 28 days postoperatively. The surgeon also has the prerogative (as an advocate for the safety of the patient) to elect not to construct an anastomosis, or to cover an anastomosis (that the surgeon is concerned about) with a proximal stoma. The informed consent process offers the surgeon the opportunity to approach the topic of a colonic anastomotic leak with the patient and reiterate the risks specific to the patient, especially, if the patient has the factors listed above.

## DIAGNOSIS

Early diagnosis of a colonic anastomotic leak and timely management are paramount in reducing associated morbidity and mortality. However, there are no fool-proof diagnostic investigations which can pick up a leak in the very early stages. A careful consideration of the overall clinical picture, laboratory parameters suggestive of sepsis, as well as cross-sectional imaging is crucial to arriving at a diagnosis. Maintaining a high degree of suspicion is important, especially in patients known to be at high risk for an anastomotic dehiscence (Table 19.1).

### Clinical findings (symptoms and signs)

The clinical findings following colonic anastomotic leak may vary from the patient seeming asymptomatic, to the catastrophic picture of sepsis and shock depending upon the site, and severity of leak and the patient's immune response. It should be remembered that the relationship between the degree of leak and clinical picture is not exactly linear, and factors such as site of leak, the presence or absence of

a covering stoma, and the patient's response to the leak determine the clinical presentation.

On the one end of the spectrum are patients who are objectively unwell with signs of sepsis and abdominal features of generalized peritonitis, corroborated by the laboratory parameters of leucocytosis (sometimes leucopenia) and raised inflammatory markers such as C-reactive protein and procalcitonin. Toward the opposite end of that spectrum are patients whose initial postoperative recovery was uneventful, and a radiological leak is discovered much later in the postoperative period when the patient undergoes a contrast study prior to stoma closure.

Most patients lie somewhere in middle of the spectrum in terms of signs, symptoms, and laboratory parameters. It is in this subset of patients that the acumen of the clinician, coupled with an appreciation of likely technical as well as patient-related risk factors supplemented by radiological investigations, help in arriving at an early diagnosis and in guiding the nature and timing of intervention. Often, initial signs may be subtle and difficult to distinguish from other postoperative infections (pneumonia, urinary tract infections, etc.). Any unexpected abdominal pain (including increasing need for analgesia) and tenderness, tachycardia, tachypnea, fever, alteration of mental status, decreased urine output, new-onset cardiac symptoms, wound discharge, or infections, or delayed return of bowel activity should alert the clinician about a possible colonic anastomotic leak. Although the placement of drains during surgery is now on the decline, the appearance of turbid or feculent fluid in a drain (if one is present) is often pathognomonic of a colonic anastomotic leak.

Alterations in nature or volume of discharge from drains should be given due consideration as changes in drain fluids have been reported to predate frank colonic anastomotic leak.

## INVESTIGATIONS

None of the routine lab parameters (raised total leucocyte count or raised lactate) and markers, like C-reactive protein and procalcitonin, are diagnostic of a colonic anastomotic leak. Both C-reactive protein and procalcitonin are sensitive, though not specific, and have higher negative predictive values than positive predictive values and are, therefore, better at excluding rather than confirming colonic anastomotic leak.

Contrast-enhanced computed tomography scan of the abdomen and pelvis with water-soluble rectal contrast (in-rectal resection-anastomoses) remains the most important investigation commonly used for the detection of a colonic anastomotic leak. Oral contrast administration may not contribute much to the diagnosis, and presents a risk for aspiration in a patient with an ileus, however, it helps determine if there is distal flow of contents. Rectal contrast should be given using a soft catheter and gentle instillation of contrast. Presence of a colonic anastomotic leak may be revealed by presence of free air, active leakage of intraluminal contrast (Figure 19.1), localized fluid collection around the anastomosis, localized perianastomotic leak without significant collection (Figure 19.2), and intra-abdominal or pelvic fluid collections. The findings of the CT scan are paramount in planning treatment. An asymptomatic and contained leak with flow of contrast into the distal bowel presents an opportunity for conservative management with the placement of a percutaneous drainage catheter.

Other diagnostic investigations like flexible sigmoidoscopy may be considered in patients with low (extra-peritoneal) colorectal anastomosis to better define exact location and extent of disruption, especially when planning trans-anal management techniques (vide infra).

## PREVENTING COLONIC ANASTOMOTIC LEAK

Considering the devastating consequences of a colonic anastomotic leak, it is worthwhile to consider if anything can be done to prevent the leak from happening, or at least mitigating the effects of the leak if it occurs. Some fundamental principles include the following:

### Preoperative interventions

- Cessation of smoking and alcohol at least two weeks preoperatively.

- Nutritional supplementation in those with >10% weight loss, or with clinical evidence of malnutrition.

- Tapering of steroids as much as feasible in patients with Crohn's disease.

- Waiting for at least six weeks after bevacizumab administration prior to elective surgery.

### Intraoperative and immediate postoperative considerations

- Ensure that the anastomosis is fashioned between two well vascularised loops of bowel.

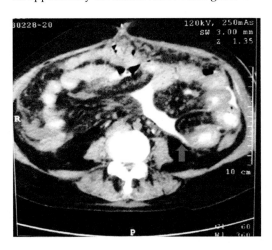

**Figure 19.1** Axial post-oral and rectal contrast CT section demonstrating free intraperitoneal contrast leak (blue arrow).

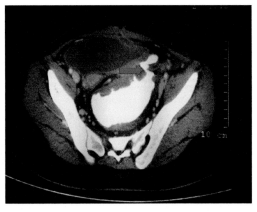

**Figure 19.2** Axial post-oral and rectal contrast CT section demonstrating a perianastomotic localized leak (blue arrow).

■ Tools like Doppler flowmetry and intraoperative fluorescence vascular angiography for assessing vascular perfusion of bowel ends are useful but are not routinely available.

■ Perfusion of the bowel ends and hence oxygenation is likely to be impaired in the setting of:

  • Intraoperative hypotension

  • Tension at the suture/staple line due to inadequate mobilization

  • Rough dissection with damage to marginal arterial supply

  • Emergency/damage control surgery

  • Preoperative radiation

■ Marginal arterial supply from the middle colic is usually good enough if descending or transverse colon are being used for a colorectal/coloanal anastomosis, but it may be insufficient for the sigmoid colon. If the sigmoid colon is used for anastomosis, then the left colic artery should be preserved. There is some data to suggest that it is not just the point of arterial ligation but the site of transection in the colon that impacts the blood supply at the anastomosis. Especially in patients who have received preoperative radiation, it may be necessary to remove the sigmoid and mobilize the descending colon to the pelvis. The splenic flexure should be completely mobilized and the greater omentum dissected off the transverse colon. Also, the retroperitoneal attachments at the tail of pancreas should be completely freed. The inferior mesenteric vein must be ligated just lateral to the ligament of Treitz, as this allows gain of length of several centimeters. For a transverse colon anastomosis, both hepatic and splenic flexures should be mobilized.

■ If the cut edge of the mesentery of the bowel, as it passes over the pelvic brim, allows a finger to slip behind easily then tension at the anastomosis is unlikely.

■ If the basic tenets of a safe anastomosis are adhered to then the choice of technique – namely hand sewn vs staples, single layer vs double layer, and monofilament vs polyfilament sutures – has not been shown to affect the development of colonic anastomotic leak.

■ Diverting stoma: Perhaps the most effective tool in the armamentarium of the surgeon to reducing the clinical consequences of a leak is the creation of a proximal stoma to divert the fecal stream away from the anastomosis.

■ The use of pelvic drains to prevent presacral collections of fluids to rupture into the anastomotic line is widely practiced but has not been proven to alter the incidence of colonic anastomotic leak.

■ Air leak test: Immediate testing of anastomotic integrity can be performed for colorectal or left-sided resections by this technique. It adds minimal time, cost, and risk to the procedure and should be done whenever feasible (by placing the patient in reverse Trendelenburg position, filling the pelvis with saline, ensuring all visible bubbles have been cleared, occluding the proximal bowel, and instilling air transanally with a syringe). A proximal stoma should be constructed if the test is positive after attempts to reinforce the site of suspected leak.

## MANAGEMENT

There are no specific guidelines for management of colonic anastomotic leak. Because of the absence of randomized controlled trials (which would be difficult to conduct because of the overall relatively low incidence and involvement of multiple factors), individual surgeons need to rely on information from large retrospective studies from high volume centers or analysis of large national databases.

There has been an attempt to classify the grade/severity of anastomotic leaks by The International Study Group of Rectal Cancer to better assist decision making and help compare results of treatment. It was suggested that severity of anastomotic leaks should be graded based on the impact of the leak on clinical management [3].

**Grade A:** Anastomotic leaks requiring no active therapeutic intervention

These are radiological leaks (usually revealed on a postoperative contrast study). Such leaks are usually not seen after colonic anastomoses and are more often seen patients with colorectal anastomoses.

**Grade B:** Anastomotic leaks requiring active therapeutic intervention but manageable without relaparotomy

Management usually involves administration of antibiotics and/or radiological placement of drains.

**Grade C:** Anastomotic leaks requiring relaparotomy

Since the grading is based on the treatment/intervention required and can be done only after the treatment, it is not of much help in decision making.

The fundamental goal of immediate and early treatment is to treat the sepsis by obtaining source control and minimizing further contamination. Depending upon the clinical situation (the general condition of the patient, the severity of the leak, as well as the presence of a stoma) this may be feasible (singly or in combination) by:

- No specific measures except waiting for spontaneous healing

- Medical means alone: Administration of intravenous broad-spectrum antibiotics, intravenous fluids, bowel rest, and nutritional supplementation

- Percutaneous aspiration and/or drainage of collections: Radiological (ultrasound or CT-guided) placement of single or multiple drains in fluid collections

- Surgical exploration (laparoscopic or open) with the procedure performed determined by the operative assessment of peritoneal contamination and degree of anastomotic dehiscence.

  - Lavage and drainage in all

  - Creation of proximal diverting stoma

  - Revision of anastomosis with proximal diverting stoma

  - Dismantling of anastomosis and exteriorization of both ends as stoma and mucus fistula (or a Hartman-like procedure for a colorectal anastomosis)

- Transanal drainage and techniques like endoluminal vacuum assisted early transanal closure

Figure 19.3 lists the three scenarios (1, 2, and 3) highlighting the management algorithm for each of them.

Waiting for spontaneous healing is appropriate in patients in whom the leak is discovered late, on a contrast study done prior to closure of a proximal stoma fashioned at the time of resection and anastomosis (Figure 19.3: Scenario 3). The patient is generally otherwise well with no signs or symptoms related to the leak. Waiting for another two to three weeks would allow spontaneous healing when the stoma can be closed. The problem of a chronic sinus has been alluded to in studies dealing with low colorecrtal/anal anastomoses. The first step may be to give more time, and repeat the contrast study after another three to four weeks. However, a definite percentage of patients with these low leaks do not heal (especially in patients who have received neo-adjuvant radiotherapy) and the choices in that case are to not close the temporary stoma, undertake a redo anastomotic pull-through procedure, or carry out an inter-sphincteric resection with permanent colostomy.

For patients with obvious signs of peritonitis or severe sepsis (Figure 19.3: Scenario 1), relaparotomy/relaparoscopy should be performed immediately following resuscitation. The choice of procedure would be determined by the extent of anastomotic disruption, the site of previous anastomosis, the degree of contamination, and whether a proximal stoma is already present or not. The site of the anastomosis determines the ease of access as well as the likelihood of free peritoneal contamination. A low colorectal anastomosis following an anterior resection may be difficult to access at relaparotomy, and a proximal stoma with additional placement of pelvic drains may be all that is possible. In contrast, for a leaking ileocolic anastomosis, it may be relatively simple to take the anastomosis down and exteriorize the ends as ileostomy and mucus fistula. Thorough peritoneal lavage with warm saline should be performed in all patients.

For patients falling somewhere in between the two extremes, (Figure 19.3: Scenario 2), the clinical picture along with findings of contrast-enhanced computed tomography scan should guide the clinician in decision making. Patients who do not have obvious peritonitis but have features of sepsis and are shown to have significant collection/s on contrast-enhanced computed tomography which are accessible radiologically, placement of percutaneous drainage catheters under radiological guidance may be considered. In case the collections are multiple or inaccessible and the patient is showing evidence of sepsis, reoperation is indicated. The clinical course thereafter should be monitored carefully for resolution; in case the patient deteriorates or fails to improve, reoperation should not be delayed.

Though extensive experience with endoscopic covered stent placement for postoperative colonic anastomotic leak is lacking, there are reports of successful resolution following temporary placement of removable stents. Stent migration remains a problem and patients have required multiple stent placements, with use of endoclips to hold the stents in place. In patients with significant comorbidities, in whom a second surgical insult may be associated with

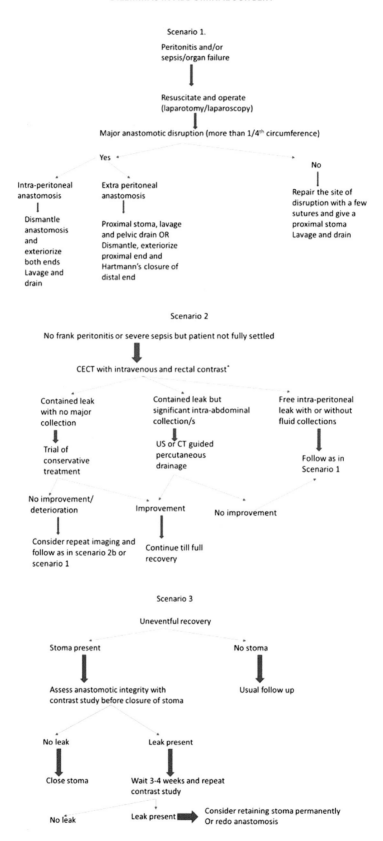

**Figure 19.3** Suggested algorithms for the management of colonic anastomotic leak.

a high risk, if expertise is available, endoscopic stenting may be an option to consider.

Transanal drainage works best for low colorectal anastomotic disruptions in the absence of generalized peritoneal contamination. A minimally invasive treatment method utilizing vacuum-assisted drainage along with early transanal closure of anastomotic disruption has been reported to be successful in patients with leaking ileal pouch anal anastomosis for ulcerative colitis and familial adenomatous polyposis, as well as low colorectal anastomosis after anterior resection for rectal cancer [4]. Acceptable rates of anastomotic healing and stoma reversal have been reported with this treatment strategy which involves endoscopic-guided placement of one or two open-pored polyurethane endosponges into the presacral abscess cavity and connected to a low-vacuum suction. Endosponges are changed every three or four days until the cavity is clean and filled with healthy granulation tissue. At this time, transanal closure of anastomotic defect is done surgically.

## KEY MESSAGES

- Colonic anastomotic leak is a significant complication associated with morbidity, mortality as well as compromised long-term prognosis. It is therefore important to understand the risk factors for colonic anastomotic leak to make informed operative decisions.
- Creation of a proximal diverting stoma is an effective tool to reduce the risk and clinical consequences of a colonic anastomotic leak.
- Early diagnosis and proper management can minimize the morbidity and mortality resulting from colonic anastomotic leak. It is important to have a high index of suspicion and tailor the management approach to the clinical presentation.
- Contrast-enhanced computed tomography scans of the abdomen and pelvis with or without rectal contrast should be used as they not only help in diagnosis, but also aid in the planning of treatment.
- A significant number of patients can be managed non-operatively so long as the contamination is contained, the patient is hemodynamically stable, enteral nutrition is feasible, and there is flow of enteric stream past the site of leak into the distal bowel loops.

## REFERENCES

1. Phitayakorn R, Delaney CP, Reynolds HL et al. Standardized algorithms for management of anastomotic leaks and related abdominal and pelvic abscesses after colorectal surgery. *World J Surg* 2008 Jun;32(6):1147–1156.
2. Davis B, Rivadeneira DE. Complications of colorectal anastomoses: Leaks, strictures, and bleeding. *Surg Clin North Am* 2013 Feb;93(1):61–87. Review.
3. Rahbari NN, Weitz J, Hohenberger W et al. Definition and grading of anastomotic leakage following anterior resection of the rectum: A proposal by the International Study Group of Rectal Cancer. *Surgery* 2010 Mar;147(3):339–351.
4. Borstlap WAA, Musters GD, Stassen LPS et al. Vacuum-assisted early transanal closure of leaking low colorectal anastomoses: The CLEAN study. *Surg Endosc* 2018 Jan;32(1):315–327.

# 20 Toxic Megacolon in Crohn's Colitis

*Dayan de Fontgalland*

## CONTENTS

## CASE SUMMARY

A previously fit and healthy 21-year-old woman, 20 weeks pregnant, presented to the emergency department in a regional hospital with acute onset generalized abdominal pain, fever, and diarrhea. She was assessed and discharged home with advice to increase her oral fluid intake, and was given a prescription for anti-diarrheal medications. She presented 24 hours later, significantly dehydrated with associated plum-colored bleeding per rectum mixed with the diarrhea. A diagnosis of infective colitis was made and she was transferred to a tertiary center for further management. On presentation, the woman was tachycardic, dehydrated, and was in acute renal failure. She was in excruciating abdominal pain with a labile blood pressure. She was resuscitated with fluids but not commenced on antibiotics. Stool specimens were sent off for microscopy and culture sensitivity. Her serum C-reactive protein was 160 mg/L at the time of her presentation to the tertiary center. She was admitted under the medical gastroenterology team. The obstetric team was consulted to monitor fetal heart sounds with ongoing surveillance for monitoring fetal distress.

Over the course of the next two days she became more unwell, had further abdominal distension, and had worsening per rectal bleeding necessitating blood transfusions. She was transferred to the intensive care unit (ICU) and commenced on inotropic support. At this time, a plan was made for a magnetic resonance imaging (MRI) scan of the abdomen and pelvis, as well as a flexible sigmoidoscopy. At sigmoidoscopy, the patient was noted to have significant colitis involving the rectum and distal colon extending up to the mid transverse colon (Figure 20.1). Biopsies were taken and the patient was sent for the MRI scan. The MRI scan demonstrated features of florid colitis from the mid transverse colon to the anus, with proximal colonic dilatation proximally to the cecum (Figure 20.2). The cecum to the proximal/mid transverse colon did not appear grossly inflamed, but the cecal diameter was approximately 10 cm with a transverse colon diameter of 6 cm. There was no free perforation. At this point, a surgical consultation was sought for assessment of the need for surgery.

The patient was commenced on high dose intravenous hydrocortisone (100 mg) four times a day for suspected colitis due to inflammatory bowel disease. Over the next 48 hours there was some clinical improvement. The colonic biopsies were suggestive of an indeterminate inflammatory colitis with superimposed cytomegalovirus infection. Stool cultures confirmed the presence of *Clostridium difficile* colitis. She was commenced on intravenous valaciclovir, oral vancomyin, and metronidazole. Serial abdominal X-rays revealed worsening of the megacolon, now including the descending colon with clinical signs of right-sided peritonism. There was ongoing need for transfusions of packed red blood cells, potassium transfusions, and her serum albumin dropped to as low as 18 g/L. At this point, the decision was made to perform a laparotomy and a total

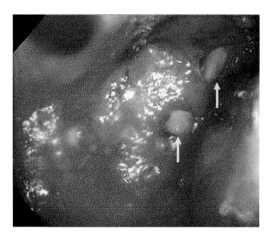

**Figure 20.1** Aphthous ulcers (yellow arrows) seen in the less-inflamed segment of the transverse colon on flexible sigmoidoscopy, reflecting likely Crohn's disease.

colectomy. The patient and her partner were informed of the plan and the risk benefit profile of surgery clearly explained (informed consent for surgery). Although there was no evidence of fetal distress, this first acute presentation of inflammatory bowel disease (likely Crohn's disease) had resulted in fulminant colitis, recalcitrant to high-dose steroids, antibiotics, and antivirals. The stomal therapist was involved in her care with counseling and stoma siting. The risk of fetal loss was difficult to quantify

but the patient was counseled appropriately by both the surgical and obstetric teams.

## BACKGROUND OF THE PATHOLOGY

Toxic megacolon is a condition traditionally characterized by gross colonic distension in the setting of severe colitis culminating in septic shock. It may occur as a consequence of either inflammatory bowel disease (more so in ulcerative colitis than Crohn's disease) or infective colitis (e.g. cytomegalovirus or *Clostridium difficile*) characterized by gross segmental or pancolonic distension greater than 6 cm [1]. The muco-submucosal barrier is lost with severe pancolonic inflammation resulting in colonic dysmotility, colonic dilation, fecal stasis, and bacterial translocation. This functional obstruction runs the risk of a megacolon and perforation of a thin-walled ascending colon and cecum. Often in pancolitis, diarrhea, with or without blood, prevails. Septic shock in colitis may not necessarily be accompanied by a megacolon. Hence, we tend to use the term "toxic colitis" to describe the condition of severe colitis causing shock, despite maximal antibiotic and anti-inflammatory treatment. Toxicity and the entity of a megacolon may exist independent of each other.

On imaging such as an abdominal X-ray, there is loss of the colonic haustral pattern. In the acute scenario, biopsies from flexible sigmoidoscopy often cannot distinguish between

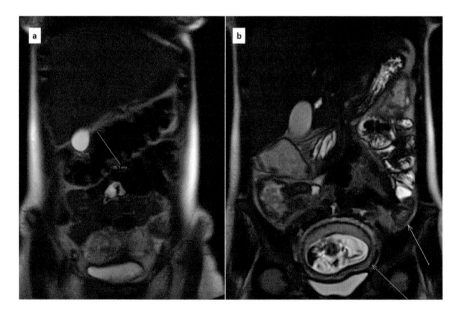

**Figure 20.2** MRI of the patient on coronal sections demonstrating: (a) Dilated transverse colon up to 6 cm. (b) Descending colitis (marked by yellow arrow) beside a live intrauterine fetus (red arrow).

ulcerative colitis or Crohn's disease. Deep ulceration and fissuring, typical of Crohn's disease can be a manifestation in severe ulcerative colitis which is usually a muco-submucosal disease. In this setting, a pathologist deems the colitis an indeterminate one.

Superimposed infection with cytomegalovirus and *Clostridium difficile* reflects severe disease necessitating surgical intervention. It is advised to test for these coinfections via stool samples and endoscopic biopsies [2]. It is unknown if cytomegalovirus and/or *Clostridium difficile* create an environment for an acute flare of inflammatory bowel disease or if the severity of inflammatory bowel disease leads to these opportunistic infections.

Surgery remains the mainstay of managing toxic megacolon due to inflammatory bowel disease and is often a life-saving procedure.

## APPROACH TO THE PATIENT
### Symptoms and signs
Physical examination findings need to be correlated with radiological evidence of disease. Plain radiographs and CT scans often reveal a severe colitis with or without a megacolon. General examination findings often reveal a tachycardic, hypotensive, oliguric, dehydrated, and febrile patient. They are often anemic, hypokalemic, and hypoalbuminemic, and may show signs of peripheral edema. They may examine with gross abdominal pain, distension, peritonism, and even obstipation from their functional obstruction. This is often confused with a patient being constipated, which is incorrect and may give the clinician a false sense of security that the colitis is settling. A patient who presents with gross bloody diarrhea, who then becomes obstipated with abdominal distension, is likely developing a megacolon. Again, it is important to note that the presence and persistence of one or more of these symptoms while a patient is on steroids heralds recalcitrance to medical management.

### Management
The initial management of a patient with suspected toxic megacolon begins with securing the airway, providing supplemental oxygen, assessing the hemodynamic stability (heart rate, blood pressure, and urine output) and cognitive state. Early insertion of large bore intravenous cannula and an in-dwelling catheter are essential components of resuscitation. Usually, patients present severely dehydrated with renal impairment. Along with intravenous

fluid resuscitation using crystalloids, the need for albumin and blood products (packed red cells) must be determined. In patients who are bleeding per rectum and in sepsis, attempts should be made to correct coagulopathy. A strict fluid balance chart and stool chart should be maintained, with stool specimens sent off for microscopy and cultures.

The abdominal examination should focus on the assessment determining the severity of the condition to guide early planning of relevant investigations and the need for surgery.

Generaized guarding and peritonism with abdominal distension and washboard rigidity suggest the possibility of a free perforation. An erect chest X-ray, with the inclusion of both domes of the diaphragm, is warranted to confirm the same before proceeding to emergency surgery (in the context of hemodynamic instability that is not responsive to aggressive resuscitation with concurrent need for inotropic support). In the absence of the clinical need for an immediate laparotomy, the investigative principles are outlined below.

### Blood investigations
Blood samples need to be drawn for an urgent hemoglobin, hematocrit, total leucocyte count, blood glucose levels, serum electrolytes, liver and renal function tests, coagulation studies, and C-reactive protein. Daily reassessment of these investigations are imperative. C-reactive protein is a good determinant of clinical improvement.

### Flexible sigmoidoscopy
Early flexible sigmoidoscopy utilizing rectal enemas if necessary, and with limited $CO_2$ insufflation, will determine severity of disease, confirm diagnosis, establish superimposed infections (biopsies needed), and act as a comparative marker for the assessment of improvement.

There are several endoscopic grading scores available for assessing the severity of inflammatory bowel disease [3]. However, in severe disease it is endoscopically difficult to differentiate Crohn's disease from ulcerative colitis. The findings of erythema, granularity, loss of submucosal vessels with deep ulceration, and spontaneous bleeding with contact or air insufflation often portends the risk for surgery (as was in the patient presented in the case summary). The efficacy of treatment may be assessed with repeat flexible sigmoidoscopies.

Biopsies for histopathology, cytomegalovirus inclusion bodies, and for *Clostridium difficile* culture need to be taken.

## Radiology

Frequent abdominal X-rays are recommended to assess the caliber of the transverse and right colon. Progressive colonic dilatation either reflects functional obstruction due to non-improvement of inflammation distally, or an evolving megacolon. Featureless thick-walled colon with worsening "thumb printing", and interval development of intramural gas mandates surgical consideration.

An abdominal and pelvic contrast-enhanced CT scan is preferable in the initial setting to evaluate distribution of colitis, presence of ischemia, perforation, or collections. CT scans are more accurate than abdominal X-rays in determining the true size of the colon. However, the aim of repeat radiographs is to monitor change in caliber, and plain X-rays are sufficient to assess this. Clinical deterioration in a patient may result in the need for repeat imaging with a CT scan.

In the setting of pregnancy, especially in the first trimester, radiologists are reticent to perform CT scans and multiple plain radiographs. An alternative to CT is an MRI of the abdomen, however, this is not advisable in the clinically unstable patient as it takes an hour to perform. CT scans are still indicated and should be performed, irrespective of pregnancy trimester, in a sick patient. Developmental delay in the fetus is a small risk and should be informed to the patient.

## The need for counseling and early involvement of colorectal surgeons

Tertiary centers often have a subspecialist colorectal surgical unit that must be involved early, should the need for surgery arise from failed medical management. Often patients look well with initial resuscitation and high dose intravenous steroid therapy. It is important to note that, like in pancreatitis, "the end of the bed test" is often not representative of the disease severity. Steroids mask symptoms and often there may be a sudden deterioration of the patient into a moribund state. This should be avoided at all costs and regular clinical review with appropriate blood tests often helps prevent this. Failure to improve often indicates failed therapy and the necessity for surgery.

These patients are often young and are mortified by the prospect of a stoma. Thus, early involvement of the stoma therapist is essential to initiate the conversation and help with the counseling around the creation of a stoma. Patients often maintain notes of their own stool chart and are aware of their daily biochemistry results if they are well educated and counseled early. This helps with acceptance for surgery.

## Involvement of obstetrics unit (when indicated)

In the case summary, the patient was is in her second trimester of pregnancy and an illness such as this puts her into a high fetal loss risk. The medications, and general inflammatory and stress response from the illness could result in preterm labor and/or intrauterine growth retardation. Should the viability of the fetus and/or the survival of the mother be compromised, the involvement of the obstetric team would help not only with the care of the fetus and the pregnant mother, but also provide guidance (along with the paediatrician) about the indication for early termination of the pregnancy and counseling on preterm delivery and information on the ability of the fetus to survive ex-utero. This would likely entail the need for a neonatal ICU admission. Hence, management of such patients should be carried out in centers equipped to manage not only the mother, but the baby as well.

## MANAGEMENT AFTER RESUSCITATION
### Medical therapy

After initial treatment with intravenous steroids, and in this case, antibiotics and antivirals, patients are assessed for disease progression. Disease progression warrants a trial of biologic therapy (monoclonal antibodies) in the absence of hemodynamic instability. Infliximab (Remicade) has the fastest onset of action with rapid recovery should the colitis be sensitive to this drug. Although the pharmaceutical advice from Janssen Immunology (J&J) reveals that it crosses the placenta and poses a theoretical risk of infections in the newborn child for six months, clinical evidence suggests that infliximab is relatively safe in pregnancy to both mother and fetus/newborn [4]. However, in the absence of a response to the first dose of infliximab, surgery should be considered urgently.

The patient presented in this case summary had superimposed cytomegalovirus and *Clostridium difficile* infections. In the setting of superimposed infection, as well as the underlying pregnancy, a decision to proceed to surgery was made. Considerations for fecal transplantation to regulate the microbiome in the colon can be considered in the setting of non-life threatening, yet medically recalcitrant, disease.

## Surgery

The surgical management of toxic megacolon in fulminant inflammatory bowel disease is an exploratory laparotomy along with a total colectomy, end ileostomy, and mucus fistula (if feasible). Whenever possible, the sites for stoma must be marked preoperatively. Other options for managing the rectosigmoid stump include oversewing and leaving it within the abdominal cavity (as was done in the patient presented in the case summary owing to the presence of a gravid uterus), or tacking the stump to the lower end of the midline wound with sutures in the event of a blowout (in which case it would lead to a controlled mucus fistula). Anywhere between 5–30% of rectal stumps leak in the setting of florid colitis supporting the performance of a mucus fistula in the emergency setting. Should the rectal stump blowout within the abdominal cavity, a pelvic abscess would result. To reduce the pressures within the rectal stump, a large three-way urinary catheter is inserted into the rectum, the balloon inflated just enough to prevent it from dislodging from the anal canal, and left in for three to five days on free drainage. Some surgeons advocate flushing the catheter with saline to prevent it from being blocked.

Laparoscopy has no role in the emergency setting, and open surgery is regarded as the gold standard. A lengthy procedure with raised intra-abdominal pressures in the setting of general anesthesia induced hypotension reduces placental perfusion and increases the risk of fetal distress.

The most common postoperative complications include wound infections, stomal dehiscence, and rectal stump leaks, and are a manifestation of poor healing consequent to the illness, malnutrition, and high-dose steroids. In the absence of complications following surgery, most patients improve rather quickly with the attendant weaning off of the steroids and their medication changed to maintenance treatment with azathioprine or biologic therapy in the ensuing four weeks.

In the patient presented in the case summary, we had the obstetric unit on stand-by in the event of fetal distress Fortunately, there were no intraoperative complications to the patient or fetus. The histopathology of the specimen demonstrated Crohn's disease with numerous granulomas and transmural inflammation observed on microscopy. The patient required total parenteral nutrition to maintain her nutritional requirements until return of adequate bowel function. She carried the pregnancy to term. At 38 weeks, she underwent an elective C-section and the colorectal surgeon was involved in this surgery to evaluate the remainder of the small bowel for Crohn's disease activity.

## KEY MESSAGES

- Acute fulminant colitis cannot be underestimated and is potentially life-threatening.
- Principles of management involve acute aggressive fluid resuscitation and maintenance of fluid, electrolytes, blood, and nutrition.
- Early diagnosis and management, with surveillance of biochemical parameters, including C-reactive protein in conjunction with clinical signs, are imperative to monitor improvement or worsening of the disease.
- Patients can exhibit deterioration despite appearing clinically well on steroids.
- Involvement of multiple subspecialist teams with constant communication is important. It is often important for a clinical lead consultant to co-ordinate efforts.
- There is a need for appropriate and early counseling of the patient for inevitable outcomes, including surgery and stoma formation, and in this patient, preterm labor and neonatal complications.
- Surgery is time-critical before septic shock intervenes [5].
- Laparoscopy has no safe role here, and laparotomy remains the gold standard approach. Ideally, a mucus fistula should be fashioned unless physically not possible, such as in the morbidly obese or, as in this case, pregnancy.

## REFERENCES

1. Sheth SG, LaMont JT. Toxic megacolon. *Lancet* 1998;351(9101):509–513.
2. Snyder C, Berk W, Genes N, Shah BJ, Dubinskey MC. Standardizing the Care of Acute Severe Ulcerative Colitis Inpatients at an Inflammatory Bowel Disease Referral Hospital. *Gastroenterology* 2019;157(1):32.
3. Mohammed Vashist N, Samaan M, Mosli MH et al. Endoscopic scoring indices for evaluation of disease activity in ulcerative colitis. *Cochrane Database Syst Rev* 2018;1:CD011450.

4. Truta B, Leeds I, Efron J et al. Pregnancy outcomes in inflammatory bowel disease pregnancy treated with infliximab: Early versus late discontinuation of therapy. *Gastroenterology* 2019;156(6):S17–S18.

5. Brown SR, Fearnhead NS, Faiz OD et al. The Association of Coloproctology of Great Britain and Ireland consensus guidelines in surgery for inflammatory bowel disease. *Colorectal Dis* 2018;20:3–117.

# 21 Colonic Perforation Pelvic Collection with Air in a Hemodynamically Stable Patient

*Varughese Mathai*

## CONTENTS

## CASE SCENARIO

A 40-year-old man was seen in the out-patient department with a seven-day history of abdominal pain, fever, and increased frequency of stool. He had an episode of acute abdominal pain seven days prior which was relieved with simple analgesia. He developed fever a few days later. The fever was high-grade and associated with chills and rigors. He had loose stools which were liquid to semisolid with associated mucus but no blood. He reported anorexia. The patient had a long-standing history of constipation. He offered no personal or family history of inflammatory bowel disease or malignancy.

## BACKGROUND OF THE PATHOLOGY

Spontaneous colonic perforation can occur from a variety of causes. The most common include:

1) Diverticular disease

2) Inflammatory bowel disease

3) Colonic cancer

4) Ischemic bowel disease

5) Trauma

6) Foreign body ingestion (e.g. fish bone)

In a 40-year-old patient, the pathology is more likely to be benign rather than malignant. Ischemia is unlikely.

### Diverticular disease

Acquired colonic diverticular disease is more prevalent in Western societies, as compared to Eastern societies, and its incidence increases dramatically with age. In patients less than 30 years of age, the incidence is less than 10% and rises to 50–60% by the age of 80. Approximately 10–25% of patients with diverticular disease will develop an episode of acute diverticulitis. Right-sided diverticuli are more frequently reported in Asian patients and tend to be true (congenital, with a genetic predisposition) diverticuli, i.e., with all the layers c.f. mucosal outpouchings of the acquired variety. Albeit, even among Asian patients, left-sided acquired diverticular disease is more common than right-sided disease. The common hypotheses for the development of left-sided diverticular disease are disordered colonic motility with high intraluminal pressure, colonic wall abnormality (related to collagen and matrix metalloproteinases), a decrease in dietary fiber, and alterations in the gut microbiome. Diverticuli occur in the areas of colonic wall weakness where the vasa recta pierce the muscle to supply the mucosa. Disordered motility with segmentation in the colon cause herniation of mucosa to form (pulsion) diverticuli that consist of mucosa with peritoneal covering. The risk of developing diverticular disease is inversely proportional to intake of insoluble dietary fiber. The Modified Hinchey Classification (Table 21.1) is used to classify the severity of acute diverticulitis complications [1].

## CLINICAL FINDINGS

A patient with a pelvic collection secondary to a colonic perforation is more likely to be febrile with tachycardia. In the event of a well walled-off collection, the patient is more often normotensive, although, in a patient with peritonitis and dehydration, the patient could present with hypotension and signs of sepsis. In the case presented above, the patient was febrile with no

## Table 21.1 Modified Hinchey Classification for Acute Diverticulitis

Stage 0    Clinically mild diverticulitis
Stage Ia    Confined pericolic inflammation and phlegmon inflammation
Stage Ib    Confined pericolic inflammation and abscess formation <5 cm in the proximity of primary inflammatory process
Stage II    Intra-abdominal abscess (pelvic or retroperitoneal) distant from the primary inflammatory process
Stage III    Generalized purulent peritonitis
Stage IV    Generalized fecal peritonitis

pallor or icterus and had a coated tongue. The abdomen was mildly distended with suprapubic tenderness and absent bowel sounds. Per rectal examination revealed a bulge anteriorly above the level of prostate. The mucosa of the rectum was normal on proctoscopy.

### INVESTIGATIONS

*Blood tests:* A complete blood picture with leucocytosis will indicate an infective pathology. Few studies have shown the presence of systemic symptoms, and leucocytosis over 12,000 per microlitre in patients with a pelvic abscess led to a higher rate of surgical intervention. Other blood tests that should be performed at presentation include renal function tests (with electrolytes) and liver function tests as these patients are likely to need some form of intervention (radiological or surgical).

*Imaging*

In addition to the routine radiology that must be performed, namely an erect chest and abdominal X-ray, a computed tomography (CT) scan of the abdomen with intravenous, oral, and rectal contrast is the preferred choice of investigation as this will not only show the diverticuli, stricture, and mass lesions but also the extraluminal abscess formation (Figure 21.2). The size and site of the abscess directly correlates to the need for intervention or surgery. Extravasation of contrast into the

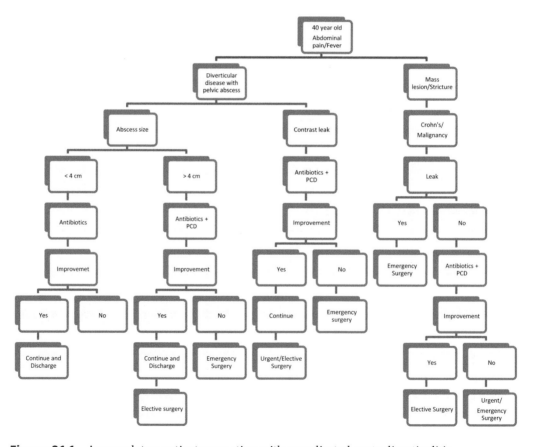

**Figure 21.1**    Approach to a patient presenting with complicated acute diverticulitis.

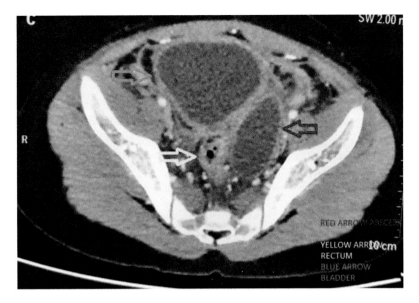

**Figure 21.2** Axial section of a CT image demonstrating a pelvic abscess secondary to perforated diverticular disease (red arrow: pelvic abscess; blue arrow: urinary bladder; yellow arrow: rectum).

abscess cavity would also indicate a need for urgent surgery. It is not always possible to rule out malignancy with a CT scan and if there is a short segment narrowing with enlarged lymph nodes, this possibility needs to be kept in mind. An abscess, if present, needs to be assessed for size, location, and the presence of air, as these are features that would steer one toward early surgery. The presence of air indicates that the perforation is likely to be large or is still leaking, and loculations would make it difficult to clear the sepsis with percutaneous drainage.

## MANAGEMENT
Abscesses <4 cm in size and in a pericolonic location are more likely to respond to conservative therapy consisting of antibiotics and keeping the patient fasted, and then steadily progressing the oral intake guided by the patient's clinical condition. Abscesses >4 cm in size most often in addition require some form of drainage. The preferred from of drainage is percutaneous if a clear radiological access window is available. The other forms of drainage may include per vaginal or per rectal. The presence of a pelvic abscess, in general, indicates a large perforation in the diverticulum. As an initial step, these would require antibiotics and percutaneous drainage. If the patient improves with these measures within 48–72 hours then one persists with this treatment. If there is no improvement, or if worsening of symptoms is

noted, then an emergency surgery would need to be considered [2,3].

## SURGICAL OPTIONS

1) Emergency

2) Urgent

3) Elective

**Emergency** surgery is the least attractive option as this often involves a Hartmann's procedure. Doing an anastomosis in the presence of frank sepsis is not a good option. The reversal rate of Hartmann's is low and entails another major challenging surgery. However, despite all this, in a patient with peritonitis and signs of sepsis, a Hartmann's procedure is a life-saving operation.

**Urgent** surgery would entail surgery during same hospital admission and once the sepsis has been controlled by percutaneous drainage and antibiotics. Here, one would have the option of doing a primary anastomosis with a covering loop ileostomy, or a primary resection and anastomosis depending on the local factors. The closure of the stoma would be an easier second operation.

**Elective** surgery would be the ideal option but can be contemplated only if the leak has sealed and the patient is completely stable. In this situation, the main indications for elective surgery are recurrent attacks of complicated diverticulitis or uncertainty in the diagnosis (cancer versus inflammation). The chance of recurrence is higher in those with pelvic abscess as compared to those who have had a pericolic or paracolic collection. In this scenario, it would be possible to do a single stage resection and anastomosis of sigmoid colon. If there is a mass or stricture present in the preoperative CT, it would be prudent to do a mucosal assessment in the form of a colonoscopy or sigmoidoscopy before embarking on the operation. In a study of long-term outcomes of diverticular abscesses, approximately 39% of patients with pelvic abscesses required surgery during their first admission. A further 51% went on to require surgical intervention on follow-up, thus making the overall surgical intervention rate in pelvic abscess 71%.

The patient presented in the case summary was admitted for observation in a high-dependency ward. He was initially kept nil by mouth and started on intravenous antibiotics (piperacillin and tazobactam) and peripheral nutrition. A contrast-enhanced CT scan of the abdomen with oral and rectal contrast revealed acute sigmoid colon diverticulitis with a pericolonic abscess and a separate pelvic abscess >8 cm. No leakage of contrast was noted. An urgent percutaneous drainage of the pelvic collection was carried out by interventional radiology. Over the next few days he improved clinically, with decreasing fever spikes and an overall sense of well-being. He was continued on conservative treatment with antibiotics and pigtail drain measurements, with a steady increase in his oral nutrition. The drain output improved from 200 ml in 24 hours down to <10 ml in 24 hours by day six. A pelvic ultrasound demonstrated resolution of the collection and he was discharged on day seven. He was readmitted three weeks later for a planned sigmoid resection. Diagnostic laparoscopy was done which showed a sigmoid diverticular disease and a small residual pelvic collection. There were dense adhesions around the sigmoid colon. The sigmoid and the left colon were mobilized, the pelvis was washed out, and a sigmoidectomy was performed. The rectal

stump was closed with a linear stapler. The end of the descending colon was anastomozed to the anterior surface of the rectum using a circular stapler. The anastomozed tissues were healthy with complete donuts and a negative leak test and so the decision was made not to perform a diverting stoma. An abdominal drain was placed. The patient was started on liquids postoperatively and progressed to a normal diet by the fourth postoperative day, by which time he had passed a normal stool. The drain was removed on the fifth postoperative day and the patient was discharged home [4,5].

## SUMMARY

- Diverticular disease is a common benign condition with high prevalence after the fourth decade.

- A contrast-enhanced CT scan of the abdomen is the investigation of choice in complicated diverticulitis.

- Control of sepsis can be achieved by percutaneous drainage and antibiotics. However, in patients with peritonitis at presentation, or those in whom sepsis control cannot be achieved by percutaneous drainage, surgery is warranted in the emergency setting.

## REFERENCES

1. Soumian S, Thomas S, Mohan PP et al. Management of Hinchey II diverticulitis. *World J Gastroenterol* 2008 Dec 21;14(47):7163–7169.
2. Welbourn HL, Hartley JE. Management of acute diverticulitis and its complications. *Indian J Surg* 2014 Dec;76(6):429–435.
3. Scotts Steele SR, Boutros M, Bordinue L et al. Clinical practice guidelines for the management of Crohn's disease. *Dis Colon Rectum* 2015;58:1021–1036.
4. Feingold D, Steele SR, Lee s et al. Practice parameters for the treatment of Sigmoid diverticulitis. *Dis Colon Rectum* 2014;57(3):284–294.
5. Tochigi T, Kosugi C, Shutok Mori M et al. *Ann Gastroenterol Surg* 2017 Sep 28;2(1):22–27.

# 22 Non-Obstructing Small Bowel Neuroendocrine Tumor with Liver Metastasis

*Mufaddal Kazi, Manish S. Bhandare, Vikram A. Chaudhari, and Shailesh V. Shrikhande*

## CONTENTS

## CASE SCENARIO

A 32-year-old man presented with episodic mild abdominal pain and repeated facial flushing over a period of one year. Physical examination of the patient was unremarkable. A contrast-enhanced computed tomography (CT) scan of the abdomen revealed an enhancing mass lesion in the proximal ileum with an enhancing mesenteric nodal mass measuring 4.2 cm in greatest dimension. Multiple arterially enhancing lesions were noted in both lobes of liver, the largest in segment 8, suggesting the possibility of a metastatic small bowel neuroendocrine tumor. Serum chromogranin A (CgA) level was elevated (113 ng/mL) and urinary 5-hydrodyindoleacetic acid level was also increased (71.2 mg every 24 hours) after a serotonin-restricted diet. A gallium-DOTA scan confirmed somatostatin receptor expression in all the lesions without additional sites of disease (Figure 22.1). Biopsy from the liver lesion was performed and confirmed the diagnosis of grade 1 neuroendocrine tumor with a Ki-67 index of 2%. The cardiac function was evaluated by echocardiogram, which was normal. The case was discussed in a dedicated multidisciplinary neuroendocrine tumor clinic. The liver lesions were deemed unresectable at that time. In view of symptoms of hormone excess, he was started on long-acting preparation of somatostatin analog (Sandostatin LAR®). Transarterial embolization of the right lobe liver lesions was performed with the aim of achieving downsizing and possible resection in the future. This treatment resulted in an improvement in symptoms. However, subsequent imaging showed progression of the liver lesions. Lutetium (Lu)-177 Dotatate peptide receptor radionuclide therapy cycles were initiated while Sandostatin LAR® was continued. Unfortunately, the patient went on to develop a small bowel obstruction between the two cycles of peptide receptor radionuclide therapy due to an increase in size of the ileal mass. He underwent emergency surgery with small bowel resection with excision of the mesenteric nodal mass. He recovered well after surgery and peptide receptor radionuclide therapy was continued for a total of four cycles, which showed largely stable disease in the right lobe with complete resolution of metastases in the left lobe. In view of persistent symptoms and hormone excess, and right limited liver disease, he is planned for liver surgery (right hepatectomy).

## BACKGROUND OF THE PATHOLOGY

Small bowel is the most frequent site of primary neuroendocrine tumor (two-thirds of all cases). These neoplasms are composed

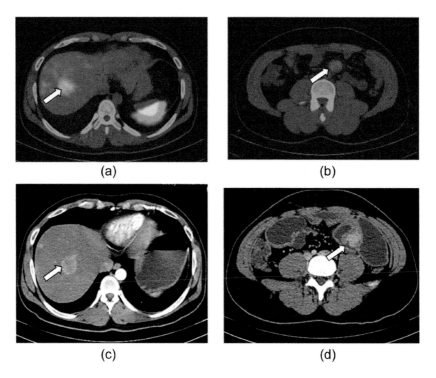

**Figure 22.1** DOTA positron emission tomography scan demonstrating the presence of a somatostatin receptor expressing lesion in segment 8 of the liver (a) and mesenteric nodal mass, (b) axial section images of an arterial contrast-enhanced CT scan confirming multiple arterially enhancing lesions in the right lobe of the liver (c and d), as well as the primary ileal mass with intense enhancement pattern (lesions marked with white arrow).

### Table 22.1 WHO Grading of Gastrointestinal Neuroendocrine Tumor

| Differentiation | Grade | Ki-67 (%) | Mitosis/10 hpf |
|---|---|---|---|
| Well differentiated | 1 | <3 | <2 |
| | 2 | 3–20 | 2–20 |
| Poorly differentiated | 3 | >20 | >20 |

of neuroendocrine cells that are scattered throughout the mucosa in the gastrointestinal tract. These cells get their name from their ability to express some proteins classically attributable to neural cells, such as neuron-specific enolase, synaptophysin, and also to their capacity to produce hormones, such as serotonin, histamine, kallikrein, substance P, and vasoactive intestinal peptide.

Among the sub-sites of the small bowel, ileum is the most common site (49.5%), followed by duodenum (12.5%) and jejunum (6.1%). The average age of patients is 66 years with no specific gender or racial predilection.

The liver is the most common site of distant metastasis and is the cause of almost all carcinoid syndromes. Unlike metastasis from adenocarcinomas, neuroendocrine tumor metastases are usually multifocal and diffuse rendering complete resection less likely. After hepatic metastasis ensue, hormone overproduction escapes first-pass metabolism by hepatocytes, and causes overt symptoms (Table 22.1).

## APPROACH TO MANAGEMENT
### Clinical findings
The clinical course for small bowel neuroendocrine tumors is variable, ranging from absence of symptoms to complaints resulting from local or metastatic tumor bulk and hormone overproduction.

Local tumor growth causes symptoms of obstruction and bleeding. Mesenteric fibrosis, elastic vascular sclerosis, and bulky nodal disease cause mesenteric angina and ischemia. More commonly, patients present with vague abdominal pain, borborygmi, and weight loss. Almost 50% of patients eventually progress to bowel obstruction if the primary tumor is left untreated.

Hormone excess leads to carcinoid syndrome, found in 80% of patients with liver metastasis. Flushing and diarrhea are the major components of carcinoid syndrome and each of them are seen with equal frequency in 60–70% of the patients. Other manifestations are wheezing from bronchospasm and heart failure from right-sided valvular dysfunction.

### Investigations
#### Laboratory tests
Baseline levels of Serum chromogranin A (CgA) and/or 24 hour urinary 5-hydroxyindoleacetic acid are recommended. If elevated, they can be used to follow treatment response, surveillance, and disease progression. The sensitivity and specificity of serum CgA for diagnosis of neuroendocrine tumors is 73% and 95%, respectively [1]. Urine 5-hydroxyindoleacetic acid levels are typically elevated in patients with liver metastasis but require 24 hour collection, a serotonin restricted diet, and a thorough review of medications consumed in the preceding days.

#### Imaging
The baseline imaging for patients with suspected metastatic disease begins with a contrast-enhanced CT of the chest, abdomen, and pelvis, preferably triple phase for better characterization of liver lesions. Carcinoids typically appear as hyperintense luminal masses due to increased vascularity. These tumors have intense desmoplasia resulting in puckering of the adjacent mesentery, giving rise to a characteristic stellate pattern on CT scan.

#### Tissue diagnosis
Obtaining a tissue diagnosis by performing a biopsy is a must prior to initiation of therapy, unless a curative resection for limited disease is planned. Minimum pathologic information needed for tailoring the treatment in neuroendocrine tumors are: the site of primary tumor; its size, grade, and mitotic index; presence of vascular and neural invasion; and presence of non-neuroendocrine components. The other important pathological aspects during histopathological examination of a resection specimen should include the number of involved, and total, nodes, as well as the status of the margins of resection. Neuroendocrine tumors are graded based on the proliferative labeling index (Ki-67) and mitosis detected per ten high-power fields. If there exists a discordance between the Ki-67 and mitotic index, the one with higher grade is assigned to the tumor. Immunohistochemistry studies are not mandatory. Specific immunohistochemistries useful to establish the diagnosis are chromogranin A, synaptophysin, and CD56.

#### Nuclear imaging
Somatostatin receptor-based imaging is recommended to assess the receptor expression of the tumors in order to determine the benefit of octreotide-based treatment. Somatostatin receptor scintigraphy with Indium-111 labeled pentreotide, also known as Octreoscan, has been supplanted by Gallium (Ga)-68 DOTA positron emission tomography scans. Somatostatin receptor expression is a predictive marker for response to peptide receptor radionuclide therapy. In poorly differentiated or grade 3 neuroendocrine tumors, somatostatin avidity decreases with concomitant increase in 18-fludeoxyglucose uptake. In such situations, a combined DOTA and fluorodeoxyglucose scan can be ordered. Figure 22.1

In suspected or established carcinoid syndrome, a cardiology consultation and echocardiogram are warranted to rule out valvular heart disease. Pulmonology consult is required if airway hyper-reactivity is demonstrated either on symptomatically by wheezing or on pulmonary function testing.

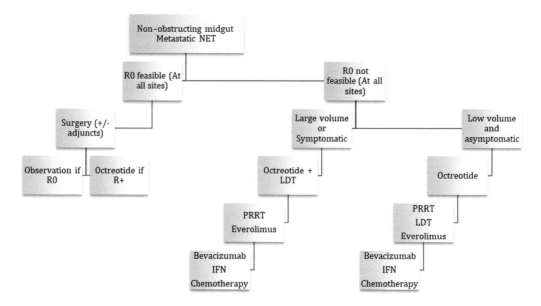

**Figure 22.2** Management algorithm.

## TREATMENT OPTIONS WITH BENEFITS AND RISKS

### Surgery for small bowel and primary liver disease

Resection of the primary tumor in the setting of unresectable liver disease is not recommended if the primary disease is asymptomatic. However, small bowel tumors rarely remain asymptomatic and the majority develop partial bowel obstruction or mesenteric ischemia. If resection is performed for any reason, a cholecystectomy is recommended since long-term treatment with somatostatin analogs is associated with gallstones and biliary symptoms.

Removal of limited metastatic disease where R0 resection is achievable at all sites, has the potential for offering long term survival. Ten-year survival after resection ranges from 40–100%. Notwithstanding complete resection, most patients eventually develop recurrent disease with nearly 100% recurrence in the remnant liver at ten years. Hepatic resection is also justified if complete cytoreduction is possible, combining surgery along with other liver directed therapies, viz. radiofrequency ablation, microwave ablation, or transarterial embolization. Subtotal resection or near complete cytoreduction is also an accepted strategy in the face of unresectable liver metastasis and hormone overproduction. Orthotopic ten-year survival data is now available from Mayo Clinic for liver transplantation and remains a viable option to venture in select patients with liver-limited, unresectable disease.

## LIVER-DIRECTED THERAPY

In case of unresectable liver metastasis (e.g. multiple bilobar lesion), with progression after somatostatin analogs and or peptide receptor radionuclide therapy, liver-directed treatments are initiated with dual goals of palliating symptoms and prolonging life. When complete resection or at least >90% debulking of the disease burden is not possible, hepatic regional therapies can be employed. These include bland embolization or embolization with chemotherapeutic or radioactive therapeutic pharmaceuticals. Overall, no form of embolization therapy has been found superior to another in terms of survival, but toxicities differ for each group. Selective internal radiotherapy, also known as transarterial radioembolization using Yttrium-90 microspheres has emerged as a promising method with superior tumor response rates, symptom control, and toxicity profile. Lastly, hepatic arterial delivery of somatostatin analogs labeled with radioactive therapeutic agents is a novel technique with good short-term results.

## MANAGEMENT OF CARCINOID SYNDROME

Somatostatin analogs remain the backbone in the treatment of metastatic neuroendocrine tumors with carcinoid syndrome. Long-acting release preparations are most often used with short acting preparations given as rescue doses. Lanreotide has similar actions and was shown to require lesser rescue doses in the ELECT trial when compared to octreotide [2]. Somatostatin analogs are supplemented with proton pump inhibitors and antimotility-antisecretory agents for breakthrough symptoms.

In those patients with symptoms uncontrolled by octreotide, a tryptophan hydroxylase inhibitor can be used. Teltoristat is the first drug in this class, administered at a dose of 250 mg thrice a day, and then titrated according to symptom (diarrhea) control. Dose-limiting side effects include nausea and elevation of liver enzymes [3].

59% of patients will have carcinoid heart disease, and majority will have tricuspid valve insufficiency. Echocardiogram suspicion should lead to early involvement of a cardiologist in the overall patient care.

For patients with unresectable metastatic disease without symptoms of hormone excess, treatment with octreotide can be considered in the initial phase, based on the PROMID study [4]. Time to progression was increased with octreotide to 14.3 months versus six months on placebo, although the overall survival was unchanged. Similarly, the CLARINET study led to the approval of lanreotide for metastatic G1-G2 neuroendocrine tumors following an improvement in progression-free survival [5].

## PEPTIDE RECEPTOR RADIONUCLIDE THERAPY

Peptide receptor radionuclide therapy has the potential to change the landscape of therapy in metastatic neuroendocrine tumor. Lutetium (Lu)-177 DOTATATE therapy selectively targets tissues with overexpression of somatostatin receptor. Data from the NETTER-1 trial comparing peptide receptor radionuclide therapy versus octreotide in metastatic unresectable somatostatin receptor-expressing midgut carcinoids showed significant improvement in progression-free survival in the peptide receptor radionuclide therapy arm [6]. In this trial, patients with well-differentiated, metastatic midgut neuroendocrine tumors were randomized to octreotide long-acting repeatable alone arm (administered intramuscularly at a dose of 60 mg every four weeks) and peptide receptor radionuclide therapy arm (Lu-177 DOTATATE given four doses every eight weeks plus best supportive care, including octreotide long-acting release administered intramuscularly at a dose of 30 mg).

The results showed a progression-free survival of 65.2 months, compared to 10.8 months with long-acting release octreotide. Other parameters including interim overall survival and quality of life also showed significant benefit. The only significant toxicities that have emerged are irreversible myelotoxicity (3.7%), myelodysplasia (2%), and acute leukemia (0.5%) of the patients.

## SYSTEMIC THERAPY

Everolimus, a mammalian target of rapamycin inhibitor, is an option in patients with progressive advanced neuroendocrine tumors. Stand-alone everolimus (RADIANT-4) [8], or everolimus in combination with octreotide (RADIANT-2) [7], when compared to placebo, has shown significant improvements in progression-free survival.

No difference in outcome was found when interferon alfa was compared to bevacizumab for patients with progressive advanced neuroendocrine tumors in a randomized controlled trial wherein both the arms received octreotide [9].

Cytotoxic chemotherapy has been shown to have a very modest response in neuroendocrine tumors. Various chemotherapeutic agents in use are capecitabine, 5-fluorouracil, streptozocin, dacarbazine, doxorubicin, and temozolomide. They, however, remain frontline therapy in poorly differentiated and high-grade neuroendocrine tumors, especially those without somatostatin receptor expression.

These recommendations are consistent with ENETS (European Neuroendocrine Tumor Society) and NANETS (North American Neuroendocrine Tumor Society) guidelines, and are also reflected in the ICMR (Indian Council of Medical Research) neuroendocrine tumor guidelines [1].

Tyrosine kinase inhibitors like imatinib and sunitinib can similarly restrict tumor growth and provide stability. However, these are observations from phase II studies, and in the absence of randomized trials, their routine use is not recommended.

In the case discussed above, surgery for the primary bowel lesion was not offered to begin with because of absence of symptoms such as pain, obstruction, or bleeding. After complete evaluation, the diagnosis of grade 1, functional small bowel neuroendocrine tumor with liver-limited metastasis (bilobar unresectable) was made. Since somatostatin receptor expression was present, long-acting release octreotide was offered as first-line treatment for control of symptoms as well a disease burden. For achieving downsizing and offering a possible future curative resection (for small bowel as well as liver), transarterial embolization of right lobe lesions was also performed. For control of liver disease, options range from resection, cytoreduction, ablation, and transarterial therapies besides octreotide and peptide receptor radionuclide therapy. The choice is based on the possibility of achieving R0 resection with surgery with anatomical and size criteria. Subsequently, peptide receptor radionuclide therapy was offered in view of disease progression. Although peptide receptor radionuclide therapy was also an option in the beginning, considering the dramatic responses and upcoming evidence in favor of the same, the exact sequence of peptide receptor radionuclide therapy and long-acting release somatostatin analogues is still uncertain. As of today, peptide receptor radionuclide therapy can be used as reserve therapy in refractory disease as well as first-line therapy in cases with high disease burden. Later, small bowel surgery had to be performed in emergency as he developed symptoms of obstruction, which he tolerated well. He went on to complete the planned peptide receptor radionuclide therapy and finally as there was a complete response in left lobe liver lesions, making it a right limited liver disease, liver resection (right hepatectomy) is planned with curative intent.

## FOLLOW-UP

Patients with advanced and metastatic disease are kept under follow up every three months with serum CgA or 24 hour urine 5-hydroxyindoleacetic acid levels and triphasic CT scans. Follow-up interval can be prolonged for indolent, slow-growing tumors. Somatostatin receptor-based imaging is performed in case of suspected recurrences and before initiating or escalating therapies. Evaluation for carcinoid heart disease is performed by echocardiogram every two or three years. Follow-up continues lifelong, as late recurrences beyond 20 years are also known.

### KEY MESSAGES

- Surgery is the treatment option of choice in resectable metastatic disease

in cases of gasteroenteropancreatic neuroendocrine tumors.
- For unresectable disease treatment may begin with octreotide and/or peptide receptor radionuclide therapy. Approved subsequent lines of therapy are everolimus, bevacizumab, and interferon. Chemotherapy is used as last resort in well differentiated neuroendocrine tumors or as first line in poorly differentiated/grade 3 tumors without somatostatin receptor expression.
- Various liver directed therapies, including cytoreduction, are employed for control of high-volume or symptomatic unresectable metastases.
- Peptide receptor radionuclide therapy is being increasingly used in progressive disease, this may change the landscape and prognosis of advanced neuroendocrine tumors.

## REFERENCES

1. ICMR GEP NET Consensus document, Dec 2019. https://www.icmr.nic.in/sites/default/files/guidelines/Consensus_2.pdf.
2. Vinik AI, Wolin EM, Liyanage N et al. Evaluation of lanreotide depot/autogel efficacy and safety as a carcinoid syndrome treatment (elect): A randomized, double-blind, placebo-controlled trial. *Endocr Pract Off J Am Coll Endocrinol Am Assoc Clin Endocrinol* 2016 Sep;22(9):1068–1080.
3. Kulke MH, Hörsch D, Caplin ME et al. Telotristat ethyl, a tryptophan hydroxylase inhibitor for the treatment of carcinoid syndrome. *J Clin Oncol Off J Am Soc Clin Oncol* 2017 Jan;35(1):14–23.
4. Rinke A, Müller H-H, Schade-Brittinger C et al. Placebo-controlled, double-blind, prospective, randomized study on the effect of octreotide LAR in the control of tumor growth in patients with metastatic neuroendocrine midgut tumors: A report from the PROMID study group. *J Clin Oncol Off J Am Soc Clin Oncol* 2009 Oct 1;27(28):4656–4663.
5. Caplin ME, Pavel M, Ćwikła JB et al. Lanreotide in metastatic enteropancreatic neuroendocrine tumors. *N Engl J Med* 2014 Jul 17;371(3):224–233.

6.  Strosberg J, El-Haddad G, Wolin E et al. Phase 3 trial of 177Lu-dotatate for midgut neuroendocrine tumors. *N Engl J Med* 2017 12;376(2):125–135.

7.  Pavel ME, Hainsworth JD, Baudin E et al. Everolimus plus octreotide long-acting repeatable for the treatment of advanced neuroendocrine tumours associated with carcinoid syndrome (RADIANT-2): A randomised, placebo-controlled, phase 3 study. *Lancet* 2011 Dec 10;378(9808):2005–2012.

8.  Yao JC, Fazio N, Singh S et al. Everolimus for the treatment of advanced, non-functional neuroendocrine tumours of the lung or gastrointestinal tract (RADIANT-4): A randomised, placebo-controlled, phase 3 study. *Lancet* 2016 Mar 5;387(10022):968–977.

9.  Yao JC, Guthrie KA, Moran C et al. Phase III prospective randomized comparison trial of depot octreotide plus interferon alfa-2b versus depot octreotide plus bevacizumab in patients with advanced carcinoid tumors: SWOG S0518. *J Clin Oncol Off J Am Soc Clin Oncol* 2017 May 20;35(15): 1695–1703.

# PART 5
# RECTUM

# 23 Transsphincteric Fistula-in-Ano with External Opening 3 cm from Anal Verge

*Parvez Sheikh and Atef Baakza*

## CONTENTS

## CASE SCENARIO

A 35-year-old man presented to the clinic with a history of repeated episodes of developing what he described as a painful perianal boil that would rupture with ensuing discharge over the past year. Nine months prior, he underwent surgery for fistula-in ano (ligation of intersphincteric fistula tract with video-assisted anal fistula treatment). Despite these surgeries, within two months his symptoms recurred. On clinical examination he was noted to have what appeared to be the external opening of the fistula over the right ischiorectal fossa (Figure 23.1) and an internal opening in the midline at the dentate line. A clinical diagnosis of a recurrent posterior transsphincteric anal fistula was made which was confirmed on pelvic magnetic resonance imaging (MRI).

After a detailed discussion with the patient on the risks involved in operative intervention, a decision was made to proceed with surgery. Since he had undergone a prior sphincter-saving procedure without success, a decision was made to attempt a sphincter-cutting procedure since this has a lower failure rate. The patient underwent a fistulectomy with primary sphincter repair uneventfully. The entire fistula tract was excised along with the posterior internal opening after dividing the lower part of the internal and external sphincters. The ano-rectal ring was preserved. The divided sphincters were primarily repaired with 2-0 polydioxanone, and the mucosa was sutured with 3-0 polyglactin. Postoperatively, the patient underwent regular supervised dressings and the wound healed after 75 days.

## BACKGROUND OF THE PATHOLOGY

A fistula-in-ano is a hollow tract lined with granulation tissue connecting a primary opening inside the anal canal to a secondary opening in the perianal skin, through which an abscess has been drained or has spontaneously ruptured. Evaluation and treatment of perianal fistula disease requires a thorough understanding of the anatomy of the anal canal and related spaces to determine the origin of the fistula and to understand subsequent course of this disease process.

Cryptoglandular infection is responsible for almost 90% of all anal fistulae. The dentate line is the site of the anal valves. Proximal to each anal valve is an anal crypt or sinus, which macroscopically appears as a small pit. The anal glands, which lie in the intersphincteric plane, empty into these anal crypts, which is the site for the internal opening of an anal fistula. Thus, all anal fistulae of cryptoglandular origin have their primary internal opening at the dentate

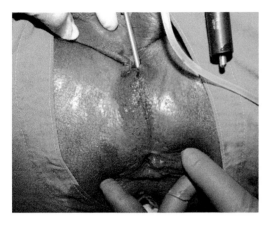

**Figure 23.1** Clinical photograph demonstrating a probe inserted through the external opening of the fistula-in-ano.

line. An anal fistula which is 3 cm away from the anal verge traverses the external sphincter and thus, by definition, is a transsphincteric anal fistula (Figure 23.2). Transsphincteric fistula are further subdivided as follows:

1) **Anterior transsphincteric:** Internal opening around the anterior midline

2) **Posterior transsphincteric:** Internal opening around the posterior midline

3) **Lateral transsphincteric:** This is uncommon and the internal opening is laterally situated

Each of the above can be either:

a) Low transsphincteric

b) High transsphincteric

c) Any of the above with a high intersphincteric extension

## APPROACH TO MANAGEMENT
### Clinical examination
A detailed history needs to be elicited from the patient. Previous anal surgery may result in scarring and distortion of the anal canal, thereby rendering subsequent surgery technically more challenging. A history of flatus and fecal incontinence should specifically be enquired in all patients with fistula-in-ano, and more so in those who have undergone prior surgery for the disease. This history is also relevant in ladies who have undergone vaginal delivery in the past as this history will guide the choice of therapy (sphincter-preserving procedures being preferred). Bowel habits should be enquired in detail, especially history suggestive of inflammatory bowel disease or a malignancy.

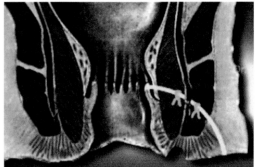

**Figure 23.2** Diagrammatic representation of a transsphincteric fistula.

Thorough examination of the perianal area should be performed to look for any induration, external opening, or abscess. Sometimes there may be more than one external opening and it is advisable to ask the patient to point out all the external openings or sites of pain. Digital rectal examination should be performed to feel for an internal opening as well as intra-anal induration which could represent intersphincteric tracts. The internal opening is situated at the dentate line and most commonly around the midline. It may be felt as an induration, a puckered spot, or one may see pus emerging from it. If an external opening is situated posteriorly, then the internal opening is also most likely to be situated in the posterior midline. However, that is not applicable to anterior openings – they can have the internal opening situated anteriorly or posteriorly. Thus Goodsal's rule is usually true for posterior fistulas. Any signs of inflammation of the rectal mucosa should alert the clinician to the possibility of inflammatory bowel disease.

Sigmoidoscopy should be performed in all patients with symptoms suggestive of anal fistula in order to locate the internal opening and to rule out other pathologies like proctitis or neoplasia. Presence of symptoms suggestive of inflammatory bowel disease or neoplasia necessitate a detailed workup including a colonoscopy and imaging modalities such as computed tomography (CT) scans and/or MRI of the abdomen and pelvis.

### Imaging
The various imaging modalities available to assess fistula-in-ano include endoanal ultrasound, CT fistulography, and MRI of the pelvis. The conventional fistulogram is now abandoned as it does not provide spatial information. MRI "is the most accurate method for determining the presence and course of anal fistulae" [1] (Figure 23.3). The success of

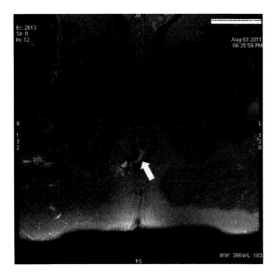

**Figure 23.3** MRI of a fistula-in-ano, marked by a white arrow.

MR imaging for preoperative classification of fistula-in-ano is a direct result of the sensitivity of MR for tracts and abscesses, combined with high anatomic precision and the ability to image in surgically relevant planes. Intravenous contrast studies are more specific and can attain similar results of local MRI fistulogram, so it should be routinely included in MRI protocols of anal fistula examination, even with no abscess or collection seen at the pre-contrast images. It is not necessary to image all fistulas as simple low fistulae can easily be diagnosed clinically.

## SURGICAL APPROACH

After the clinical examination and imaging, the surgeon should obtain a reasonable assessment of the type and course of the anal fistula. If the surgeon is still unsure, then it is advisable to seek the help of an experienced colleague. The type of surgery undertaken will depend on the type and extent of the fistula as well as the surgeon's experience. The two most important complications that need to be discussed with the patient prior to surgery include the risk of incontinence (flatus and feces) and that of recurrence [2].

## LOW TRANSSPHINCTERIC ANAL FISTULA

A low transsphincteric anal fistula crosses the external sphincter either between its superficial and subcutaneous parts or through the subcutaneous sphincter. Most colorectal surgeons agree that the best surgical option for these fistulas is to lay them open by performing a fistulotomy. Since the sphincter involved

is essentially only the subcutaneous part of the external sphincter, one need not worry about causing incontinence. It is important to curette the tract and send the material for histology. The success rate for this procedure is very high with little chance of recurrence or incontinence.

## HIGH TRANSSPHINCTERIC ANAL FISTULA

The high transsphincteric anal fistula crosses the external sphincter between its deep and superficial parts. Thus, it is still below the anorectal ring (Figure 23.2). There has been no consensus on surgical options for treating this type of fistula. The existing options have not yielded satisfying results. Hence the need to discover new options. Recurrence of the fistula and incontinence are the two major factors that warrant attention when deciding the best option for the patient. The newer techniques aim to be less invasive and more sphincter friendly, but at the cost of increased recurrence rate.

## SURGICAL OPTIONS

The current popular surgical options for treating transsphincteric fistulae include:
Sphincter-saving procedures:

1) Advancement flap

2) Ligation of intersphincteric fistula tract (LIFT)

3) Video-assisted anal fistula treatment (VAAFT)

4) Anal fistula plug

5) Light amplification by stimulated emission of radiation (LASER)

6) Draining seton

Sphincter-cutting procedures:

1) Fistulotomy/fistulectomy

2) Fistulotomy/fistulectomy with primary sphincter repair

3) Cutting seton

## ADVANCEMENTS FLAPS

Advancements flaps consisting of mucosa, submucosa, and part of internal sphincter can be used to close the internal opening in fistula. The success rates with this technique range from 59–72% [3] and are lower in patients with Crohn's-related fistulae. It is believed that the success of the procedure may increase with increasing attempts (up to 90% success rate) although it may result in incontinence in 9–14% of patients.

## LIGATION OF INTERSPHINCTERIC FISTULA TRACT

This procedure involves the water-tight ligation and disconnection of the fistula tract in the intersphincteric space along with the curettage of the remaining tract (Figures 23.2 and 23.4). The success rates vary from 68-94% with healing taking place over six or seven weeks. LIFT, due to its simplicity, is the most popular sphincter saving technique for trans-sphincteric fistulas worldwide. Adding VAAFT & LASER to it has not increased its success rate significantly.

## VIDEO-ASSISTED ANAL FISTULA TREATMENT

The video-assisted anal fistula treatment (VAAFT) procedure consists of diagnostic fistuloscopy performed with a specially designed scope that is passed through the external fistulous opening up to the internal opening (Figure 23.6). A unipolar electrode is then used to cauterize the tract while an endobrush is used to extract the ensuing necrotic material. The internal opening is then stapled off using a linear or semicircular stapler. The procedure has the advantage of preventing sphincter injury thereby avoiding incontinence. Primary healing has been noted in up to 74% of patients at 12 weeks follow-up.

## ANAL FISTULA PLUG

A biological plug has been used to treat fistula-in ano. This plug is derived from the porcine small intestinal submucosa. The procedure involves curetting and irrigating the track with saline and hydrogen peroxide, and then railroading the plug into the tract. Thereafter, one of the plugs is secured to the internal sphincter and the other end to the skin. The mucosa of the internal fistulous opening is closed with a polyglactin suture. The success rates are highly variable and range from 54–85% [3]. Extrusion of the plug is believed to contribute to the lower success rates.

## SETON

A thread (seton) made of polypropylene, nylon, rubber, or similar material is passed through the fistula tract, with an aim to keep the internal and external openings patent. By permitting complete drainage, a seton prevents accumulation of secretions and abscess formation. Setons may be used to allow a phased cutting of the sphincter (cutting seton) or to permit maturation of the tract to allow another definitive surgery (draining seton). It must be appreciated that cutting setons are associated with some fecal incontinence (5.6% if the sphincter is preserved and up to 25% if the sphincter was not preserved), and recurrence rates approach 5% for cutting setons.

## LASER

A radial emitting disposable laser probe called FiLaC™ developed by Biolitec (Germany) has been used to ablate and obliterate the epithelial lining of the fistulous tract. Early success has been reported in up to 69% of patients [4]. Further results are awaited.

## FISTULECTOMY WITH PRIMARY SPHINCTER RECONSTRUCTION

High transsphincteric fistulae have a fixed pattern of spread, namely they always cross the external sphincter between the deep and superficial parts of the external sphincter. Thus, if one were to lay open or excise such a tract, one would still not be dividing the deep part of the external sphincter and the anorectal ring. Fistulotomy/ fistulectomy was traditionally not performed for high fistulae due to perceived high incontinence rates. Primary suturing of sphincters, unlike delayed repair, results in good continence.

Thus, fistulectomy with primary suturing of sphincters seems to have the combined advantage of a low recurrence rate and a satisfying continence score, and would be a useful option even in patients with prior incontinence with complex fistula-in-ano as the previously

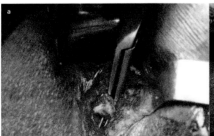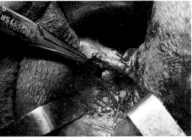

**Figure 23.4** Clinical photographs depicting: (a) the isolation of the fistula tract in the intersphincteric space, (b) ligation and division of the track.

damaged sphincters can also be repaired. The success rates are more than 90% for this procedure [5].

## HIGH INTERSPHINCTERIC EXTENSION

Trans-sphincteric fistulas may have an additional high inter-sphincteric extension going up to the anorectal ring or into the supralevator space (Figure 23.7). Access to this space may be difficult if one were to use a conservative sphincter-saving procedure. If a fistulotomy or fistulectomy is done then one can easily visualize this extension, which can either be excised by an inter-sphincteric dissection or curetted thoroughly.

### SALIENT FEATURES

- Thorough clinical examination can provide great information about the type and extent of the fistula.
- Preoperative imaging, like MRI, can be done in recurrent or high fistulas to enable the surgeon to plan their surgeries.
- Low fistulas are best treated by fistulotomy or fistulectomy.
- High fistulas have several surgical options. The sphincter-saving procedures lower success rate but have low incontinence; whereas the sphincter cutting procedures have a high success rate but can be associated with higher incontinence, unless the sphincter is primarily repaired.
- There is certainly no ideal surgery, as yet, for anal fistula. The surgeon has to decide the procedure based on their past experience and the type of fistula they are dealing with.

## REFERENCES

1. Lunniss PJ, Armstrong P, Barker PG et al. Magnetic resonance imaging of anal fistulae. *Lancet* 1992;340(8816):394–396.
2. Sheikh P. Controversies in fistula in ano. *Indian J Surg* 2012;74(3):217–220.
3. Sheikh P, Baakza A. Management of fistula-in-ano-the current evidence. *Indian J Surg* 2014;76(6):482–486.
4. Wilhelm A, Fiebig A, Krawczak M. Five years of experience with the FiLaC laser for fistula-in-ano management: Long-term follow-up from a single institution. *Tech Coloproctol* 2017;21(4):269–276.
5. Ratto C, Litta F, Donisi L et al. Fistulotomy or fistulectomy and primary sphincteroplasty for anal fistula (FIPS): A systematic review. *Tech Coloproctol* 2015;19(7):391–400.

# 24 Familial Adenomatous Polyposis

## 19-Year-Old Patient with Severe Rectal Involvement

*Paul Kolarsick and Steven D. Wexner*

## CONTENTS

## CASE SCENARIO

A 19-year-old female presented for evaluation. She had a family history significant for colon cancer (in her father at the age of 35 associated with colonic polyposis). She was asymptomatic. She underwent screening colonoscopy and was found to have more than 100 polyps throughout her colon with extensive rectal involvement. Multiple biopsies were taken; each demonstrated tubulovillous adenomas without dysplasia or malignancy.

## BACKGROUND OF THE PATHOLOGY

Familial adenomatous polyposis (FAP) syndrome results from a mutation in the *adenomatous polyposis coli* (APC), a tumor suppressor gene located on chromosome 5q21. Familial adenomatous polyposis confers a nearly 100% lifetime risk of developing colorectal cancer, mostly by forty years of age. Autosomal dominant in its inheritance pattern, FAP affects 1:10,000 individuals but accounts for <1% of all colorectal cancer [1].

There is no evidence that the adenoma-to-carcinoma sequence is accelerated in FAP; rather, it is the early onset and large quantity of polyps that increase the risk for malignant transformation [2]. While family history is helpful to identify at-risk individuals with germline mutation in APC, it is also important to recognize that FAP may be due to a de novo mutation in up to 30% of affected individuals [3]. A family history of polyposis is therefore not required to pursue genetic testing.

*Adenomatous polyposis coli* encodes a protein in the *Wnt* pathway, which signals the ubiquination and degradation of the β-catenin oncoprotein. In the absence of the APC protein product, β-catenin accumulates in the nucleus leading to unregulated cell proliferation. In addition, the APC protein product

functions in microtubule stabilization during cell division; a defective gene leads to abnormal chromosomal segregation and aberrant mitosis [1].

The APC gene consists of 15 coding sections with exon 15 accounting for 75% of the coding section and, correspondingly, for the most common site of germline and somatic mutations. More than 1,100 unique germline mutations have been reported with the majority consisting of truncating mutations in which a nonsense mutation leads to a shortened protein lacking the amino acid repeats involved in binding to and regulating β-catenin. The most common APC mutation occurs in codon 1,309 and is noteworthy in that it correlates with a more profuse and aggressive polyposis phenotype [1].

## APPROACH TO MANAGEMENT
### Clinical findings

There are a range of clinical phenotypes associated with the FAP syndrome. Patients with classic FAP typically display hundreds to thousands of polyps throughout the colon and rectum (Figure 24.1). These typically begin in the rectosigmoid region in adolescence. On average, colorectal cancer develops at 35 years of age with nearly all patients developing colorectal malignancy by 50 years of age [1, 3]. The rectum is typically affected in classic FAP [2].

Attenuated familial adenomatous polyposis (AFAP) syndrome is a phenotypic variant in which less than one hundred synchronous adenomas are detected (Figure 24.2). Attenuated familial adenomatous polyposis is associated with a later onset of polyposis, frequently a right-sided polyp distribution, and a lower lifetime colorectal cancer risk (up to 70%). Average age of colorectal cancer diagnosis is also later, generally greater than 50 years of age. However,

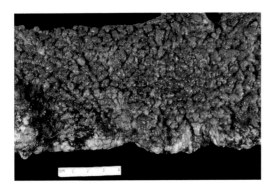

**Figure 24.1** Classic familial adenomatous polyposis gross colon specimen.

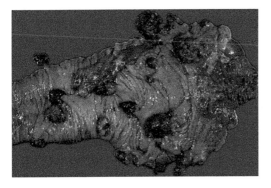

**Figure 24.2** Attenuated familial adenomatous polyposis gross colon specimen.

there are a number of other disorders that can yield a similar phenotype to AFAP, such as *MYH*-associated polyposis syndrome, Lynch syndrome, polymerase proofreading-associated polyposis, or simply multiple sporadic adenomas. The diagnosis of AFAP is made based on clinical findings including adenoma number (typically ranging from 20 to 100, with an average of 30 adenomatous polyps), family history, and results of genetic testing [3]. Upper gastrointestinal findings and the risk of duodenal cancer are similar to classic FAP.

Also described is a profuse or aggressive FAP phenotypic variant characterized by a greater number of polyps and younger age at onset, with corresponding earlier malignant transformations. Profuse FAP is most commonly associated with mutations in codons 1,309 and 1,324 [1]. Mutations in codon 1,309 account for 17% of all germline APC mutations [1].

There is evidence that these phenotypic variations of FAP correlate with the type of mutation in the APC gene (Figure 24.3). Attenuated familial adenomatous polyposis tends to be associated with mutations near the 5′ and 3′ end of the gene. Mutations in FAP between codons 1,250–1,464 typically correlate with a more aggressive phenotype. Classic FAP phenotype is associated with mutations in the remainder of the gene [1].

The APC mutational site has also been shown to be associated with the numerous extra-colonic manifestations of FAP (Figure

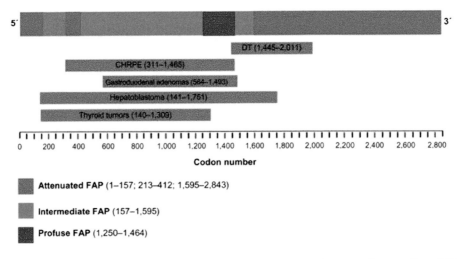

**Figure 24.3** Genotype-phenotype correlations of *adenomatous polyposis coli* gene. (Leoz ML, Moreira L. The genetic basis of familial adenomatous polyposis and its implications for clinical practice and risk management. 2015:95-107. Reused with permission © Dove Press.) (*Abbreviations:* DT – desmoid tumors; congenital hypertrophy of retinal pigment epithelium, congenital hypertrophy of the retinal pigment epithelium; FAP – familial adenomatous polyposis.)

24.1) [1]. Congenital hypertrophy of retinal pigment epithelium, found in 70–80% of patients with FAP, is a benign finding of brown to black, round to oval retinal lesions. Also common are dental abnormalities, including supernumerary teeth, found in up to 80% of patients, osteomas found in 50–90%, and soft tissue lesions, such as epidermoid cyst and fibromas, found in 50% of patients with FAP [1].

Patients with FAP are at increased risk for a number of extracolonic malignancies as well. The lifetime risk of developing duodenal cancer is around 4–12%, while the risk of gastric cancer is around 1–2%. Familial adenomatous polyposis also confers an elevated risk of desmoid tumors (10–20%), thyroid papillary cancer (2–3%), pancreatic cancers (<1%), hepatoblastomas (1%), and central nervous system tumors, including medulloblastomas (<1%) [3]. In AFAP, the risk of duodenal and thyroid cancer are similar to classic FAP, though other extracolonic manifestations, such as desmoid tumor formation and congenital hypertrophy of retinal pigment epithelium, are unusual [3].

After colorectal cancer, duodenal cancer and desmoid tumors are the most common causes of death in patients with FAP [2]. Familial adenomatous polyposis confers a nearly 100% lifetime risk of duodenal adenomas with a predilection for the second and third portion of the duodenum, particularly in the periampullary region. Patients have a 5% overall lifetime risk of developing duodenal cancer [1]. Gastric polyps mainly consist of benign fundic gland polyps found in 20–80% of patients. These lesions are generally considered non-neoplastic, but cases of high-grade dysplasia and carcinoma have been reported. Gastric adenomas are less common, found in 10% of patients, and tend to be localized to the antrum, though recent data does suggest that the incidence of gastric cancer is increasing [2].

Desmoid tumors are mesenchymal in origin and are locally invasive but generally lack metastatic potential. These tumors are demonstrate a high local recurrence even following complete resection and tend to occur after surgery [1]. Half of desmoid tumors occur intra-abdominally, often in the mesentery or pelvis, intraperitoneal, or in the retroperitoneum. They can also occur in the anterior abdominal wall or extra-abdominally in the chest, head, neck, or extremities. Desmoid tumors account for a major cause of death due to their locally invasive nature (Figure 24.4). In addition, the risk of desmoid tumor development influences surgical timing and extent. This risk can be estimated to some extent by family history and genotype.

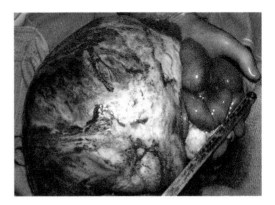

**Figure 24.4** Desmoid tumor involving mesentery of small intestine. (*Gordon and Nivatvongs' Principles and Practice of Surgery for the Colon, Rectum, and Anus*, 4th Edition. Reused with permission © Thieme Publishers.)

### Investigations

Generally, any patient with more than 20 lifetime adenomas is considered high risk for harboring an underlying polyposis syndrome and should undergo genetic testing. Current guidelines from the National Comprehensive Cancer Network recommend pursuing genetic testing in select patient with more than ten lifetime colorectal adenomatous polyps [3].

When a polyposis phenotype is discovered, a multi-gene panel is often used for initial DNA analysis [2]. This is particularly useful for AFAP as there are multiple other mutations capable of producing a similar phenotype, as mentioned above. Direct genetic sequencing is considered the gold standard method of germline testing of the APC gene and is recommended for the proband. Once a mutation is identified, family screening for that specific mutation can proceed [1]. Results of germline genetic testing carry implications for prognosis and clinical management. It is recommended that patients meet with a genetic counselor prior to undergoing testing.

Prior to surgical treatment, patients should undergo complete colonoscopy as well as upper endoscopy to evaluate extent of rectal involvement and rule out foregut neoplasia. It is our practice to screen, with computed tomography (CT), patients with family history, genetic variant, or clinical signs that put them at higher risk for desmoid tumor or pancreatic neoplasm.

### Management

Surgical options to treat FAP include total proctocolectomy with end ileostomy, total abdominal colectomy with ileorectal anastomosis, or total proctocolectomy with ileal pouch-anal

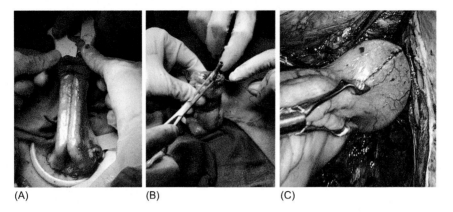

(A)              (B)                (C)

**Figure 24.5** (A–C) Intraoperative photographs of a total proctocolectomy with ileal pouch-anal anastomosis showing: (A) Second firing of 100 mm gastrointestinal anastomosis stapler, (B) securing purse string around anvil of end-to-end stapler, (C) laparoscopic view of the creation of the anastomosis.

anastomosis with either stapled or hand-sewn anastomosis with mucosectomy (Figure 24.5A-C). Surgical treatment must be individualized to the patient to optimize quality of life while reducing risk of neoplasia. Complete proctectomy minimizes the risk of malignancy but must be weighed against quality of life concerns, including postoperative bowel function as well as the potential for sexual dysfunction and fertility issues associated with the pelvic dissection.

The risk of neoplasia development in the remnant rectum is associated with the quantity of colonic and rectal polyps, as well as the specific mutational defect. In a meta-analysis of 12 non-randomized studies, factors favoring total abdominal colectomy with ileorectal anastomosis included relative rectal sparing and desire to avoid pelvic dissection. Factors favoring total proctocolectomy with ileal pouch-anal anastomosis included the presence of rectal cancer or large rectal polyp burden, defined as greater than 20 synchronous adenomas, large adenomas (>30 mm), adenomas with high-grade dysplasia, or severe familial phenotype [4]. Church et al. noted that of 165 FAP patients who underwent rectal-sparing surgery, the incidence of rectal cancer was 1.6% in patients with <20 polyps, and 10.8% in those with >20 polyps. Of those with >20 rectal polyps, 35% ultimately required proctectomy [5]. Also important to consider is the reliability of the patient to comply with surveillance of remaining rectum if total abdominal colectomy with ileorectal anastomosis is planned.

Endoscopic surveillance of patients treated with total abdominal colectomy with ileorectal anastomosis should occur every six to twelve

months depending on polyp burden. Patients treated with total proctocolectomy with ileal pouch-anal anastomosis should undergo surveillance endoscopy every one to three years unless high-grade dysplasia or large polyp burden dictates more frequent surveillance. It is our practice to use the nonsteroidal anti-inflammatory drug (NSAID) sulindac as chemoprevention in patients with retained rectum. Although not approved by the Food and Drug Administration for polyp suppression, sulindac has been shown to reduce colorectal adenoma formation. It is unknown whether chemoprevention reduces the incidence of cancer [1].

For the patient mentioned in the case study, we would recommend laparoscopic total proctocolectomy with ileal pouch-anal anastomosis, given the extensive rectal polyp burden and correspondingly increased likelihood of developing cancer without proctectomy. For patients in their reproductive years it is important to discuss the possible adverse impact of pelvic dissection on fertility. Reduced female fecundity following ileal pouch anal anastomosis has been reported, however, most of these studies were performed on patients with ulcerative colitis. A Dutch study addressed this question using a questionnaire of 138 female patients from the national FAP registry and found that one in six patients indicated having reduced fertility due to surgery. The prevalence of fertility problems was similar among those who underwent total proctocolectomy with ileal pouch-anal anastomosis, total abdominal colectomy with ileorectal anastomosis, and total abdominal colectomy with end ileostomy, though patients reporting fertility issues were significantly younger on average at age of diagnosis (20 vs 27 years) and age of first surgical procedure (22 vs 28 years) [6]. Postsurgical fertility issues are thought to arise from anatomic changes related to pelvic adhesion formation with tubal disruption. There is evidence that a laparoscopic approach to restorative proctocolectomy improves pregnancy rates [7].

## KEY MESSAGES

- Patients with greater than 20 lifetime adenomatous colorectal polyps should be considered to be at high risk for a polyposis syndrome.
- Up to 30% of familial adenomatous polyposis patients harbor a de novo germline mutation in *adenomatous polyposis coli* and therefore have no family history of polyposis.
- Select patients with less than 20 rectal polyps can be considered for a rectum-preserving approach to surgical prophylaxis.
- Genotype is associated with polyposis phenotype as well as extra-colonic manifestations, and has implications for clinical management.
- Patients with mutations of *adenomatous polyposis coli* associated with aggressive or profuse phenotype, such as at codon 1,309, are better served with prophylactic total proctocolectomy.

## REFERENCES

1. Leoz ML, Carballal S, Moreira L, Ocaña T, Balaguer F. The genetic basis of familial adenomatous polyposis and its implications for clinical practice and risk management. *Appl Clin Genet.* 2015;8:95–107.
2. Herzig D, Hardimann MDK, Weiser MDM et al. The American society of colon and rectal surgeons. (Table 1). 881–894. doi:10.1097/DCR.0000000000000912.
3. Clinical N, Guidelines P, Guidelines N. Genetic / Familial High-Risk Assessment : Colorectal. 2018.
4. Aziz O, Athanasiou T, Fazio VW et al. Meta-analysis of observational studies of ileorectal versus ileal pouch – Anal anastomosis for familial adenomatous polyposis. 2006:407–417. doi:10.1002/bjs.5276.
5. Church J, Burke C, McGannon E et al. Predicting polyposis severity by proctoscopy: How reliable is it? *Diseases Colon Rectum* 2001;44(9):1249–1254. http://www.ncbi.nlm.nih.gov/pubmed/11584194.
6. Marry Nieuwenhuis, Kirsten Douma, Eveline Bleiker et al. Female fertility after colorectal surgery for familial adenomatous polyposis: A nationwide cross-sectional study. *Ann Surg* 2010;252(2):341–344. doi:10.1097/SLA.0b013e3181e9829f.
7. Bartels SAL, D'Hoore A, Cuesta MA et al. Significantly increased pregnancy rates after laparoscopic restorative proctocolectomy: A cross-sectional study. *Ann Surg* 2012;256(6):1045–1048. doi:10.1097/SLA.0b013e318250caa9.

# 25 Management of Rectal Cancer in a Young Woman

*Dayan de Fontgalland*

## CONTENTS

## CASE SCENARIO

A fit and healthy 27-year-old woman presented to her general practitioner on more than one occasion complaining of bright rectal bleeding, increasing constipation and non-specific lower abdominal pain. She reported no constitutional symptoms of weight loss or lethargy, nor was there a family history of inflammatory bowel disease or colorectal cancer. She had recently been married and was planning to have children. After the initial failed conservative management of her abdominal complaints with increased fiber in her diet, the general practitioner organized a referral to a gastroenterologist for a colonoscopy. The gastroenterologist who performed the colonoscopy encountered an obstructing rectosigmoid lesion. A referral was made immediately to the colorectal surgeon.

## BACKGROUND OF THE PATHOLOGY

There has a troubling global rise in the incidence of young-onset colorectal cancer [1] highlighting a global phenomenon requiring re-education of general practitioners and re-evaluation of colorectal cancer screening guidelines [2]. This rise in incidence is paralleled by a significant proportion of these patients exhibiting node positive disease with overall reduction in survival compared to age and stage matched cohorts [3, 4].

Although there is a trend for genetic microsatellite instability as a cause for the young-onset rectal cancer patients, there is currently no conclusive evidence of an obvious etiology. Current colorectal cancer screening guidelines target people above the age of 50 years. However, given the alarming trend in incidence of rectal cancer in the young, there is a suggestion to bring down the age of screening to commence at 40 years of age [5].

Young-onset rectal cancer carries its own set of issues including delays in diagnosis, the interference of therapy with reproductive health, and mental health issues not only due to the cancer but the possibility of dealing with a stoma. Thus, young-onset colorectal cancer is an area in colorectal medicine that warrants investment of time and focus to better help this cohort of patients.

## APPROACH TO THE PATIENT

### Initial consultation

It is imperative that a detailed history and clinical examination, including a digital rectal examination, be performed in all patients presenting with new onset per rectal bleeding with or without constipation. Patients without hemorrhoids or fissure-in-ano disease must be considered for further investigation including the possibility of a colonoscopy. Important symptoms to guide further investigation include painless bleeding per rectum with clots or blood mixed in with the stool, associated weight loss, abdominal pain, a personal and/or family history of colorectal polyps, cancer or inflammatory bowel diseases, clinical anemia, and a palpable lump in the abdomen (which would also warrant abdominal imaging).

At the initial consult, one must conduct a detailed assessment of the symptoms for the primary cancer to determine the need for expedient management (bleeding tumors or those causing a bowel obstruction). It is also important to obtain a thorough medical and surgical history (including medical comorbidities, the use of antiplatelets and anticoagulants, and also history of previous abdominal surgery). Finally, it is essential to counsel the patient and the family on the diagnosis and provide a clear plan of management that would be determined following the multidisciplinary team meeting. In rectal cancer, there are numerous variations in terms of the options, as well as the timing of each intervention based on the disease *per se*, as well as the patient's comorbidities and wishes.

### Initial investigations to consider

1) Blood tests

   a) Full blood examination (hemoglobin in particular).

   b) Renal function tests, including electrolytes, and liver function tests.

   c) Coagulation profile.

   d) Serum carcinoembryonic antigen – this is mainly used as a baseline test to aid in surveillance.

   e) Iron studies – iron deficiency anemia is present in >30% of patients with colorectal cancer, especially in patients with anemia. In this setting, an iron infusion is indicated.

2) Colonoscopy (and biopsy)

   Colonoscopy and biopsy remain the "gold standard" for the diagnosis of rectal cancer. The reason for performing a complete colonoscopy is to rule out a proximal obstruction as well as synchronous lesions that may be found in 5% of patients with colorectal cancer. If a patient cannot have a complete colonoscopy because of an obstructing lesion, it must be performed within six months of surgery.

3) Staging contrast-enhanced computed tomography (CT) scan of the chest, abdomen, and pelvis

   a) Confirms the site and extent of the primary tumor (including the invasion of surrounding organs).

   b) Determines the presence, or absence, of regional as well as distant metastatic disease (liver lesions may need further characterization by MRI).

   c) Helps to confirm, or rule out, proximal colonic obstruction.

4) Magnetic resonance imaging (MRI) of the pelvis

   a) To determine the distance of the tumor from anal verge and its relation to the peritoneal reflection, circumferential resection margin, and extramural venous invasion.

   b) To evaluate the presence of nodal disease to determine if neoadjuvant chemoradiotherapy is indicated.

   c) To assess adjacent structure involvement (other organs/pelvic side wall) in T4 disease.

5) Positron emission tomography scan of the whole body – for the assessment of metastatic lesions suspected clinically or on other imaging.

The patient presented in the case summary had iron deficiency anemia and her CT scan demonstrated an upper rectal cancer (Figure 25.1) straddling the peritoneal reflection extending to the distal sigmoid with only partial colonic obstruction. There was no evidence of metastatic disease. MRI revealed a T3 upper rectal/distal sigmoid lesion. There were a few prominent mesorectal, inferior mesenteric artery, and presacral lymph nodes. These locoregional nodes were not pathological according to radiological criteria. The serum carcinoembryonic antigen and the rest of the blood tests were normal.

## MANAGEMENT
### Multidisciplinary team meeting

Once all the required investigations have been obtained and the patient's tumor can be staged, it is imperative that all patients be discussed in a dedicated colorectal cancer multidisciplinary team meeting to decide on the best plan of care for that particular patient.

The principles of management of non-metastatic, rectal cancer are based on local control of disease and prevention of systemic spread. Radiotherapy is the mainstay of treatment for T3 mid to low rectal cancers, especially those infiltrating the mesorectum and threatening the circumferential resection margin, with or without mesorectal node positivity suggested on MRI (N1 or N2). Patients whose tumors

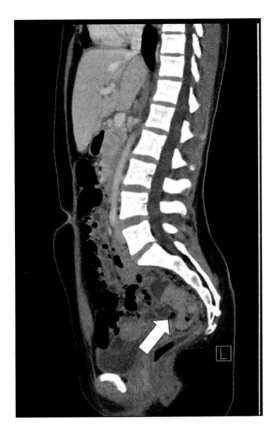

**Figure 25.1** Sagittal section of a CECT scan of the abdomen and pelvis demonstrating a large tumor involving the proximal rectum (white arrow).

demonstrate extramural venous invasion will also benefit from neoadjuvant chemoradiotherapy. The time interval to surgery, after radiotherapy, has a bearing on pathological complete response but one must be clear that there is no difference in overall survival or local recurrence of tumor with either the short-course radiotherapy or the long-course chemoradiotherapy regime [6].

In the patient presented in the case summary, owing to the near complete obstruction with an upper rectal cancer, and no lymph node positive disease suggested on imaging, the decision of the multidisciplinary team was to proceed directly to surgery.

### Fertility considerations and psychological counseling

Prior to surgery or even neoadjuvant chemoradiotherapy, it is important to advise patients on the effects of the treatment on their fertility as well as their sexual and urinary function. Prior to embarking on chemotherapy, which

chemically sterilizes a premenopausal woman, the patient must be offered the opportunity for egg harvest and cryopreservation to address fertility issues. Similarly, male patients must be warned about the potential risk of erectile dysfunction resulting from involvement of the hypogastric nerve plexus by the tumor or its inadvertent damage during surgery. They must also be offered the option of sperm heart.

### Operative considerations

a) Restoration of bowel continuity, with or without proximal diversion

b) Technique (open, laparoscopy or robotic)

c) Early Recovery After Surgery (ERAS) pathways

### Restoration of bowel continuity, with or without, proximal diversion

Upper rectal cancers often pose a dilemma in management, especially when they are large and involve the distal sigmoid colon. The question arises: Should they be managed as a colon cancer with a 5 cm margin, or as a rectal cancer with a minimum of a 1 cm margin? Traditional teaching dictates that the patient be offered an anterior resection with a >1 cm distal margin, a clear radial margin to include the surrounding mesorectum and intact mesorectal envelope (total mesorectal excision), and anastomosis in the mid-to low-rectum (between 6 cm and 10 cm from the anal verge) with preservation of the anal sphincter, and maintenance of sexual and urinary function by preservation of the hypogastric nerve plexi. The next decision would be whether to cover the anastomosis with a loop ileostomy. The indications for a covering loop ileostomy include: a positive air leak test (performed in reverse Trendelenburg position with saline in the pelvis covering the anastomosis and approximately 100–150 mL of air insufflated gently with a Toomey syringe while the bowel above the anastomosis is gently compressed), anastomosis below the peritoneal reflection, incomplete doughnut(s), patients who are at high risk from their comorbidities, and anastomosis performed on unprepared bowel. It must be reiterated here that while a covering loop ileostomy does not prevent an anastomotic leak, it helps to mitigate the sepsis that ensues should the anastomosis dehisce permitting its conservative non-operative management.

### Technique

The optimal technique for performing rectal cancer surgery is still a matter of great debate.

Some randomized controlled trials have even suggested significantly poorer outcomes with minimally invasive rectal surgery. The evidence on the topic, however, concedes that while the survival rate may not differ when comparing minimally invasive (laparoscopic and robotic) versus open surgery (although minimally invasive surgery may improve perioperative recovery), open surgery is associated with superior oncological resection rates [7].

### Enhanced Recovery After Surgery (ERAS) Society

The Enhanced Recovery After Surgery (ERAS) Society has provided their fourth updated evidence-based care pathway for the management of patients undergoing colorectal cancer surgery. These guidelines contain elements commencing pre-admission through to the postoperative period, and are designed to reduce the stress of the patient in the perioperative period while maintaining physiological function and accelerating the recovery of the patient [8].

### Postoperative advice

It is important to advise patients, prior to discharge, on the care of the ileostomy and what to expect. They need to be informed about the risk of high stomal output and how to identify and manage this situation, should it arise.

## CASE SCENARIO (CONTINUED)

For the patient presented in the case summary, a hybrid laparoscopic low anterior resection was performed with total mesorectal excision performed open via a Pfannenstiel incision. Owing to a poorly prepared bowel, an on-table colonic lavage was necessary prior to a low double-stapled anastomosis. A covering loop ileostomy was fashioned.

Postoperatively, she was taken through the ERAS pathway established by the hospital for colorectal surgery. She went on to have an uneventful recovery. She received stoma education and left the hospital seven days postsurgery.

The histopathology of the resected specimen returned as a T3b upper rectal, poorly differentiated cancer, with 3 out of 25 (N2) lymph nodes being positive, with clear resection margins. She was referred by the multidisciplinary team for adjuvant chemotherapy without adjuvant radiotherapy. She underwent six months of 5-fluorouracil, leucovorin, and oxaliplatin (FOLFOX) chemotherapy. Her ileostomy was then reversed and she remains disease free during regular surveillance.

## KEY MESSAGES

- There is a concerning global rise in the incidence of young-onset rectal cancer.
- Management of rectal cancer is complex and revolves around staging of the disease, presence of symptoms (bleeding and obstruction which may warrant early surgery), the distance of the tumor from the anal verge, and patient comorbidities.
- In non-metastatic rectal cancer, neoadjuvant chemoradiation is mainstay of treatment in tumors that are T3 and/or mesorectal node positive. In T2 or N0 disease, or if the tumor is at the upper rectum, surgery is often first-line treatment.
- All patients with rectal cancers should be discussed at the colorectal cancer multidisciplinary team to determine the appropriate management plan for that particular patient.
- In mid-low rectal cancers, a complete total mesorectal excision should be performed with the most updated evidence suggesting open rectal dissection as the preferred approach.
- Histological node positive disease mandates adjuvant chemotherapy. Adjuvant radiotherapy is necessitated if the risk of local failure is perceived to be high.
- Rectal cancer surgery should be performed by specialist colorectal surgeons in tertiary centers for better outcomes and access to radiation oncology, medical oncology, and allied health professionals, such as cancer nurse co-ordinators, stomal therapists, physiotherapists, and psychologists.
- In young patients where fertility is compromised with treatment, egg and sperm harvest/storage should be discussed and offered.

## REFERENCES

1. Vuik FE, Nieuwenburg SA, Bardou M et al. Increasing incidence of colorectal cancer in young adults in Europe over the last 25 years. *Gut* 2019;68(10):1820–1826.
2. Sung JJY, Chiu HM, Jung KW et al. Increasing trend in young-onset colorectal cancer in Asia: More cancers in men and more rectal cancers. *Am J Gastroenterol* 2019;114(2):322–329.
3. Barreto SG. Young-onset rectal cancer patients: In need of answers. *Future Oncol* 2019;15(10):1053–5.

4. Barreto SG, Chaubal GN, Talole S et al. Rectal cancer in young Indians – Are these cancers different compared to their older counterparts? *Indian J Gastroenterol* 2014;33(2):146–150.

5. Panteris V, Vasilakis N, Demonakou M et al. Alarming endoscopic data in young and older asymptomatic people: Results of an open access, unlimited age colonoscopic screening for colorectal cancer. *Mol Clin Oncol* 2020;12(2):179–185.

6. Cisel B, Pietrzak L, Michalski W et al. Long-course preoperative chemoradiation versus 5 × 5 Gy and consolidation chemotherapy for clinical T4 and fixed clinical T3 rectal cancer: Long-term results of the randomized Polish II study. *Ann Oncol* 2019;30(8):1298–1303.

7. Simillis C, Lal N, Thoukididou SN et al. Open versus laparoscopic versus robotic versus transanal mesorectal excision for rectal cancer: A systematic review and network meta-analysis. *Ann Surg* 2019;270(1):59–68.

8. Gustafsson UO, Scott MJ, Hubner M et al. Guidelines for perioperative care in elective colorectal surgery: Enhanced Recovery After Surgery (ERAS) Society recommendations: 2018. *World J Surg* 2019;43(3):659–695.

# PART 6

# GALLBLADDER AND BILIARY TREE

# 26 Acute Cholecystitis

## *Four Days Duration with a Palpable Lump*

*Takanori Morikawa and Michiaki Unno*

## CONTENTS

## CASE SCENARIO

A 60-year-old man presented to our outpatient department with a chief complaint of recurrent upper abdominal pain that was worsened with food intake. The patient had a medical history of hypertension, angina pectoris, non-alcoholic fatty liver disease, hyperuricemia, sleep apnea syndrome, and no history of abdominal surgery. On physical examination, he was found to have a soft abdomen without epigastric tenderness and Murphy's sign, and magnetic resonance imaging (MRI) revealed gallbladder and common bile duct stones (Figure 26.1). Endoscopic lithotripsy with sphincterotomy was then performed. His right upper abdominal pain recurred four days after its onset, and he was again referred to our department. His abdomen was soft, but right-upper abdominal pain and Murphy's sign were remarkable, and a right-upper quadrant mass was slightly palpable. Computed tomography (CT) demonstrated dilatation and wall thickening of the gallbladder with surrounding fat stranding and calculi within it (Figure 26.2).

## BACKGROUND OF THE PATHOLOGY

Acute cholecystitis is one of the common diseases that requires emergent treatment, and presents in 3–9% of all patients with acute abdominal symptoms who visit the emergency department [1]. The primary etiology of acute cholecystitis is gallstones (90–95% of the cases). However, only 10% of the patients with gallstones experience acute cholecystitis. The mechanism of acute calculous cholecystitis is bile stasis and activation of inflammation due to obstruction of the cystic duct by an impacted gallstone [2]. Less commonly, patients may develop acute cholecystitis in the absence of stones. This entity, referred to as acalculous cholecystitis, is encountered in critically ill patients, especially related to trauma, surgery, burn, long intensive care unit (ICU) stays, and prolonged fasting. Acute acalculous cholecystitis is defined as an acute necro-inflammatory disease of the gallbladder, accounts for 3.7%–14% of acute cholecystitis [3], and is reported to result from bile stasis and/or ischemia due to the underlying disease state [4].

## APPROACH TO MANAGEMENT
### Clinical symptoms

Most of the patients with acute cholecystitis present with right-upper quadrant abdominal pain lasting several hours, with or without pyrexia. They may have varying degrees of nausea, anorexia, jaundice, and abdominal pain with radiation to the right shoulder or interscapular area. On clinical examination, right-upper quadrant tenderness with arrest of respiration by deep palpation at the tip of the ninth costal cartilage at the height of inspiration (Murphy's sign) is a pathognomonic sign. As the disease process advances with local adhesions, a right-upper quadrant mass may be palpable. In general, diagnosis of acute cholecystitis is determined using the combination of clinical symptoms, blood tests, and radiological findings. In addition, it is very important to confirm the duration from the onset of the symptoms to the first visit because that is needed to determine the therapeutic strategy.

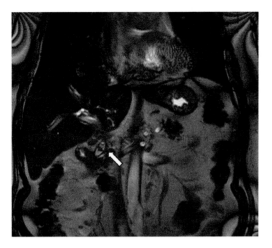

**Figure 26.1** MRI showed signal voids within the high signal intensity (white arrow) in the common bile duct which indicated common bile duct stones.

In cases with acute acalculous cholecystitis, the patient is usually critically ill and may have no ability to present their symptom due to sedated, intubated, and/or unconscious status. Therefore, it is very difficult to diagnose acute acalculous cholecystitis in the early stages, and high clinical suspicion for this disease is warranted in all critically ill patients [4].

### Blood investigations

In patients with acute cholecystitis, inflammatory findings such as elevation of white blood

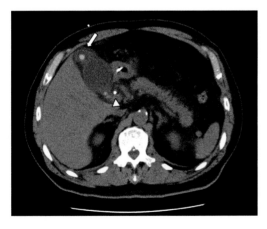

**Figure 26.2** Axial CT images demonstrating gallbladder wall thickening with pericholecystic fat stranding and calcification in the gallbladder (white arrow), which suggested acute cholecystitis, and also demonstrated endoscopic nasobiliary tube (arrowhead) in the common bile duct.

cell count, neutrophil count, and C-reactive protein and slight elevation of liver enzymes (alanine aminotransferase, aspartate amino-transferase, gamma-glutamyl transpeptidase, and alkaline phosphatase) are often detected in blood investigations. However, there is no single laboratory test with sufficient diagnostic accuracy to establish the diagnosis of acute cholecystitis. In addition, elevation of liver bio-chemical enzymes and bilirubin levels are also used as diagnostic tests for acute cholecystitis with common bile duct stones, but they are not specific either.

### Radiological investigations

The most common modality performed for the patients who are suspected to have acute cholecystitis is abdominal ultrasound, due to its lower cost, easy availability, and non-invasive nature [3]. Ultrasound findings of acute chole-cystitis are described below, although there is no single ultrasound feature that is useful in the diagnosis of acute cholecystitis.

1) Enlargement of the gallbladder

2) Thickening of the gallbladder wall

3) Subserosal edema of the gallbladder wall

4) Pericholecystic fluid

5) Linear shadow in the fat tissue around the gallbladder

6) Calcification or retained debris in the gallbladder

The accuracy of an abdominal ultrasound is limited by the patient's body habitus and the expertise of the sonographer. In case of doubt, contrast-enhanced CT scan of the abdomen can be performed. CT helps in the identification of acute cholecystitis-related complicationa such as emphysema of the gallbladder, abscess for-mation, and perforation; however, its diagnostic accuracy has not been proven to supersede abdominal ultrasound. Magnetic resonance cholangiopancreatography (MRCP) is preferred for the assessment of patients with gallstones and suspected common bile duct stones (derangement of liver function tests including an elevated serum bilirubin). Hepatobiliary iminodiacetic acid scintigraphy is reported to yield higher diagnostic accuracy compared with ultrasound, but it is not recommended due to limited availability and its time-consuming nature. Endoscopic retrograde cholangio-pancreatography is a useful modality as both diagnostic and therapeutic tool for common bile duct stones with cholangitis. It is fraught with the inherent risk of inducing an attack of acute pancreatitis (<5%).

Differential diagnosis of acute cholecystitis are presented in Table 26.1.

## MANAGEMENT

There are two options for the treatment of acute cholecystitis after initial medical treatment, namely surgery, and conservative therapy.

### Initial medical treatment

After diagnosis of acute cholecystitis is confirmed, initial treatment includes monitoring of respiration and hemodynamics, intravenous fluid resuscitation, intravenous antibiotics, and analgesics should be performed [5]. Antimicrobial therapy is recommended as the primary therapy in patients either undergoing surgical or conservative treatment in complicated cholecystitis. In cases with bacteremia or septic shock, appropriate antimicrobial therapy should be administered within one hour empirically and continued until systemic inflammation is subsided. It should be kept in mind that source control (i.e. cholecystectomy or cholecystostomy) is an essential part of the treatment of acute cholecystitis and antimicrobial agents should be adjusted once causative microorganism and susceptibility testing result are available. For patients with mild or moderate cholecystitis, antimicrobial therapy should

## Table 26.1 Differential Diagnosis of Acute Cholecystitis

*Biliary tract*
Chronic cholecystitis
Acute cholangitis
Gallbladder cancer
Cholangiocarcinoma
*Pancreas*
Acute pancreatitis
Pancreatic cancer (Courvoisier sign)
*Liver*
Liver abscess
Liver tumor
Fitz-Hugh–Curtis syndrome
*Gastrointestinal*
Acute gastritis
Gastroduodenal ulcer
Acute appendicitis
Diverticulitis of the ascending colon
Ulcerative colitis
Intestinal obstruction
Irritable bowel syndrome
Colon cancer
*Other organs*
Ischemic heart disease
Aortic dissection
Urolithiasis
Pyelonephritis

be administered within six hours of diagnosis and continued until surgery or drainage.

### Surgery

Surgery is the gold standard for the treatment of the acute cholecystitis, and early laparoscopic cholecystectomy is strongly recommended [5]. Especially in the patients with complicated cholecystitis, early laparoscopic cholecystectomy should be performed by surgeons with adequate expertise in laparoscopic surgery. Early laparoscopic cholecystectomy is defined as that performed within one to seven days after the onset of acute cholecystitis. It is often difficult to perform early cholecystectomy because of delayed diagnosis, incorrect determination of disease onset, lack of availability of operation theater space, and staff. However, the Tokyo guidelines 2018 suggested consideration for cholecystectomy as soon as a diagnosis has been made [5], and the 2016 World Society of Emergency Surgery guideline documented that laparoscopic cholecystectomy should be completed within ten days of onset of symptoms [3], so long as expertise in advanced laparoscopy is available.

In the patients with severe acute cholecystitis, the rate of complications such as bile leakage, bile duct injury, and bowel injury is reported to be higher than mild or moderate acute cholecystitis. In such cases, laparoscopic subtotal cholecystectomy as a bail-out procedure is recommended is access to the Calot's and hepatocystic triangles is hampered by inflammation in the porta hepatis. Furthermore, if the cystic duct cannot be closed clipped, then the use of endoloops needs to be considered. If there is a failure to progress during laparoscopic cholecystectomy due to technical or anatomical reasons, conversion to an open procedure through a Kocher incision must be performed.

### Conservative treatment

Although several patients may experience alleviation of symptoms only by antimicrobial therapy, antibiotics should be considered as supportive care. Most of the patients who initially responded with antimicrobial therapy and continue observational treatment suffer recurrence of symptoms and eventually require an unplanned surgery [3].

In case of patients who are not be suitable for emergent surgical treatment due to severe comorbidities or the severity of cholecystitis, due consideration for a percutaneous cholecystostomy or percutaneous transhepatic gallbladder drainage, should be considered as an alternative treatment to surgery if their disease

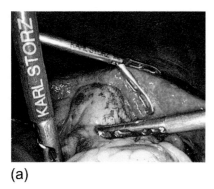 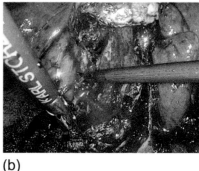

(a)                              (b)

**Figure 26.3**  Intraoperative photographs demonstrating the gallbladder with dense omental adhesions. (a) Although conversion to laparoscopic partial cholecystectomy was commenced due to abscess formation, (b) around the gallbladder, continuing laparoscopic surgery was unable due to abrupt bleeding at the neck of gallbladder.

does not respond to conservative measures [5]. Percutaneous transhepatic gallbladder drainage has been reported to have comparable outcomes to cholecystectomy in literature when performed for the appropriate indications. It may also be used as a bridge to surgery at the hospitals where complicated surgeries are difficult and/or surgeons at work do not have expertise in managing severe acute cholecystitis.

In this case, the patient was taken up for a laparoscopic cholecystectomy. Intraoperative findings confirmed acute cholecystitis with dense omental (Figure 26.3a) and duodenal adhesions that were dissected sharply to reveal gangrenous changes in the gallbladder along with abscess formation. The Calot's triangle could not be dissected safely. In this patient, persisting laparoscopically was not done owing to severe pericholecystic fibrosis (Figure 26.3b) and bleeding at the neck of gallbladder. The decision was made to convert to open cholecystectomy and hemostasis was achieved. A subtotal cholecystectomy was performed. The postoperative course was uneventful.

### KEY MESSAGES

- Diagnosis of acute cholecystitis is determined using a combination of clinical symptoms, blood tests, and radiological findings. The most common imaging modality is abdominal ultrasound.
- It is very important to confirm the duration from the onset of the symptoms to the first visit because that is needed to determine therapeutic strategy.

- In critically ill patients, clinical suspicion for acute acalculous cholecystitis is necessary to make an early diagnosis.
- Surgery is the gold standard for the treatment of the acute cholecystitis, and early laparoscopic cholecystectomy is strongly recommended as soon as possible after diagnosis of acute cholecystitis.
- In the case of high risk of bile duct injury, conversion to open surgery with subtotal cholecystectomy as a bail-out procedure should be considered. Conversion to open surgery should not be considered a complication of the operation.

### REFERENCES

1. European Association for the Study of the Liver (EASL). EASL clinical practice guidelines on the prevention, diagnosis, and treatment of gallstones. *J Hepatol* 2016;65(1):146–181.
2. Kimura Y, Takada T, Strasberg SM et al. TG13 current terminology, etiology, and epidemiology of acute cholangitis and cholecystitis. *J Hepatobil Pancreat Sci* 2013;20(1):8–23.
3. Ansaloni L, Pisano M, Coccolini F et al. 2016 WSES guidelines on acute calculous cholecystitis. *World J Emerg Surg* 2016;11:25.
4. Huffman JL, Schenker S. Acute acalculous cholecystitis: A review. *Clin Gastroenterol Hepatol* 2010;8(1):5–22.
5. Okamoto K, Suzuki K, Takada T et al. Tokyo guidelines 2018: Flowchart for the management of acute cholecystitis. *J Hepatobil Pancreat Sci* 2018;25(1):55–72.

# 27 Intraoperative Cholangiogram Shows <1 cm Stone at the Lower End

*Michael Cox*

## CONTENTS

## CASE SCENARIO: Part one

A 69-year-old woman presented with several episodes of typical biliary pain. More recently, she had two episodes of jaundice; the most recent was associated with rigors and night sweats. The symptoms resolved spontaneously over the next 12 hours. An ultrasound revealed multiple gallstones in the gallbladder and a dilated common bile duct (Figure 27.1). The liver function tests revealed elevated transaminases and alkaline phosphatase, but the bilirubin was normal. An elective laparoscopic cholecystectomy was organized a week after the initial consultation. The routine intraoperative cholangiogram was performed and revealed a distal common bile duct stone (Figure 27.2).

## BACKGROUND OF PATHOLOGY

Common bile duct stones are classified as either primary or secondary stones. Primary common bile duct stones form due to stasis in a dilated biliary tree. The stasis may be idiopathic, or secondary to ampullary stenosis, a biliary stricture, or a duodenal diverticulum (compressing the lower end of the common bile duct). Primary common bile duct stones usually have a brown pigment (calcium bilirubinate), are soft stones and are easily fragmented with the consistency of mud. Secondary common bile duct stones have formed in the gallbladder and migrated down via the cystic duct. The majority are cholesterol stones formed by

combination of super saturation of bile with cholesterol, biliary stasis, accelerated nucleation, and mucin hypersecretion of the gallbladder. Less often, secondary common bile duct stones may be black pigment stones arise from increased levels of either unconjugated bilirubin (as seen in patients with cirrhosis or alcohol-related hepatitis), or elevated conjugated bilirubin (as seen in patients with various forms of intravascular hemolysis).

There are several clinico-pathological scenarios that may occur with common bile duct stones (Table 27.1). Each of these have a specific clinical presentation. Common bile duct stones may be completely asymptomatic. Obstruction by the common bile duct may simply cause biliary pain and associated with an acute elevation of liver enzymes (Table 27.2). A higher grade of obstruction may be associated with clinical jaundice; however, bilirubin levels seldom exceed 120 umol/L (normal range 3–15) with obstructive stone disease. Common bile duct obstruction may be associated with secondary bacterial infection (*Escherichia coli* or other gram-negative bacteria) with associated acute cholangitis. Cholangitis may range in severity from mild infection with minimal systemic response to severe overwhelming sepsis. Severity is graded according to the Tokyo guidelines and the severity determines subsequent management (Table 27.3).

Simultaneous obstruction of the common bile duct in the pancreatic duct or passage of

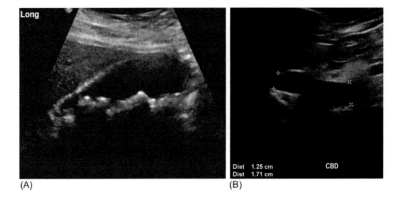

**(A)**  **(B)**

**Figure 27.1** (A) Ultrasound demonstrating multiple stones in the gallbladder with a normal gallbladder wall and no evidence of acute cholecystitis. (B) Ultrasound demonstrating a dilated common bile duct (1.1–1.2 mm) but no stones were seen in the common bile duct.

a stone across the ampulla may result in acute biliary pancreatitis with the main biochemical findings being an elevated lipase and amylase in addition to other changes in liver function tests (Table 27.2).

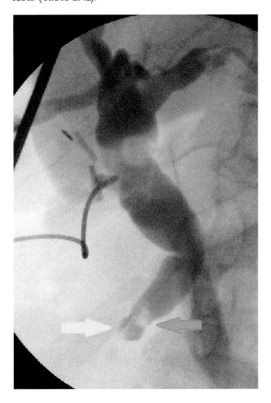

**Figure 27.2** Intraoperative cholangiogram revealing dilated common bile duct (12 mm) and a distal common bile duct stone that was 8 mm and faceted. The cystic duct was 4–5 mm in diameter. There was no flow into the duodenum, suggesting an impacted stone in the distal common bile duct.

**Table 27.1 Clinicopathological Scenarios Associated with Common Bile Duct Stones**

Silent / asymptomatic
Biliary pain with normal liver function tests
Biliary pain with elevated liver function tests
Obstructive jaundice
Cholangitis
Biliary pancreatitis

## APPROACH TO MANAGEMENT

The approach to management for suspected or proven common bile duct stones is dependent in part upon the clinical presentation, patient comorbidities, available expertise, equipment, and previous surgical interventions. A patient presenting with recurrent biliary pain and gallbladder stones on imaging without any risk factors for common bile duct stones (Table 27.4) shall proceed to laparoscopic cholecystectomy with routine intraoperative cholangiogram. The role of routine intraoperative cholangiogram is constantly debated. However, the author performs routine intraoperative cholangiogram to ensure that no stones are overlooked, to ensure that the interpretation of the operative dissection is correct, and to facilitate the management of any postoperative symptoms [1].

A patient presenting with biliary pain and positive risk factors for common bile duct stones (Table 27.4) are managed with laparoscopic cholecystectomy and routine intraoperative cholangiogram. When the common bile duct stone is found, the treatment is to clear the stone either at the time of laparoscopic cholecystectomy or with a subsequent endoscopic approach (Table 27.5).

## Table 27.2 Pattern for Liver Function Tests

| Pathology | Bilirubin | AST/ALT | GGT | ALP | Amylase/Lipase |
|---|---|---|---|---|---|
| Silent | N | N - ↑ | N - ↑ | N | N |
| Acute obstruction | N - 120 | ↑↑↑ | ↑↑ | N - ↑ | N - ↑ |
| Chronic obstruction | N - 50 | ↑ | ↑↑ or ↑↑↑ | ↑↑ - ↑↑↑ | N |
| Acute biliary pancreatitis | N - 50 | ↑↑ or ↑↑↑ | ↑ - ↑↑ | ↑ | ↑↑ - ↑↑↑ |

N = Normal
AST = Aspartate amino transferase
ALT = Alanine amino transferase
GGT = Gamma glutamyl transferase
ALP = Alkaline phosphatase
↑ = Mild elevation, 0.5–1 times normal
↑↑ = Moderate elevation, 1–3 times
↑↑↑ = Markedly elevated, greater than 3 times

## Table 27.3 Classification for the Severity of Cholangitis Adapted from the Tokyo Guidelines [5]

| Grade | Definition | Treatment |
|---|---|---|
| III—Severe | Acute cholangitis with severe dysfunction in at least one organ system: Cardiovascular, respiratory, renal, neurological, hepatic, or hematological. | Emergency endoscopic biliary drainage (ERCP) |
| II—Moderate | No organ dysfunction but at least two of the following: WCC >12,000, fever >39, age >75, bilirubin >75 umol/L, albumin <30 g/L. | Antibiotics. If settles early LC. If does not settle or worsens emergency ERCP |
| I—Mild | None of the above criteria. | Antibiotics and early LC when resolved |

**Abbreviations:** WCC – white cell count, LC – laparoscopic cholecystectomy, ERCP – endoscopic retrograde cholangiopancreatography.

## Table 27.4 Clinical, Common Laboratory and Radiological Factors Indicating Possible Common Bile Duct Stones

History of obstructive jaundice

History of acute biliary pancreatitis

Elevated bilirubin

Elevated AST/ALT

Elevated GGT

Elevated ALP

Dilated CBD on ultrasound greater than 6 mm

Stone seen in CBD on ultrasound (Figure 27.3)

**Abbreviations:** AST – aspartate aminotransaminase, ALT – alanine aminotransaminase, GGT – gamma glutamyl transferase, ALP – alkaline phosphatase, CBD – common bile duct.

Patients with obstructive jaundice but no associated cholangitis may require additional imaging to determine the underlying cause of the jaundice prior to any intervention. The intervention would be dependent on the certainty of a common bile duct stone as the cause of the jaundice and the degree of clinical suspicion of a malignant biliary obstruction or Mirizzi syndrome.

Patients presenting with cholangitis are managed according to the likelihood of the diagnosis (Table 27.6) and the severity of cholangitis (Table 27.3). Grade I cholangitis can be managed with intravenous antibiotics and when settled proceed to an early laparoscopic cholecystectomy with intraoperative cholangiogram and subsequent management of any stone found. Although, some surgeons may perform preoperative endoscopic retrograde cholangiopancreatography and clear the duct as the initial procedure and the laparoscopic cholecystectomy as the second procedure, this is associated with a higher overall morbidity. Therefore, the preference of the author is to go directly to laparoscopic cholecystectomy and intraoperative cholangiogram. Grade II cholangitis that settles with antibiotics may be managed as for grade I cholangitis with an early laparoscopic cholecystectomy and intraoperative cholangiogram and subsequent management of any bile duct stones.

## Table 27.5 Options of Treatment of a Common Bile Duct Stone Found on Routine Intraoperative Cholangiogram

Laparoscopic transcystic exploration

Transcystic stenting and postoperative ERCP

Laparoscopic choledochotomy and CBD exploration

Conversion to open surgery with choledochotomy and CBD exploration

Complete LC with no additional procedure and postoperative ERCP

**Abbreviations:** CBD – common bile duct, IOC – intraoperative cholangiogram, ERCP – endoscopic retrograde cholangiopancreatography, LC – laparoscopic cholecystectomy.

## Table 27.6 Criteria for the Diagnosis of Acute Cholangitis, Adapted from the Tokyo Guidelines [5]

| Criteria | Definition |
|---|---|
| A = Inflammation | Fever >38 and/or rigors<br>WCC >16,000 or CRP >50 |
| B = Cholestasis | Clinical jaundice<br>Elevated LFT (Table 27.2) |
| C = Imaging | Dilated CBD >8 mm<br>Pathology noted such as: Stone, stricture, or biliary stent |
| Suspected acute cholangitis | One item in A and one in either B or C |
| Confirmed cholangitis | One item in each of A, B, and C |

Patients with grade II cholangitis that does not settle or accompanied by clinical deterioration, and patients with grade III cholangitis require urgent endoscopic biliary drainage with endoscopic retrograde cholangiopancreatography, sphincterotomy, stone extraction, and possible biliary stenting. These patients then need a laparoscopic cholecystectomy, which should be performed as an early laparoscopic cholecystectomy once the organ failure has recovered. A delay in laparoscopic cholecystectomy results in a more difficult laparoscopic cholecystectomy in a similar fashion to delayed surgery for acute calculous cholecystitis.

Patients with mild biliary pancreatitis should have an early laparoscopic cholecystectomy and intraoperative cholangiogram once the pain has resolved, during the same admission for the acute biliary pancreatitis. Delayed surgery results in up to 30–35% of patients representing within three months. Patients with moderately severe or severe biliary pancreatitis should proceed to cholecystectomy when the complications of the acute pancreatitis (acute fluid collection, infected necrosis, or pseudocysts) have resolved on imaging or have been treated (Table 27.7).

Patients who have had a prior cholecystectomy that present with common bile duct stones require an endoscopic retrograde cholangiopancreatography to treat these stones. Patients with a previous cholecystectomy and Billroth I partial gastrectomy may still be able to have an endoscopic retrograde cholangiopancreatography. However, patients with a partial gastrectomy and Roux-en-Y anastomosis, a total gastrectomy, or gastric bypass bariatric surgery will not have endoscopic access to the ampulla. If these patients present with cholangitis (grade II or III) the biliary tree can be drained with a percutaneous biliary drain to resolve the sepsis. The definitive management of the common bile duct stone, whether percutaneous drainage is required or not, shall be either a laparoscopic or an open exploration of the common bile duct. There remains the possibility of performing a laparoscopic, transgastric endoscopic retrograde cholangiopancreatography via the gastric remnant in a patient who has had a previous Roux-en-Y gastric bypass for obesity. The advantage of this procedure is that it can be done synchronously with the laparoscopic cholecystectomy. However, this is a difficult complex procedure and should only be attempted by experienced

## Table 27.7 Management of Gallbladder Stones in Acute Biliary Pancreatitis

| Severity | Management |
|---|---|
| Mild | LC and IOC in same admission |
| Moderately severe | LC once local complication resolves or has been treated |
| Severe | LC once local complication resolves or has been treated |

**Abbreviations:** SIRS – systemic inflammatory response syndrome, LC – Laparoscopic cholecystectomy, IOC – intraoperative cholangiogram.

laparoscopic surgeons with endoscopic expertise or in association with an experienced medical endoscopist.

## CLINICAL FINDINGS
### History

*Biliary pain:* Biliary pain is often called "biliary colic" which is a misnomer as the pain is constant, not colicky. Biliary pain is usually a sudden onset in the epigastrium, lower central chest, right upper quadrant, or across the upper abdomen. It frequently radiates to the right subscapular area or to the central back. It may happen at any time of the day and can wake the patient from sleep. The pain may occur two to three hours after meals, but not always. The pain is severe and the patient is usually unable to get comfortable and feels quite agitated with the pain. The pain may be associated with nausea and vomiting. The duration can be anything from 15 minutes to 8 hours. Pain lasting beyond eight hours is usually associated with a complication of gallstone disease such as acute cholecystitis or cholangitis. Biliary pain arises due to the obstruction at the neck of the gallbladder or the distal common bile duct. The pain description is the same regardless of whether the obstruction is of the gallbladder or of the common bile duct.

*Obstructive jaundice:* The level of jaundice in common bile duct stone disease is normally accompanied by a bilirubin below 120 umol/L and hence may go unnoticed by the patient. The patient may, however, notice dark urine. Pruritus and steatorrhea are uncommon with common bile duct obstruction due to stones unless the obstruction is particularly long standing.

*Fevers and night sweats:* Patients with biliary pain that complain of fever and night sweats may have either acute cholecystitis or cholangitis. The author's clinical experience would be that this is more commonly associated with acute cholecystitis as it is a more common problem.

*Rigors:* The occurrence of rigors is associated with biliary pain is usually due to cholangitis. Indeed, the presence of rigors should be considered cholangitis until proven otherwise.

### Clinical signs

*Normal examination:* The patient with biliary pain that has resolved may have no clinical signs at all.

*Tenderness and Murphy's sign:* The patient may be tender in the epigastrium or the right upper quadrant. In some patients, there may be minimal tenderness, but they experience an arrest of respiration while taking a deep breath and the right upper quadrant is being deeply palpated simultaneously. This sign, referred to as "Murphy's sign" is due to the inflamed gallbladder descending down during deep inspiration to the point of the deep palpation.

*Gallbladder mass:* A palpable gallbladder mass in the right upper quadrant is associated with a distended gallbladder. This is more often associated with gallbladder specific pathology such as a mucocele due to a stone impacted in the gallbladder neck and a phlegmon formed from adherent omentum and colon, rather than a common bile duct stone. In the presence of progressive, painless jaundice, it may indicate a malignant distal common bile duct obstruction (Courvoisier's sign).

*Jaundice:* Scleral icterus may be subtle or it may be obvious. The presentation of jaundice indicates probable biliary obstruction. The more frequent cause is a stone in the common bile duct and a less frequent cause is Mirizzi syndrome.

*Systemic inflammatory response syndrome:* The presence of systemic inflammatory response syndrome indicates either acute cholecystitis or cholangitis. In cholangitis, this will indicate either grade II or grade III cholangitis.

### Investigations

*Ultrasound:* Transabdominal ultrasound should be the initial imaging performed when the clinical diagnosis is gallstone disease (Figure 27.1). The features suggesting associated common bile duct stones are a dilated common bile duct greater than 7 mm, or the presence of stones in the common bile duct.

*Liver function tests:* Liver function tests may be elevated with either acute biliary obstruction or long-standing common bile duct stone disease (Table 27.2).

The majority of patients presenting with symptomatic gallstone disease with confirmation of gallstones on ultrasound require no further investigation prior to proceeding to surgical intervention (laparoscopic cholecystectomy and intraoperative cholangiography). The exception to this is in the case of patients with obstructive jaundice where there is concern about a malignant cause for the jaundice, a suspicious thickening or mass in the gallbladder, or the possibility of Mirizzi syndrome. In such cases, a magnetic resonance cholangiopancreatography (MRCP) may be helpful in planning further management. The routine use of computed tomography (CT) cholangiogram or MRCP is not required to diagnose common bile duct stones as in the absence of cholangitis the appropriate management is to proceed to laparoscopic cholecystectomy and intraoperative cholangiographyand treat the subsequent stones at the time of laparoscopic cholecystectomy. Although, some surgeons would perform an ERCP and clear the CBD as the initial procedure, as noted previously, performing the endoscopic retrograde cholangiopancreatography first is associated with a higher morbidity compared to performing the laparoscopic cholecystectomy first [2,3].

## Treatment options for the stone found at intraoperative cholangiography

The author's preference for managing a common bile duct stone found at laparoscopic cholecystectomy (Figure 27.2) is to insert an antegrade transcystic biliary stent, complete the laparoscopic cholecystectomy and perform a postoperative endoscopic retrograde cholangiopancreatography. This technique is used in all cases unless there has been previous surgery the prevents endoscopic access to the ampulla (see above). Other techniques that can be used include laparoscopic transcystic duct exploration, laparoscopic choledochotomy, and common bile duct exploration, conversion to open surgery, or completing the laparoscopic cholecystectomy without a transcystic biliary stent, and performing a postoperative endoscopic retrograde cholangiopancreatography.

### Transcystic exploration

The technique of transcystic exploration [3] allows for removal of the common bile duct stone disease in up to 65% of cases. It has the benefit of clearing the duct at the time of the laparoscopic cholecystectomy, avoiding a second procedure, and avoiding a sphincterotomy. This technique may be used when previous surgery prevents endoscopic access to the ampulla. This technique does require special equipment and a reasonable amount of technical expertise with laparoscopic biliary surgery. The potential disadvantage in the case presented is the stone is 3 mm larger than the cystic duct and is faceted, making it more difficult to remove back through the cystic duct. Nonetheless, the stone could be attempted to be removed transcystically with a basket and possibly the addition of balloon dilatation of the cystic duct. Cases where laparoscopic transcystic extraction is unlikely to be effective include: very large stones, stones impacted in the distal end, multiple stones, and stones above the cystic duct confluence or in the intrahepatic ducts.

If the transcystic exploration fails there needs to be a "ramp-up approach" adopted [3]. This may be with the insertion of a transcystic stent with subsequent postoperative endoscopic retrograde cholangiopancreatography, laparoscopic choledochotomy, and duct exploration, or conversion to open surgery with open common bile duct exploration.

### Transcystic stenting of postoperative endoscopic retrograde cholangiopancreatography

The insertion of a transcystic stent to lie across the sphincter of Oddi and then subsequent endoscopic retrograde cholangiopancreatography and duct clearance [4] has been the author's routine management of this clinical scenario for over 20 years [2]. The only contraindication is where there has been previous gastric surgery that prevents endoscopic access to the ampulla. It has the advantage of achieving common bile duct clearance in greater than 90% of cases at endoscopic retrograde cholangiopancreatography and greater than 99% of cases at a subsequent endoscopic retrograde cholangiopancreatography. The stent ensures successful common bile duct cannulation and avoids the risk of postoperative endoscopic retrograde cholangiopancreatography acute pancreatitis with a low instance (less than 0.5%) of either perforation or bleeding [2]. Transcystic stenting can be used when transcystic stone extraction has been unsuccessful. Transcystic stenting has advantages over laparoscopic choledochotomy and common bile duct exploration in that it is technically more easy to perform and can be done by most general surgeons. Furthermore, it has a much lower morbidity than either laparoscopic or open common bile duct exploration.

### Laparoscopic choledochotomy and common bile duct exploration

While technically possible, a laparoscopic choledochotomy and subsequent duct exploration [3] is a more complex laparoscopic procedure that many general surgeons may not have the competency or technical skill to perform. Although this has a high success rate, it is associated with a much higher morbidity compared to transcystic exploration or transcystic stenting. Furthermore, it has a higher morbidity than postoperative endoscopic retrograde cholangiopancreatography, particularly postoperative endoscopic retrograde cholangiopancreatography facilitated by transcystic stenting.

*Open common bile duct exploration*

There are two clinical scenarios that conversion to open exploration of the common bile duct is appropriate:

1) An isolated practice where there is no access to endoscopic retrograde cholangiopancreatography, which in the majority of high-income countries, is unusual.

2) Previous gastric surgery where endoscopic access is not possible and laparoscopic clearance cannot be achieved. However, open common bile duct exploration is associated with a much higher postoperative morbidity in terms of respiratory complications, wound infection, length of stay, and return to normal activities.

When either laparoscopic or open exploration of the common bile duct is performed, clearance of the common bile duct must be checked using direct visualization with a choledochoscopy. Where a choledochoscope is not available, an intraoperative cholangiography through a T-tube inserted into the choledochotomy can be used. At both laparoscopic and open exploration of the common bile duct, there are three options for closure of the choledochotomy. Firstly, the traditional approach is to close the choledochotomy over a T-tube. This has problems associated with fluid and electrolyte loss, early dislodgement, and leakage at the time of removal if a good tract has not developed. Secondly, where it is certain that the common bile duct has been cleared at choledochoscopy, the choledochotomy can be closed and a drain left adjacent to the closure. Thirdly, if there is concern that the common bile duct is not cleared or the distal common bile duct is edematous, an antegrade stent may be inserted to ensure biliary drainage a the choledochotomy closed.

*Postoperative endoscopic retrograde cholangiopancreatography*

Throughout the world the most common practice when confronted with a distal common bile duct stone (Figure 27.2) is to close the cystic duct, complete the laparoscopic cholecystectomy and refer the patient for postoperative endoscopic retrograde cholangiopancreatography. Although this is common practice, it is associated with a failed endoscopic retrograde cholangiopancreatography cannulation rate of 2–8%, failed removal of stones in up to 15%, the need for repeat endoscopic retrograde

cholangiopancreatography in up to 20% of cases and post endoscopic retrograde cholangiopancreatography pancreatitis in 1–5% of cases. The reason the author prefers to insert the transcystic stent is it facilitates the subsequent endoscopic retrograde cholangiopancreatography. The stent-facilitated endoscopic retrograde cholangiopancreatography is associated with a higher initial cannulation rate, a higher rate of stone clearance, reduced need for a second endoscopic retrograde cholangiopancreatography and a reduced morbidity from postoperative endoscopic retrograde cholangiopancreatography pancreatitis [2]. The stent kits are easily available, the technique is not difficult to perform [4], and with the better outcomes the author would encourage surgeons to use this technique, rather than cystic duct closure and refer for an endoscopic retrograde cholangiopancreatography.

### CASE SCENARIO: Part two

A transcystic stent was inserted to lie across the sphincter of Oddi (Figure 27.3). Two days later,

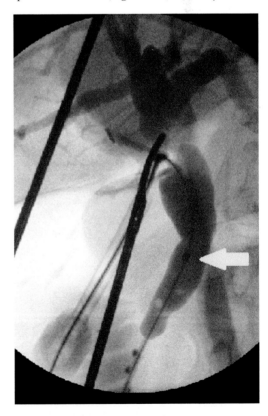

**Figure 27.3** A transcystic stent placed in the Case Scenario patient to lie across the sphincter of Oddi to facilitate a subsequent endoscopic retrograde cholangiopancreatography and sphincterotomy and stone removal.

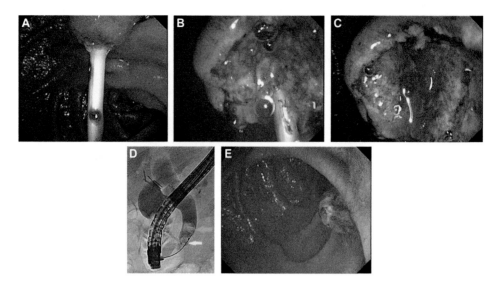

**Figure 27.4** (A) Endoscopic view of the transcystic stent across the ampulla in good position. (B) The completed endoscopic sphincterotomy using a needle knife over the stent. Note the swelling of the ampulla, prior to the removal of the stent. (C) The complete endoscopic sphincterotomy after removal of the stent with a snare. (D) The cholangiogram demonstrating the large more proximal stone (green arrow) and some smaller more distal stenos (yellow arrow). (E) The stone removed from the common bile duct in the third part of the duodenum at the conclusion of the procedure.

an endoscopic retrograde cholangiopancreatography was performed. The stent was in the correct position (Figure 27.4A) and a complete sphincterotomy was performed using a needle knife sphincterotome over the stent (Figure 27.4B). The stent was removed with a polypectomy snare (Figure 27.4C), the common bile duct cannulated, and a cholangiogram performed confirming the common bile duct stone (Figure 27.4D). The stone was then removed with a balloon trawl and the patient discharged home later that day (Figure 27.4E).

## KEY MESSAGES

- Patients with possible common bile duct stones and gallbladder in situ usually only require preoperative ultrasound and liver function tests for assessment.
- They can be managed by laparoscopic cholecystectomy and intraoperative cholangiogram with either transcystic stone extraction or transcystic stenting and postoperative endoscopic retrograde cholangiopancreatography.
- Preoperative endoscopic retrograde cholangiopancreatography is only required for the treatment of grade II cholangitis that does not resolve or grade III cholangitis.

- Laparoscopic common bile duct exploration or open common bile duct exploration should be performed when endoscopic access to the common bile duct is not possible.
- Surgeons that would normally close the cystic duct and refer for postoperative endoscopic retrograde cholangiopancreatography should consider insertion of a transcystic stent to improve the cannulation and clearance rates and reduce the risk of post endoscopic retrograde cholangiopancreatography pancreatitis.

## REFERENCES

1. Rangelova EPR. Intraoperative cholangiography. In: Cox MR, Eslcik GD, Padbury RTA, editor. *The Management of Gallstone Disease: A Practical Evidence Based Approach*. Springer, Cham, Switzerland; 2018. p. 249–262.
2. Cox MR. Transcystic stenting and post-operative ERCP for CBD stones at laparoscopic cholecystectomy. In: Cox MR, Eslcik GD, Padbury RTA, editor. *The Management of Gallstone Disease: A Practical Evidence-Based Approach*. Springer, Cham, Switzerland; 2018. p. 307–326.
3. Nathanson L. Laparoscopic bile duct exploration. In: Cox MR, Eslcik GD, Padbury RTA,

editor. *The Management of Gallstone Disease: A Practical Evidence-Based Approach*. Springer, Cham, Switzerland; 2018. p. 291–306.

4. Gomez D, Cox MR. Laparoscopic transcystic stenting and postoperative ERCP for the management of common bile duct stones at laparoscopic cholecystectomy. *Ann Surg* 2018;267(5):e86–ee8.

5. Kiriyama S, Kozaka K, Takada T et al. Tokyo guidelines 2018: Diagnostic criteria and severity grading of acute cholangitis (with Videos). *J Hepatobil Pancreat Sci* 2018;25(1):17–30.

# 28 Incidentally Detected 7 mm Gallbladder Polyp

*Nisar Hamdani and V.K. Kapoor*

## CONTENTS

## CASE SCENARIO

A 60-year-old Caucasian man was referred by his general practitioner with an abdominal ultrasound report suggestive of a 7 mm polyp in the gallbladder (Figure 28.1). The patient had presented a few days earlier to the general practitioner with persistent right upper abdominal pain. The general practitioner had ordered a battery of tests as well as an abdominal ultrasound. The liver and kidney function tests were within normal limits. However, the patient, who happened to be a hypertensive and chronic smoker, was also noted to have a high serum cholesterol level (254 mg/dL). He had had no prior surgery on his abdomen.

## BACKGROUND OF PATHOLOGY

The term "polypoidal lesion of the gallbladder" is used to describe a mucosal outgrowth presenting as a protuberant lesion into the lumen of the gallbladder. Gallbladder polyps are uncommon lesions with an estimated prevalence of 0.3–9.5%. They are usually detected as an incidental finding on imaging performed for right upper quadrant abdominal pain, or on histological examination of cholecystectomy specimens.

The vast majority (95%) of polyps are benign. Polypoidal lesion of the gallbladder is a mucosal outgrowth presenting as a protuberant lesion into the lumen of the gallbladder. The nomenclature or classification of polypoidal lesion of the gallbladder is confusing. The first attempt at classifying these lesions was done by Christensen and Ishak in 1970 [1]. However, we find this classification to be non-comprehensive and inadequate. We propose a new classification system for *polypoidal lesions of the gallbladder* in Table 28.1.

Male sex, obesity, hyperlipidemia, hepatitis B surface antigen positivity, and hereditary polyposis syndromes (Peutz-Jeghers and Gardner's syndrome) increase the risk of development of polyps, while gallstones have an inverse relationship.

Polyps that demonstrate local infiltration should be considered as harboring malignancy and should be treated similarly to gallbladder cancer. People of Indian heritage are at an increased risk of malignant transformation in their polyps. Thus, in them, surgical treatment of gallbladder polyps is recommended. Risk factors for harboring malignancy in polyps can be remembered by the six Ss, namely sixty years of age, size >6 mm, sessile, solitary, (coexistence of) (gall)stones, and/or (primary) sclerosing cholangitis.

## CLINICAL SYMPTOMS

While most gallbladder polyps are clinically silent (90% are asymptomatic), patients may present with right upper abdominal pain, nausea, dyspepsia, and even jaundice. The underlying causes for symptoms could be the presence of associated gallstones or polyps detaching and behaving like gallstones. In the absence of gallstones or the presence of small polyps, it is important that the clinician thoroughly investigates the patient to rule out other causes for patient's complaints.

As mentioned above, the possibility of large/infiltrative polyps harboring an underlying malignancy needs to be remembered and symptoms interpreted in this context.

Should the patient be referred with a diagnosis of a gallbladder polyp, the clinician must enquire about risk factors including ethnicity (Indian origin), hepatitis B status,

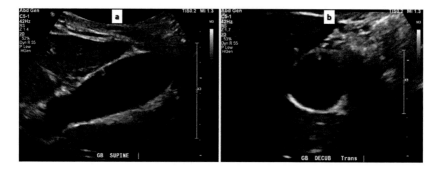

**Figure 28.1** Abdominal ultrasound images of the patient demonstrating an anti-dependent echogenic focus measuring approximately 7 mm arising from the wall of the gallbladder: (a) longitudinal view, (b) transverse sectional view.

## Table 28.1 Classification of Polypoidal Lesions of the Gallbladder (PLGB)

| Benign polypoidal lesions of the gallbladder | Malignant polypoidal lesions of the gallbladder |
|---|---|
| **A) Pseudopolyps (95% of all PLGBs)** | **A) Primary tumors of the gallbladder** |
| Cholesterol polyps (most common PLGB) | *Epithelial* |
| Adenomyomatosis (2nd common after cholesterol) | Adenocarcinoma (most common primary tumor) |
| Inflammatory polys | Squamous cell carcinoma |
| Tumefactive sludge/Sludge balls | Adenosquamous carcinoma |
| Heterotopias | |
| Biliary hamartomas (rarely malignant) | *Mesenchymal* |
| | Carcinoid (1% of GIT carcinoids) |
| **B) Tumors** | Sarcoma including Kaposi's sarcoma[r] |
| *Epithelial* | Rhabdomyosarcoma[r] |
| Adenoma (most common benign tumor) | Leiomyosarcoma[r] |
| • Pyloric type | Malignant fibrous histiocytoma[r] |
| • Intestinal type | Angiosarcoma[r] |
| | Carcinosarcoma[r] |
| *Mixed* | Melanoma[r] |
| Adenomyoma | Lymphoma |
| | |
| *Mesenchymal* | **B) Metastatic tumors to the gallbladder[r]** |
| Hemangioma | Gastrointestinal malignancy |
| Lipoma | Renal cell carcinoma |
| Leiomyoma[r] | Melanoma |
| Neurofibroma[r] | Bronchogenic carcinoma |
| Inflammatory myofibroblastic tumor (IMT)[r] | Lymphoma |
| Fibroma | Myeloma |
| | Hepatocelluar carcinoma[r] |
| | Cholangiocarcinoma[r] |

[r] = rare
**Abbreviations:** GIT – gastrointestinal tract.

hyperlipidemia, primary sclerosing cholangitis, and hereditary polyposis syndromes, such as Peutz-Jeghers syndrome or Gardner's syndrome.

### APPROACH TO MANAGEMENT
#### Blood investigations
In a patient with a gallbladder polyp on imaging, there are no specific findings in routine blood investigations, such as a complete blood count, and liver and renal function tests, and in most patients, they would be within normal limits. In the event that the polyp(s) is/are associated with gallstones, due to which the patient

develops acute cholecystitis, the findings in the blood tests would reflect the pathology.

Additional blood investigations that should be performed specifically in these patients include lipid profile and hepatitis B surface antigen. There is no role for routine tumor marker (carbohydrate antigen 19-9 or CA19-9) in polyps <10 mm and without concerning features on imaging (see below).

#### Radiological investigations
In addition to the presence of symptoms and underlying risk factors, the management of a gallbladder polyp is largely determined on its size.

The most common modalities employed in the imaging of gallbladder polyps are transabdominal ultrasound and/or endoscopic ultrasound.

A recent Cochrane review [2] has confirmed that ultrasound is good at discriminating between the presence and absence of gallbladder polyps although its accuracy drops in its ability to differentiate between a true versus, a pseudo polyp, or determining its malignant nature. In the latter situations, a contrast-enhanced computed tomography (CECT) scan of the abdomen is a better investigation to further characterize a polyp "suspicious" of harboring an underlying malignancy. "Suspicious" features include polypoidal lesions >10 mm, infiltration into the liver, diffuse asymmetric thickening of the gallbladder wall, and/or "displaced" (lifted from the wall by the focal thickening) or "floating" (neither settling nor wall adherent) stones [3]. Imaging of gallbladder cancer will be dealt within the appropriate chapters. The Cochrane review was also unable to demonstrate a significant advantage of endoscopic ultrasound over ultrasound. Thus, if there is concern about a polyp detected on ultrasound with a need to further characterize it, then the treating clinician may opt to proceed to an endoscopic ultrasound if the lesion is less than 10 mm, or a CECT scan of the abdomen for lesions >10 mm in size.

## MANAGEMENT

The two options in the management of a polypoidal lesion of the gallbladder are surgery (cholecystectomy) and ultrasound surveillance.

### Surgery

The indications for cholecystectomy (generally performed laparoscopically) include:

1) Polyps ≥10 mm in size (if there is even the slightest doubt of underlying malignancy, the patient must be referred to a hepatobiliary surgeon for further management)

2) Symptomatic polyps

3) Presence of risk factors in a polyp ≥6 mm, such as:

   a) Indian ethnicity

   b) Age >50 years

   c) Sessile polyps (including focal wall thickening >4 mm)

   d) Associated gallstones

   e) Associated primary sclerosing cholangitis

4) Polyp that increases by ≥2 mm or reaches 10 mm in size (even if asymptomatic) while on surveillance

The only contraindications for surgery are patients unfit for surgery or refusing consent for surgery despite being explained the risks.

In patients with polyps who are offered surgery in the absence of gallstones, and in those in whom the presenting symptoms are not typically biliary, during the informed consent process it is important to discuss the post-cholecysectomy symptoms, such as persistence of their presenting symptoms, dyspepsia, and diarrhea.

Any lesion in the gallbladder which is suspicious for gallbladder cancer should be further evaluated and managed as a *"suspected gallbladder cancer"* at a hepatopancreatobiliary center and laparoscopic cholecystectomy should not be attempted in such cases.

### Surveillance

Ultrasound is generally the preferred form of surveillance. The optimal timing of ultrasound surveillance [4] is determined by the size of the lesion. For lesions <6 mm, surveillance is recommended at one-, three- and five-year intervals. For polypoidal lesions of the gallbladder <6 mm but with associated high-risk factors, and in polyps that are 6–9 mm, more frequent follow-ups are recommended (six months, and one-, two-, three-, four-, and five-year intervals).

In a recent study [5] in which patients with polyps were followed up to 11 years, the authors noted that while the polyps persisted in 52% of patients, in the remaining 48%, they actually disappeared. In the latter, no further surveillance is warranted.

The patient presented in the **Case Scenario** was offered a laparoscopic cholecystectomy in view of the high-risk features of age >50 years, size >6 mm, and symptoms. The patient proceeded to have his surgery. Histopathological examination of the surgically resected gallbladder (Figure 28.2) confirmed cholesterolosis with a cholesterol polyp of the gallbladder.

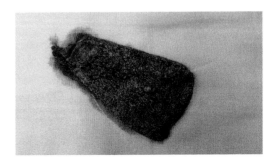

**Figure 28.2** Photograph of the opened gallbladder specimen demonstrating a 7 mm polyp.

## KEY MESSAGES

- Polypoidal lesions of the gallbladder are uncommon lesions that are generally asymptomatic.
- A new classification system has been proposed by us for polypoidal lesion of the gallbladder.
- Polyps ≥10 mm in size or demonstrating features of infiltration must be referred to a hepatobiliary surgeon as they are at risk of harboring an underlying malignant process.
- Age (>50 years), ethnicity (Indian), size, the presence of symptoms, and associated diseases such as primary sclerosing cholangitis, are risk factors that should prompt early surgery.
- A "safe laparoscopic cholecystectomy" by a well-trained experienced hepatobiliary surgeon is safer and more economical than the burden of follow-up on the patient in this selected subgroup of patients with polypoidal lesion of the gallbladder size of 7 mm, as surgery is the only method to know the nature of polypoidal lesion of the gallbladder with 100% accuracy (on histopathological examination).
- Ultrasound surveillance is feasible in most other patients with polyps <6 mm, asymptomatic, or without risk factors.

## REFERENCES

1. Christensen AH, Ishak KG. Benign tumors and pseudotumors of the gallbladder. Report of 180 cases. *Arch Pathol* 1970;90(5):423–432.
2. Wennmacker SZ, Lamberts MP, Di Martino M et al. Transabdominal ultrasound and endoscopic ultrasound for diagnosis of gallbladder polyps. *Cochrane Database Syst Rev* 2018;8:CD012233.
3. Shukla PJ, Barreto G, Neve R et al. Can we do better than 'incidental' gallbladder cancer? *Hepatogastroenterology* 2007;54(80):2184–2185.
4. Wiles R, Thoeni RF, Barbu ST et al. Management and follow-up of gallbladder polyps: Joint guidelines between the European Society of Gastrointestinal and Abdominal Radiology (ESGAR), European Association for Endoscopic Surgery and other Interventional Techniques (EAES), International Society of Digestive Surgery - European Federation (EFISDS) and European Society of Gastrointestinal Endoscopy (ESGE). *Eur Radiol* 2017;27(9):3856–3866.
5. Heitz L, Kratzer W, Grater T et al. Gallbladder polyps - A follow-up study after 11 years. *BMC Gastroenterol* 2019;19(1):42.

# 29 Gallbladder Cancer with Obstructive Jaundice and Periportal Lymph Node

*Arindam Mondal, Vikram A. Chaudhari, Manish S. Bhandare, and Shailesh V. Shrikhande*

## CONTENTS

## CASE SCENARIO

A 55-year-old woman presented with complaints of dyspepsia for three months, right upper quadrant pain for one month, and yellowish discoloration of eyes for two weeks. She reported no loss of weight, though her appetite was reduced. On clinical examination, she was found to be icteric with a hard, palpable gallbladder on abdominal examination. Her serum bilirubin level was 8 mg/dL and serum carbohydrate antigen 19-9 (CA 19-9) levels were elevated at 811 U/ml. A contrast-enhanced CT scan of her abdomen revealed a gallbladder replaced by a 4 × 3 cm mass with a 3 cm liver infiltration in the region of gallbladder fossa. A few enlarged periportal lymph nodes were noted, the largest measuring 2 × 2.1 cm in size. The malignant mass extended up to the common bile duct, resulting in local narrowing and secondary biliary obstruction with upstream intrahepatic biliary radical dilatation. The adjacent organs (duodenum, colon, and pancreas) appeared uninvolved. There was no evidence of liver metastases, ascites, or retroperitoneal lymphadenopathy on the scan.

### Background of the pathology

Gallbladder cancer is the fifth most common malignancy of the gastrointestinal tract. The cancer demonstrates marked geographic variations with the highest incidence reported in South America (Chile and Bolivia) and India. Gallbladder cancer is more common in women (4:1 ratio), and the main risk factors include gallstone disease, gallbladder polyps, and abnormal pancreaticobiliary duct junction. Gallbladder cancer is associated with low five-year survival rate. The poor prognosis is largely due to two factors: The absence of specific symptoms early in the course of the disease, and absence of a submucosa in the gallbladder permitting the cancer to invade deeper tissues with a high propensity for adjacent organ involvement and nodal spread, even for relatively small-sized tumors. On the flip side, around 50–70% of patients with gallbladder cancer are detected incidentally on histopathology following simple cholecystectomy for presumed benign conditions.

Less than 10% of patients with gallbladder cancer have disease limited to the gallbladder wall on presentation. More than 50% of patients have lymph nodal spread, and the rest present with metastatic disease. More than 60% of the patients present with locally advanced disease with invasion of the liver and/or adjacent organs.

Surgery is the only option of treatment with the promise of cure. However, most patients with gallbladder cancer need chemotherapy during the course of their treatment.

### Clinical presentation

While world literature generally suggests gallbladder cancer as a disease affecting patients in their sixth or seventh decades of life, in countries like India, the disease has been known to affect younger women. As noted above, incidental gallbladder cancer is encountered following 0.3–1.87% of cholecystectomies. Gallbladder cancer may mimic a polyp (this has been covered in Chapter 28 on gallbladder polyps). More commonly though, patients are diagnosed with a symptomatic mass in an advanced stage with associated features of anorexia and loss of weight. Dyspepsia and persistent right upper quadrant pain are common complaints. A palpable abdominal mass, abdominal distension (ascites), and jaundice are signs of advanced disease.

Patients with gallbladder cancer develop jaundice usually due to direct involvement of biliary ducts by the primary tumor or occasionally due to a pericholedochal or periportal lymph node mass externally compressing the biliary tract. Obstructive jaundice in gallbladder cancer is regarded as an ominous sign as most patients harbor advanced stage disease.

## INVESTIGATIONS

*Ultrasound*: Is the first-line investigation in patients with right upper quadrant pain or obstructive type of jaundice. It may raise the suspicion of malignancy and guide further evaluation. It helps detect the level of biliary block in jaundiced patients. Ultrasound can also detect advanced disease states like ascites and liver metastasis in many patients. It is limited in its ability to detect lymph nodal or peritoneal disease and fails to provide any more definitive information.

### Computed tomography (CT) scan and magnetic resonance imaging (MRI)

Triple phase contrast-enhanced CT scan of the chest, abdomen, and pelvis remains the most important investigation for diagnosis, staging, and preoperative planning in gallbladder cancer patients. Local extent of disease, nodal involvement, distant metastases, adjacent organ, and vascular involvement can be detected with sensitivity and specificity exceeding 80%. Metastasis to liver and lung can be reliably demonstrated. MRI is regarded as equivalent to CT scan in terms of its overall efficacy in the evaluation of gallbladder cancer. It is used selectively as an adjunct to CT scan in patients with jaundice to ascertain the level of obstruction and aid in biliary drainage. Perihilar blocks are preferably drained by a percutaneous approach and distal blocks near the ampulla can be drained by an endoscopic approach.

### Fluorodeoxyglucose positron emission tomography (FDG PET) scan

Most gallbladder cancers are fluorodeoxyglucose avid. Positron emission tomography CT has been found to have an accuracy of 95.9% for diagnosing the primary lesion, 85.7% for lymph node involvement, and 95.9% for metastatic disease in gallbladder cancers. It can result in change in management in up to 25–30% of patients [1]. False positivity remains a concern in early postoperative period in the case of incidental gallbladder cancers, inflammatory pathologies like Xanthogranulomatous cholecystitis, and in patients with undrained obstructive jaundice with high bilirubin levels, cholecystitis or cholangitis.

Selective use of PET CT in gallbladder cancer is likely to provide a higher yield in detection of metastatic disease. PET scan would detect metastatic lesions more frequently in patients with large primary lesions with liver infiltration, periportal lymph nodes, obstructive jaundice, suspicious aortocaval nodal metastasis, or high CA 19-9 levels.

*Tumor markers*: Serum CA 19-9 and carcinoembryonic antigen are commonly used tumor markers in gallbladder cancer patients. They are predictors of overall prognosis, response to chemotherapy, and postoperative recurrence. Sensitivity and specificity of these markers is around 70% and they have no diagnostic value. Both markers are known to be falsely elevated in obstructive jaundice and values should be reassessed after biliary drainage and normalization of liver functions tests [2].

*Tissue diagnosis*: In a clearly resectable, radiologically suspected gallbladder cancer, preoperative biopsy should not be performed as this aggressive cancer is known to spread across needle tracts. Suspected gallbladder cancer patients with locally advanced or metastatic disease would need tissue diagnosis before administration of neoadjuvant or palliative intent chemotherapy, respectively.

*Role of staging laparoscopy*: Staging laparoscopy identifies metastatic peritoneal disease in around 23% of patients of gallbladder cancer, with an accuracy 94.1%. The yield is more for locally advanced disease as compared to early disease (25% vs 10.7%). It prevents a non-therapeutic laparotomy and reduces the associated morbidity. A large proportion of gallbladder cancer patients have advanced disease at the time of presentation. Locally advanced inoperable and metastatic gallbladder cancer patients usually don't require any palliative surgical procedure and therefore staging laparoscopy is routinely recommended in all gallbladder cancer prior to exploration for definitive surgery [2].

## MANAGEMENT

For the patient described in the Case Scenario, a positron emission tomography CT scan was performed which did not reveal any evidence of metastatic disease. A magnetic resonance cholangiopancreatography was performed which revealed a type II communicating

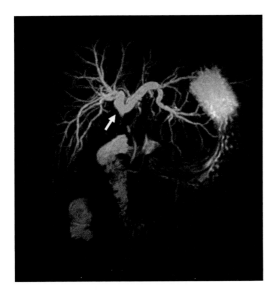

**Figure 29.1** Magnetic resonance cholangiopancreatography image demonstrating a type II communicating block (marked with a white arrow) with intrahepatic biliary ductal dilatation.

type of block (Figure 29.1). And so, the patient underwent an endoscopic retrograde cholangiopancreatography (ERCP) with the placement of a self-expanding metal stent placement for biliary drainage. An ultrasound-guided fine-needle aspiration cytology from the primary lesion was performed which was suggestive of a poorly differentiated carcinoma. Staging laparoscopy ruled out metastatic peritoneal disease. In view of the locally advanced nature of the disease, she was planned for neoadjuvant chemotherapy after proper counseling and consent. Her chemotherapy regimen consisted of

three cycles of gemcitabine and cisplatin, which was followed by repeat imaging for response assessment.

Post-chemotherapy response assessment contrast-enhanced CT scan showed significant reduction in the size of the primary tumor, as per response evaluation criteria in solid tumors (RECIST) criteria, suggestive of a partial response to chemotherapy (Figure 29.2, Figure 29.3). Repeat serum CA 19-9 level was 35 U/mL.

After adequate preoperative evaluation and optimization, the patient was taken up for surgery. On exploration, the tumor was found to infiltrate the middle of the common bile duct and there were enlarged periportal lymph nodes. She underwent an extended (radical) cholecystectomy encompassing extrahepatic biliary tract excision, with a margin-negative liver wedge excision and complete lymphadenectomy. Intraoperative frozen section examination confirmed negative proximal and distal biliary duct margins. Her postoperative recovery was uneventful. The final histopathology report showed residual viable moderately differentiated adenocarcinoma in a sclerotic stroma (tumor regression grade – 3/5) with liver infiltration. Liver and bile duct cut margins were negative, and one out of seven lymph nodes dissected showed viable tumor. The patient's cancer was finally staged—ypT3ypN1, stage IIIB (post-chemotherapy). She went on to complete three more cycles of gemcitabine and cisplatin, and remains disease-free on regular follow-up.

## Clinical dilemma

This patient had locally advanced gallbladder cancer with associated obstructive jaundice which is known to have poor prognosis.

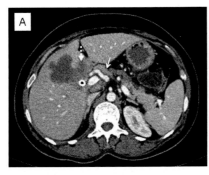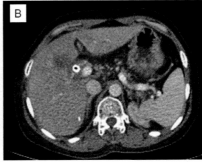

**Figure 29.2** Contrast-enhanced CT scan sections of the abdomen. (A) Pre-chemotherapy: Axial post-contrast image showing a gallbladder neck mass (dashed arrow) with liver infiltration and periportal LN (white arrow). (B) Pre-chemotherapy: Axial post-contrast image demonstrating a significant reduction in size of the tumor and lymph nodes suggestive of partial response to neoadjuvant chemotherapy.

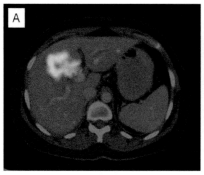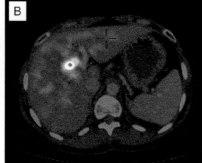

**Figure 29.3** Positron emission tomography CT images of the abdomen corresponding to Figure 29.2. (A) Pre-chemotherapy: Axial image showing metabolic activity in the gallbladder mass. (B) Post-chemotherapy: Axial image demonstrating a reduction in size of the tumor and extent of liver infiltration.

However, in the absence of distant metastases on positron emission tomography CT, an aggressive approach with the intent to cure was pursued. This Case Scenario highlights the need to consider treatment with a curative intent in well selected patients with locally advanced gallbladder cancer presenting with obstructive jaundice by employing the use of neoadjuvant chemotherapy.

### Discussion

Development of jaundice in patients with gallbladder cancer is considered an indicator of advanced disease and portends a poor prognosis. In a study by Hawkins et al., among 240 patients with gallbladder cancer, 34% presented with jaundice, and 96% of these jaundiced patients had advanced-stage disease. Only six (7%) jaundiced patients could be resected with curative intent, and only four (5%) had negative surgical margins. The median disease-specific survival in patients presenting with jaundice was six months and there were no disease-free survivors at two years [3]. These patients with advanced CAGB develop jaundice secondary to involvement of the bile duct or due to nodal disease pressing against the common bile duct. For higher blocks, relieving jaundice entails placement of a percutaneous transhepatic biliary drainage tube followed by stenting using a percutaneous or rendezvous technique. Conventional wisdom regarded presence of jaundice as a contraindication for surgical exploration. However, a number of recent reports have shown encouraging results especially for patients with an R0 resection and outcomes comparable to patients without jaundice. In a study evaluating 110 GBC patients with jaundice by Regimbeau et al. showed that the resectability was 45%, and the one- and three-year survival of these resected

patients was 48% and 19%, respectively, which was significantly higher than the unresectable population [4]. Hence, jaundice should not be considered as a contraindication to surgery and all jaundiced patient with gallbladder cancer should be assessed for curative intent treatment once metastatic disease has been ruled out with extensive staging workup.

The ABC 02 trial (Valle et al.) has demonstrated the benefit of gemcitabine in combination with Cisplatin in advanced biliary tract cancers. The use of palliative chemotherapy for advanced gallbladder cancer, and adjuvant chemotherapy for stage II and beyond, in curatively resected gallbladder cancers is well established. Neoadjuvant chemotherapy in patients with locally advanced gallbladder cancer is being increasingly evaluated, and a few retrospective studies have been published. Locally advanced gallbladder cancer remains a heterogeneous group of patients with a variety of disease extents and treatment intents. Our own experience with locally advanced gallbladder cancer led us to propose clinicoradiologic criteria (TMH criteria) to define locally advanced or borderline resectable gallbladder cancer. Disease spread beyond the gallbladder, T3/T4 disease, node positivity, jaundice, residual disease in incidentally detected gallbladder cancer patients were the factors used to identify patients at "high risk" of recurrence and possibly poor outcome. These patients were treated with neoadjuvant chemotherapy. Response rate and clinical benefit rate were 52.5% and 70%, respectively. A total of 41% of patients could undergo curative intent resection. Patients who underwent definitive surgery after favorable response to neoadjuvant chemotherapy experienced good survival [5]. The jury is still out, though, with regard to neoadjuvant chemotherapy and neoadjuvant chemotherapy with radiation therapy for locally advanced gallbladder cancer, as a systematic review by Hakeem et al. did not find any benefit of neoadjuvant chemotherapy or neoadjuvant chemotherapy with radiation therapy in advanced gallbladder cancer, since only one-third of these patients underwent an R0 resection [6]. The problem is that most studies club all biliary tract cancers together, despite the fact that they behave differently. The regimens which have shown the maximum benefit are gemcitabine/cisplatin or gemcitabine/oxaliplatin. Well planned studies with strict inclusion criteria focusing on gallbladder cancer alone, rather than clubbing all biliary tract cancers together, is needed to conclusively answer this question. Having said this, the use of neoadjuvant chemotherapy in patients with locally advanced gallbladder cancer deemed unresectable on initial evaluation, is worth considering. Chemotherapy may aid in better patient selection in terms of which patients should be offered a trial of surgery. In these patients, the use of staging laparoscopy is imperative before embarking on neoadjuvant chemotherapy as even positron emission tomography CT may miss peritoneal (metastatic) disease [1]. Surgery in these patients may likely culminate in extended resections with the attendant risk of morbidity. Hence, careful patient selection for treatment with curative intent remains the cornerstone of success.

## KEY MESSAGES

- Jaundice in the context of gallbladder cancer raises the concern for unresectable disease and poor outcomes. These patients warrant a detailed assessment to rule out metastatic disease.
- A small proportion of gallbladder cancer patients with jaundice may be amenable to treatment with a curative intent so long as the initial assessment conclusively rules out metastatic disease.
- In this select cohort of patients, neoadjuvant chemotherapy may be considered with a planned response evaluation. For patients who are locally advanced and unlikely to withstand chemotherapy, palliative options need to be considered.

- Endoscopic retrograde cholangiopancreatography with self-expanding metal stent or percutaneous transhepatic biliary drainage with stent are useful to reduce jaundice.
- If the disease demonstrates objective radiological response to neoadjuvant chemotherapy, then the role for surgery in high-volume hepatobiliary surgical centers merits consideration.
- Surgery is associated with an increased risk of morbidity and hence patient selection is of utmost importance.
- Surgery should be attempted if there is a realistic possibility of achieving a margin negative resection.
- There is no role for palliative or margin positive surgery in locally advanced gallbladder cancer.
- Neoadjuvant therapy needs to be studied prospectively in locally advanced gallbladder cancer in the setting of prospective controlled trials.

## REFERENCES

1. Shukla PJ, Barreto SG, Arya S et al. Does PET–CT scan have a role prior to radical re-resection for incidental gallbladder cancer? *HPB* 2008 Dec 1;10(6):439–445.
2. Shukla PJ, Neve R, Barreto SG et al. A new scoring system for gallbladder cancer (aiding treatment algorithm): An analysis of 335 patients. *Ann Surg Oncol* 2008 Nov 1;15(11):3132–3137.
3. Hawkins WG, DeMatteo RP, Jarnagin WR et al. Jaundice predicts advanced disease and early mortality in patients with gallbladder cancer. *Ann Surg Oncol* 2004;11(3):310–315.
4. Regimbeau JM, Fuks D, Bachellier P et al. Prognostic value of jaundice in patients with gallbladder cancer by the AFC-GBC-2009 study group. *Eur J Surg Oncol* 2011;37(6):505–512.
5. Chaudhari VA, Ostwal V, Patkar S et al. Outcome of neoadjuvant chemotherapy in "locally advanced/borderline resectable" gallbladder cancer: The need to define indications. *HPB* 2018 Sep 1;20(9):841–847.
6. Hakeem AR, Papoulas M, Menon KV. The role of neoadjuvant chemotherapy or chemoradiotherapy for advanced gallbladder cancer–A systematic review. *Eur J Surg Oncol* 2019 Feb 1;45(2):83–91.

# 30 Mid Common Bile Duct Cholangiocarcinoma Involving the Portal Vein and Right Branch of the Hepatic Artery

*Charles W. Kimbrough and Timothy M. Pawlik*

## CONTENTS

## CASE SCENARIO

A 58-year-old man presented to his primary physician with vague abdominal pain and new onset jaundice. Laboratory evaluation was remarkable for an elevation of the total bilirubin. Cross-sectional imaging showed both intrahepatic and extrahepatic biliary ductal dilation with a proximal common bile duct mass extending cephalad toward the hepatic hilum. The mass appeared to involve the main portal vein and right hepatic artery (Figure 30.1). Brushings obtained from endoscopic retrograde cholangiopancreatography confirmed adenocarcinoma. The patient was diagnosed with an extrahepatic cholangiocarcinoma and offered an extended right hepatectomy. On exploration, the tumor was noted to invade the main portal vein and required vein resection with primary reanastomosis. The right hepatic artery was divided close to the bifurcation and taken en bloc with the specimen. A lymphadenectomy was also performed. Pathology confirmed a 2.8 cm, moderately differentiated adenocarcinoma with local invasion into the portal vein and right hepatic artery; three out of six nodes had the presence of metastatic disease.

## BACKGROUND OF THE PATHOLOGY

Cholangiocarcinoma is a rare malignancy that arises from the biliary tract epithelium. Broadly speaking, these tumors can be classified as either intrahepatic or extrahepatic. Extrahepatic tumors can be further classified into perihilar or distal cholangiocarcinoma. Perihilar cholangiocarcinoma is the most common variant, and accounts for 50–60% of all cholangiocarcinomas. However, many tumors demonstrate microscopic extension up to 2 cm or more from the primary tumor, which can sometimes complicate exact classification. Given the tendency for aggressive infiltration, true mid-duct tumors are rare and are commonly managed as either distal or perihilar cholangiocarcinoma, depending upon both location and growth pattern.

Overall, cholangiocarcinoma accounts for approximately 3% of gastrointestinal malignancies. The incidence is relatively low among Western nations and is highest in Southeast Asia. The majority of tumors develop sporadically and most known risk factors are associated with chronic inflammation of the biliary tract. Primary sclerosing cholangitis represents a major risk factor in the West, as up to 20% of patients can develop cholangiocarcinoma. Additional risk factors include chronic choledocholithiasis, hepatolithiasis, choledochal cysts, parasitic liver flukes, and exposure to certain hepatotoxins. Cholangiocarcinoma is also linked to genetic disorders such as Lynch syndrome and biliary papillomatosis.

Historically, the diagnosis of cholangiocarcinoma carries a dismal prognosis, and surgery remains the only potentially curative therapy. Long-term outcomes are largely dependent on stage at presentation and the ability to achieve a margin-negative resection. Given the anatomic location and aggressive biology, only one-third of patients are resectable at presentation. Following surgery, risk factors associated with survival include resection margin status, nodal involvement, tumor differentiation, and vascular invasion. While overall survival among patients with unresectable disease is generally less than one year, patients with

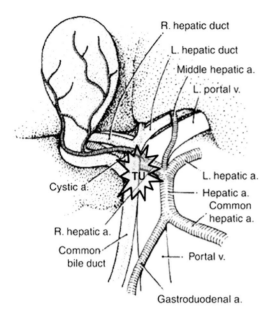

**Figure 30.1** Anatomy of the biliary tree and porta hepatis. The common bile duct, hepatic arteries, and portal vein run in close proximity within the porta hepatis. In this scenario, tumor (TU) arising from the mid bile duct invades both the right hepatic artery and main portal vein. (Adapted from: Weinberg J.A., Fabian T.C. (2015) Vascular Injuries of Porta Hepatis. In: Ivatury R. (eds) *Operative Techniques for Severe Liver Injury*. Springer, New York, NY.)

margin-negative resection and no evidence of lymph node involvement can have a five-year survival rate of up to 60%. As the only risk factor potentially controlled by surgeons, the impact of margin status underscores the importance of good surgical technique. Lymph node involvement reflects aggressive systemic disease, and five-year survival drops to approximately 20% among patients with nodal disease. Ultimately, three-quarters of patients will recur following surgery, including almost all patients with metastatic disease in the lymph nodes.

## CLINICAL FINDINGS

Most patients present with painless jaundice, with cholangitis being much less common. Biliary obstruction can also lead to pruritis, acholic stools, and dark urine. Other symptoms are usually non-specific and include anorexia, weight loss, vague abdominal pain, or fatigue. Elevated serum bilirubin and alkaline phosphatase levels will be present with biliary obstruction. While the tumor marker carbohydrate antigen 19-9 (CA 19-9) may also be elevated, it is not specific for cholangiocarcinoma and has

poor sensitivity to identify patients with early-stage, resectable disease. Ultimately, CA 19-9 is more helpful for surveillance after resection or as a prognostic biomarker.

## PREOPERATIVE INVESTIGATIONS

Patients suspected of cholangiocarcinoma require comprehensive and multidisciplinary evaluation. The evaluation entails determination of resectability, with careful consideration of anatomic, oncologic, and physiologic factors.

Anatomic resectability refers to the technical ability to achieve complete resection with microscopic margins. High quality imaging is essential to define the local extent of the tumor and its relationship to critical anatomic structures. Contrast-enhanced cross-sectional imaging using multidetector computed tomography (MDCT), magnetic resonance imaging (MRI), or magnetic resonance cholangiopancreatography (MRCP) is preferred to evaluate tumor extension and any vascular or biliary involvement. Compared with MDCT, MRI and MRCP may better demonstrate biliary infiltration but can be less indicative of vascular invasion. In addition to tumor features, careful attention should be given to imaging for any variations in native vascular and biliary anatomy.

Oncologic resectability refers to weighing the underlying tumor biology against both the morbidity and benefits expected from surgery. A full staging workup is necessary, as the presence of metastatic disease precludes operation in these patients. Careful review of imaging should also evaluate overall tumor burden, including subtle signs of peritoneal disease or lymphadenopathy. A subset of patients who undergo surgical exploration are ultimately not candidates for curative resection due to advanced disease that was not evident on imaging. To decrease the chance of unnecessary laparotomy, staging laparoscopy can be considered for selective use in patients at high risk for metastatic or unresectable disease.

Tissue diagnosis is not always required in patients when there is a high clinical suspicion for cholangiocarcinoma, although it may be pursued in instances of diagnostic uncertainty or when considering neoadjuvant therapy. Both endoscopic retrograde cholangiopancreatography and percutaneous transhepatic cholangiography provide biliary decompression, permit cholangiography to further delineate anatomy, and allow brushings or biopsies to assist diagnosis. Cytology from brushings can have a high false-negative rate and should be interpreted with caution, although accuracy can be increased with cytologic techniques including fluorescent in situ hybridization. Endoscopic ultrasound with fine-needle aspiration may be considered for any suspicious lymphadenopathy. Transperitoneal biopsy of extrahepatic lesions should be avoided in order to minimize the risk of peritoneal dissemination.

Physiologic resectability refers to a patient's ability to safely tolerate major surgery. Severe comorbidities, poor functional status, inadequate nutrition, or underlying liver disease may indicate that a patient will not tolerate major oncologic resection. In the case of hepatic resection for perihilar cholangiocarcinoma, patients must have adequate future liver remnant to avoid postoperative hepatic insufficiency. Most patients with normal liver function require a future liver remnant of at least 20%, but this may increase to 40–50% in cases of fibrosis/cirrhosis or chemotherapy-induced liver dysfunction. CT or MRI volumetry can be used to assess the future liver remnant preoperatively, while portal vein embolization is a common strategy to increase future liver remnant prior to resection. For jaundiced patients, preoperative biliary drainage improves coagulopathy and may decrease morbidity from hepatic surgery. Most surgeons recommend a maximum total bilirubin level of 2–4 mg/dL.

## APPROACH TO MANAGEMENT

A thorough understanding of the tumor's anatomic location and the relationship to critical structures dictates the operative approach. While distal cholangiocarcinoma is often managed with pancreaticoduodenectomy, more proximal or hilar lesions require hepatic resection (Table 30.1). The goal of curative resection is to achieve microscopically negative margins while maintaining vascular inflow/outflow, biliary-enteric drainage, and an adequate future liver remnant.

Historically, contraindications to hepatic resection included involvement of the main portal vein, bilateral involvement of the portal venous or hepatic arterial branches, extensive ductal spread with contralateral involvement of the vascular inflow, or bilateral involvement up to the second-order biliary radicals. However, advances in surgical technique have expanded the indications for resection in highly selected patients.

The standard strategy for hepatic resection entails either extended right or left hepatectomy with caudate lobectomy, en bloc resection of the extrahepatic bile duct, and portal lymphadenectomy. For perihilar tumors, the extent of hepatic resection is guided by the Bismuth-Corlette classification (Table 30.1). When necessary to achieve an R0 resection, evidence supports vascular resection in select patients. In one series of 305 patients, portal vein resection was performed in 15% of hepatic resections for perihilar cholangiocarcinoma. Although there was increased perioperative mortality with portal vein resection, long-term outcomes were similar to patients who underwent hepatectomy alone [1]. Additional studies support the role of portal vein resection in carefully selected patients, although hepatic artery resection and reconstruction remains more controversial [2]. In general, vascular resection is reserved for highly selected patients and should be performed by experienced surgeons in high-volume centers.

### Case scenario revisited

Applying these principles to the Case Scenario, an extended right hepatectomy with portal vein resection was performed for this tumor given its location in the porta hepatis. The surgical approach was similar to that described for a hilar en bloc resection (Figure 30.2) [3]. After

## Table 30.1 Surgical Approaches to Extrahepatic Cholangiocarcinoma

**Distal cholangiocarcinoma**

- Pancreaticoduodenectomy +/- extended extrahepatic bile duct resection with portal lymphadenectomy

**Perihilar cholangiocarcinoma**

*Bismuth-Corlette type I[#]*
- If small and isolated: Extrahepatic bile duct resection with portal lymphadenectomy and cholecystectomy (rarely performed)
- If tumor extends proximally: Partial hepatectomy
- If tumor extends distally: Pancreaticoduodenectomy

*Bismuth-Corlette type II*
- Standard hepatectomy with regional lymphadenectomy

*Bismuth-Corlette type IIIa*
- Extended right hepatectomy with regional lymphadenectomy

*Bismuth-Corlette type IIIb*
- Extended left hepatectomy with regional lymphadenectomy

*Bismuth-Corlette type IV*
- Right or left extended hepatectomy with regional lymphadenectomy
- Consider orthotopic liver transplantation if unresectable and meets criteria

# Mid common bile duct tumors can be managed similarly to Bismuth-Corlette type I tumors.

DILEMMAS IN ABDOMINAL SURGERY

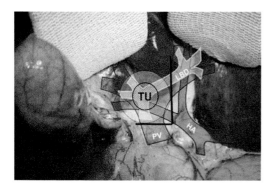

**Figure 30.2** Hilar en bloc resection. En bloc resection of the portal confluence with the resection margins marked by the bold black lines. (*Abbreviations:* HA – hepatic artery, PV – portal vein, LBD – left bile duct, TU – tumor.) (From: Neuhaus P, Thelen A, Jonas S, et al. Oncological superiority of hilar en bloc resection for the treatment of hilar cholangiocarcinoma. *Ann Surg Oncol.* 2012;19(5):1602–1608.)

laparotomy and confirmation of no metastatic disease, the right liver was mobilized with the right hepatic vein dissected and isolated. The proper hepatic artery was identified, and the right branch divided immediately beyond its origin. The distal extrahepatic bile duct was divided at the superior border of the pancreas. Retraction of the proper hepatic artery medially and elevation of the distal common

bile duct allowed exposure and dissection of the main portal vein (Figure 30.3A). The left portal vein was identified near the umbilical fissure and isolated, and both the left and main portal veins were controlled with clamps (Figure 30.3B). The main portal vein and left portal vein were divided, allowing the portal bifurcation to be removed en bloc with the specimen (Figure 30.3C). An end-to-end anastomosis was created between the left and main portal vein (Figure 30.3D), followed by parenchymal transection and removal of the specimen. Biliary enteric drainage was restored with a hepaticojejunostomy to the left hepatic duct.

While this tumor was amenable to an extended right hepatectomy, the right hepatic artery can also be involved with tumors arising from the left side of the porta hepatis. Given a similar scenario with vascular invasion from a perihilar tumor involving the left hepatic duct, resection via extended left hepatectomy has been reported. However this procedure remains controversial, as it requires simultaneous resection and reconstruction of the portal vein and right hepatic artery [4]. The left hepatic artery courses along the left border of the porta hepatis away from the biliary confluence, and is not as often invaded by tumor in patients who are candidates for resection.

### Adjuvant and neoadjuvant therapy

Even after margin-negative resection, cholangiocarcinoma is associated with high rates

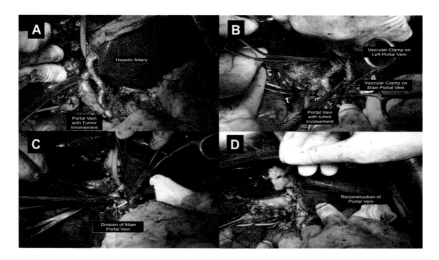

**Figure 30.3** Portal vein resection and reconstruction. (A) The main portal vein is clearly visualized with medial retraction on the proper hepatic artery and elevation of the distal common bile duct. (B) After identification of the left portal vein near the umbilical fissure, both the left and main portal veins are controlled with clamps. (C) Division of the left and main portal veins permits en bloc resection of the portal confluence. (D) Portal flow is restored with an end-to-end anastomosis between the left and main portal veins.

190

of locoregional and distant recurrence and adjuvant therapy should be considered. The National Comprehensive Cancer Network (NCCN) guidelines recommend adjuvant therapy for patients with gross residual disease (R2), microscopically positive margins (R1), or lymph node metastasis. Common regimens include fluoropyrimidine or gemcitabine-based chemotherapy, either alone or with fluoropyrimidine-based chemoradiation. Following results from the BILCAP-2 trial (NCT00363584), many patients now receive adjuvant capecitabine. While observation or adjuvant therapy are options for patients with node-negative disease and microscopically negative margins, patients should generally be referred to medical oncology for discussion of additional treatment.

Among patients with locally advanced disease, neoadjuvant chemotherapy may be considered. While the current role for neoadjuvant therapy in cholangiocarcinoma is not well defined, it may improve the rate of resection in patients who initially present with unresectable disease. There is little evidence to suggest that neoadjuvant therapy improves outcomes among patients with upfront resectable tumors.

## OTHER TREATMENT OPTIONS WITH BENEFITS AND RISKS
### Systemic therapy

In patients with unresectable locally advanced or metastatic disease, doublet therapy with gemcitabine and cisplatin is standard first-line chemotherapy on the basis of the ABC-02 trial (NCT00262769). With an improved understanding of the genetic drivers and molecular pathways involved in cholangiocarcinoma, newer targeted therapies, and immunotherapy options are being explored. All patients with advanced disease should be considered for enrollment in clinical trials in order to help develop new treatments.

### Role of transplantation

Liver transplantation is another potential strategy for unresectable perihilar cholangiocarcinoma. Careful patient selection is essential; patients with either intrahepatic or distal cholangiocarcinoma, distant metastases, or regional lymph node involvement are not eligible. Patients are generally subject to a rigorous evaluation and a strict treatment protocol, including a full course of neoadjuvant chemoradiation. Results for this heavily selected population are promising, with a five-year overall survival of 53%, and a five-year recurrence-free survival of 65% reported by the Mayo Clinic [5].

## KEY MESSAGES

- Cholangiocarcinoma is a rare malignancy of the biliary tract, and is associated with overall poor survival outcomes due to aggressive local infiltration and early systemic spread.
- Although cholangiocarcinoma represents a surgical challenge due to its aggressive nature and close proximity to critical structures, margin-negative resection provides the best opportunity for prolonged survival or cure.
- High-quality cross-sectional imaging is necessary to determine anatomic resectability and to guide surgical planning. Tissue diagnosis is not necessary when there exists a high index of suspicion in upfront resectable patients.
- Refinements in surgical technique have expanded indications to include complex vascular resection and reconstruction in highly selected patients. If complete resection is performed, overall survival in this population is comparable to patients without vascular involvement.
- Management requires a comprehensive multidisciplinary approach, as systemic chemotherapy, radiation, and even transplant are potential therapy options. Patients should be evaluated by high volume, experienced centers.

## REFERENCES

1. de Jong MC, Marques H, Clary BM et al. The impact of portal vein resection on outcomes for hilar cholangiocarcinoma: A multi-institutional analysis of 305 cases. *Cancer* 2012;118(19):4737–4747.
2. roeschl RT, Nagorney DM. Portal vein reconstruction during surgery for cholangiocarcinoma. *Curr Opin Gastroenterol* 2016;32(3):216–224.
3. Neuhaus P, Thelen A, Jonas S et al. Oncological superiority of hilar en bloc resection for the treatment of hilar cholangiocarcinoma. *Ann Surg Oncol* 2012;19(5):1602–1608.
4. Ebata T, Ito T, Yokoyama Y et al. Surgical technique of hepatectomy combined with simultaneous resection of hepatic artery and portal vein for perihilar cholangiocarcinoma (with video). *J Hepatobil Pancreat Sci* 2014;21(8):E57–E61.
5. Darwish Murad S, Kim WR, Harnois DM et al. Efficacy of neoadjuvant chemoradiation, followed by liver transplantation, for perihilar cholangiocarcinoma at 12 US centers. *Gastroenterology* 2012;143(1):88–98.

# PART 7

# LIVER

# 31 Hydatid Cyst of the Liver

*Rajeev M. Joshi, Murtaza Dadla, and Sandeep Sangale*

## CONTENTS

## CASE SCENARIO

A 55-year-old woman presented with complaints of intermittent abdominal pain over a period of seven months. She reported no fever, jaundice, or other systemic symptoms. On clinical examination, her vital parameters were normal, and a per-abdominal examination was unremarkable. Routine blood investigations were normal. An abdominal ultrasound revealed a large, well-defined cystic lesion in the right lobe of the liver with no septations or internal echoes. A contrast-enhanced CT scan of the abdomen demonstrated a $12 \times 7$ cm thin walled lesion in segment VIII of the liver with minimal wall calcification and no internal septations or solid components (Figure 31.1). Serum IgG levels for echinococcus antibodies were raised to twice the normal value. The patient was treated with oral albendazole 400 mg twice daily for a week. Following this, a laparoscopic cyst deroofing, evacuation, and omentoplasty was performed. She made an uneventful postoperative recovery. Oral albendazole was continued for a further five weeks. At six-months of follow-up, the patient remains recurrence free.

## BACKGROUND OF THE PATHOLOGY

*Echinococcus granulosus* and *Echinococcus multilocularis* (dog tape worm) infections are the most common parasitic diseases of the liver and are endemic in South America, Eastern Europe, the Middle East, Russia, and China [1]. Hydatid cyst of the liver is the most common type of hydatid cyst in humans. Dogs are the definitive hosts and sheep are the intermediate hosts (Figure 31.2). Humans are accidental dead-end intermediate hosts infected as a result of consumption of contaminated vegetables or water containing the larval stage of cestodes (flatworms) of genus *Echinococcus* and family *Taeniidae* (commonly called dog tapeworm). There is no human-to-human transmission.

With the liver being the first line of defense to portal circulation, 50–90% of the cysts occur here and are commonly seen in the right lobe (66%). Cysts may be encountered even on the left lobe (17%) or both lobes (16%). The next common site is the lungs (20–25%). Arterial system invasion (5–10%) and deposition in muscles (5%), bones (3%), kidneys, heart, brain, and spleen are rare [2].

A typical hydatid cyst appears within three weeks of infestation and by five months a mature cyst is formed. It grows at the rate of 1–1.5 mm per month and has three layers: The first, adventitia, or pericyst is the outermost thin, indistinct, inseparable fibrous tissue layer due to adventitial reaction of the liver to the parasitic infection. It helps in mechanical support and acts as a metabolic interface between host and parasite. It incorporates bile ducts and vessels in the wall as the cyst grows (which explains biliary and hemorrhagic complications associated with resection). As the cyst ages and dies, this layer calcifies and is diagnosed on ultrasound. The second, laminated membrane or ectocyst, is the outer layer formed by the parasite. It is 0.5 cm thick, bluish-white, gelatinous, elastic, and is made up of chitinous cuticular stratified cells. It can be peeled off readily from the adventitia and forms the basis for sub-adventitial cystectomy as a form of surgical treatment. The third, germinal epithelium

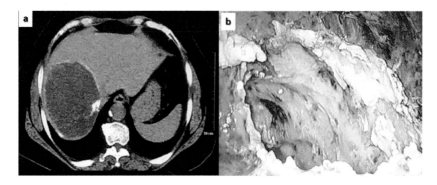

**Figure 31.1** Hydatid cyst of the liver. (a) Axial section of an abdominal CT scan demonstrating a cystic lesion with marginal calcification. (b) Intraoperative photograph depicting deroofing and cyst evacuation.

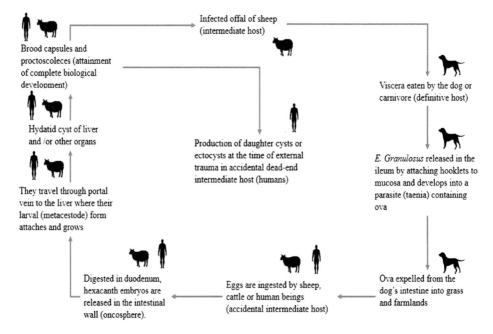

**Figure 31.2** Lifecycle of *Echinococcus Granulosus*.

or endocyst, is the only living part lining the cyst and secretes hydatid fluid, brood capsules with scolices, and is responsible for daughter cysts and ectocysts.

## CLINICAL FEATURES

Most hydatid cysts are asymptomatic (75%). In symptomatic patients, right upper quadrant and epigastric pain (85%), dyspepsia (39%), and vomiting (22%) are seen. The most common clinical signs are hepatomegaly or a palpable lump (46%), fever (8%), and jaundice (5%). Not so commonly, minor trauma can lead to an acute abdomen or anaphylaxis due to a traumatic rupture of the cyst.

The most common complication of a hydatid cyst is rupture which can be obscure (internal), free or communicant. Obscure rupture leads to multivesicular ectocyst formation and free rupture can be across peritoneal, pleural, or pericardial cavity. Intraperitoneal rupture can present as acute abdomen, anaphylactic reaction, or disseminated abdominal hydatidosis. Secondary echinococcosis in the peritoneal cavity causes abdominal distension, ascites, or intestinal obstruction gradually over years. Secondary cysts in the spleen, mesentery, retroperitoneum, and other organs may add to the symptoms. Intrathoracic rupture (0.6–16%) gives rise to an elevated hemidiaphragm and sterile pleural effusion. Empyema is rare. Rupture into a bronchiole may show daughter cysts in sputum and may form a bronchobiliary fistula. In cases of communicant rupture with the biliary radicles, a triad of biliary colic, cholangitis with obstructive jaundice, and germinative membrane in the feces may be seen. It can rupture into adjacent digestive tract (stomach) causing hydatidemesis or hydatidenteria. Hydatiduria is seen if the cyst ruptures in the urinary tract. Rupture into the blood vessels (inferior vena cave) is rare [3]. Leakage and cystobiliary communication are more commonly associated with a bacterial contamination of the cyst presenting as a pyogenic liver abscess (11–27%). Jaundice occurs due to cystobiliary communication or mass effect over biliary tree leading to portal hypertension, Budd-Chiari syndrome, and eventual liver failure due to parenchymal replacement.

## INVESTIGATIONS (ALGORITHM AS IN FIGURE 31.3)
### Blood investigations
Blood counts show eosinophilia in 35% of cases. Leucocytosis indicates superadded infection. Serum bilirubin more than 2 mg% or a raised alkaline phosphatase level with hypogammaglobulenemia may be seen.

### *Serological tests*
Infection induces an antibody response most commonly with IgG (IgG1 and IgG4), followed by IgM, IgA, and IgE. A total of 30-40% have no detectable antibody. Historically there has been an evolution from Casoni intradermal testing to the present-day enzyme-linked immunosorbent assay and indirect hemagglutination tests.

IgE: Enzyme-linked immunosorbent assay (results are positive in approximately 85% of infected patients) and radioallergosorbent tests. The enzyme-linked immunosorbent assay test results may be negative in an infected patient if the cyst has not leaked, does not contain scolices, or if the parasite is no longer viable.

Secondary laboratory tests include detection of precipitation line arc 5 in immunoelectrophoresis which is most specific and virtually diagnostic of hydatid disease. The sensitivity is 95% and specificity is 100%. Immunoblotting and polymerase chain reaction may be useful in extrahepatic hydatid disease and calcified, non-fertile liver hydatid.

### Imaging
The chest X-ray may demonstrate an elevated hemidiaphragm and concentric calcification in the cyst wall in 30% cases. Ultrasound has a specificity of 90% and is the primary imaging modality. A simple hydatid cyst appears as a well circumscribed hypodense lesion with budding signs on the cyst membrane and may contain free-floating hyperechogenic hydatid sand. A rosette appearance is seen when daughter cysts are present. They are more hypodense as compared to the mother cyst. A double contoured membrane of the cyst indicates detachment of the cyst membranes (floating membrane). Ring-like calcifications in the wall of the cyst are highly suggestive of hydatid disease and can help arrive at a diagnosis. The criteria for classification of hydatid liver cysts on ultrasound were first developed by *Gharbi et al* in 1981 and improved by the World Health Organization (WHO) in 2001 (WHO-IWGE) (Table 31.1) [4,5]. Ultrasound also helps in screening family members, planning treatment, intraoperative mapping, and in the postoperative follow-up.

CT scan is more specific than ultrasound in identifying the location of the abscess, its depth, the presence of daughter and exogenous cysts, and extrahepatic disease.

Magentic resonance imaging (MRI) of the abdomen may be useful in the evaluation of the subdiaphragmatic area and disseminated extra-abdominal involvement. It is specifically performed in patients who are jaundiced in order to visualize the biliary tree and its relation to the hydatid cyst. It permits the identification of cystobiliary communications or biliary hydatids.

Endoscopic retrograde cholangiopancreatography can identify cystobiliary communications. As a form of therapy, it can be used to drain the biliary tree before surgery or clear the common bile duct in the case of a rupture of cyst with obstructive jaundice due to plugging of the duct with scolices. It is also helpful in postoperative cases of a high output biliary fistula or a fistula lasting more than three weeks.

### Treatment

### Medical therapy
Commonly used antihelminthic agents are benzimidazoles (mebendazole and albendazole), having a success rate of 30% when used alone. Mebendazole is poorly absorbed and is inactivated by the liver. Albendazole is readily absorbed from the intestine and metabolized by the liver to an active form and is hence the drug of choice for medical therapy. The duration of therapy is at least four to six weeks, and should not exceed three months. WHO recommends albendazole to be given 4–30 days preoperatively and to continue for one month postoperatively.

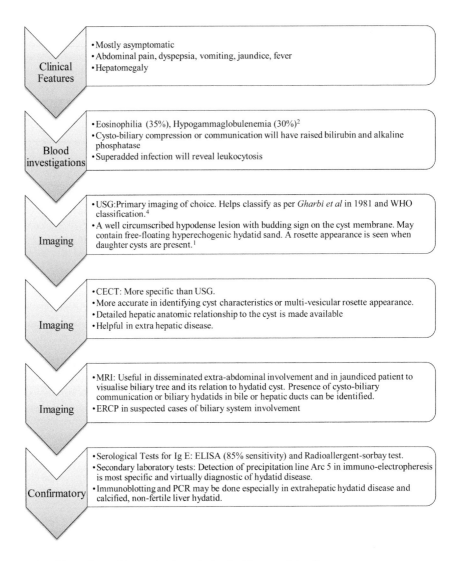

**Figure 31.3** Algorithm of investigations in hydatid cyst of the liver.

Indications for medical treatment include:

1) Small (less than 4 cm) uncomplicated cysts (CE1 and CE3a)

2) Deep-seated cyst

3) Densely calcific cyst

4) Extrahepatic manifestations of the disease

5) Alveolar form caused by *Echinococcus multilocularis*

6) Postoperative in case of spillage, partial cyst removal or biliary rupture

7) Widely disseminated disease

8) Moribund patients who are poor surgical candidates

### Percutaneous aspiration, injection, and reaspiration

Though not commonly used, the percutaneous aspiration, injection, and reaspiration technique may be indicated for unilocular and non-communicating cysts that are accessible percutaneously.

### Surgery

Hydatid disease of liver is the only parasitic disease for which the treatment is surgical. Surgical options are:

1) Conservative: Cyst deroofing and evacuation (open or laparascopic), drainage and/or obliteration of cavity (omentoplasty)

2) Radical resection: Cystopericystectomy or liver resection

## Table 31.1 Classification of Hydatid Cysts – A Comparison of the Gharbi versus the WHO Classification

| Gharbi | WHO | Description |
|---|---|---|
| | CL | Active, unilocular, no cyst wall, early stage, not fertile |
| I | CE 1 | Active, cyst wall present, hydatid sand present, fertile |
| III | CE 2 | Active, multivesicular rosette-like cyst wall, honeycombing present; fertile |
| II | CE 3a | Transitional, detaching laminated membrane, water-lily sign |
| III | CE 3b | Transitional, daughter cysts in solid matrix, beginning of degeneration |
| IV | CE 4 | Inactive, degenerative contents, no daughter cysts, not fertile |
| V | CE 5 | Inactive, thick calcified wall, not fertile |

In preparation for an operation, preoperative steroids are recommended. Epinephrine and steroids should be readily available in case of an anaphylactic reaction. During any surgical procedure on the hydatid cyst, caution must be exercised to avoid rupture of the cyst and resultant peritoneal dissemination of protoscolices. Peritoneal contamination can result in an acute anaphylactic reaction or peritoneal implantation of scolices with daughter cyst formation and inevitable recurrence. After gaining access to the abdomen, the area around the cyst should be isolated with packs soaked in 20% hypertonic saline (scolicidal agent). The cyst should be punctured and drained with due caution to avoid spillage of contents. This can be achieved by placing a purse-string suture and using a closed suction system. The membranes are then removed with a Rampley forcep. Once the cyst has been dealt with, a thorough search must be made for biliocystic communications and these should be overrun with sutures to prevent bile leaks postoperatively. The cyst cavity may then be obliterated using omentum.

Open cyst evacuation is safest with a recurrence rate of 10–30%, morbidity of 10–60%, and a mortality of 0–3%. Open surgery is preferred in multiple, central, or posterior cysts.

Radical procedures aim at complete removal of the cyst with or without hepatic resection. They are associated with greater intraoperative risks, but less frequent relapses. Pericystectomy involves complete resection of the cyst wall without entering the cyst cavity. A decreased risk of spillage and recurrence along with an increased risk of bleeding and bile duct injury is noted. Liver resection is excessive and unnecessary in most instances. It is indicated in cases where multiple cysts within proximity to a major blood vessel, cyst in segment II or III (relatively safe location), or in *Echinococcus multilocularis* involvement.

Laparoscopic management has gained ground despite the initial exaggerated fear of complications. It is indicated in peripheral or anteriorly placed cysts. Various techniques such as total pericystectomy, puncture and aspiration of contents, marsupialization, deroofing, drainage, and omentoplasty have been described. Recurrence rates of 0–10%, morbidity rates of 10–30%, and mortality rate less than 0.5% have been reported in expert hands. The most difficult part is the initial cyst puncture and aspiration of fluid. Palanivelu developed the Palanivelu hydatid system consisting of a complex system of fenestrated trocar and cannulas to avoid peritoneal spillage. The Palanivelu hydatid system not only prevents any spillage of hydatid fluid but also assists complete evacuation of the cyst content and allows intra-cystic magnified visualization for cystbiliary communication [2].

In summary, surgery maintains its place as the treatment of choice in patients with complicated hydatid cysts (rupture, cystobiliary fistulas, compression of vital organs and vessels, hemorrhage, and secondary bacterial infection). In uncomplicated cysts, a trial of medical therapy should be considered before embarking on surgery [2].

### KEY MESSAGES

- Hydatid cyst of the liver is a complex, dynamic disease with each successive active cyst stage carrying its own risks and even life-threatening complications.
- Although largely asymptomatic and detected incidentally, a variety of symptom complex from chronic and subacute to an acute presentation can occur.
- Ultrasound with serology helps clinch the diagnosis. CT scan is more specific than ultrasound in identifying location, depth, daughter, and exogenous cyst and is also helpful in extrahepatic disease.

- Treatment includes surgery in conjunction with pharmacotherapy, with oral albendazole being the drug of choice.
- For complex manifestations, no "one size fits all" approach is to be adopted, and a stage-specific and resource-specific approach is necessary.

## REFERENCES

1. Brunetti E, Kern P, Vuitton DA. Expert consensus for the diagnosis and treatment of cystic and alveolar Echinococcosis in humans. *Acta Tropica* 2010 Apr 1;114(1):1–6.
2. Anand S, Rajagopalan S, Mohan R. Management of liver hydatid cysts–Current perspectives. *Med J Armed Forces India* 2012 Jul;68(3):304.
3. Akgun V, Battal B, Karaman B et al. Pulmonary artery embolism due to a ruptured hepatic hydatid cyst: Clinical and radiologic imaging findings. *Emergency Radiol* 2011 Oct 1;18(5):437.
4. Vuitton DA. The WHO Informal Working Group on Echinococcosis. Coordinating board of the WHO-IWGE. *Parassitologia* 1997 Dec;39(4):349–353.
5. Meeting of the WHO Informal Working Group on Echinococcosis (WHO-IWGE) WHO headquarters, Geneva, Switzerland, 15–16 December 2016. https://www.who.int/echinococcosis/resources/WHO_HTM_NTD_NZD_2017.01/en/.

# 32 Pyogenic Liver Abscess

*Rajeev M. Joshi, Murtaza Dadla, and Sandeep Sangale*

## CONTENTS

## CASE SCENARIO

A 50-year-old man with a history of chronic alcohol abuse presented with right upper abdominal pain and intermittent fever for two weeks. He was offered symptomatic treatment by his family physician which settled the fever. However, the pain persisted and so he presented to the emergency department. At initial assessment, his vital parameters were within normal limits and his respiratory system was normal on auscultation. His abdomen was generally soft but tender in the right hypochondrium. There was no discernible organomegaly.

His white cell count was 31,000/mm$^3$ with normal liver function tests and coagulation profile. His chest x-ray was normal. However, an abdominal ultrasound revealed a solitary 10 × 10 × 8 cm hypoechoic loculated fluid collection in the right lobe of the liver, and so a computed tomography (CT) scan of the abdomen was performed to better characterize the lesion. The contrast-enhanced CT scan (CECT) of the abdomen confirmed a 12 × 10 × 10 cm hypoattenuated lesion with peripheral enhancement in the right lobe of the liver suggestive of a liver abscess.

Since the collection was predominantly liquefied on ultrasound, intravenous antimicrobial therapy followed by ultrasound-guided percutaneous drainage with a pigtail catheter was carried out. The patient responded well to this combination of antibiotics and radiological intervention.

## BACKGROUND OF THE PATHOLOGY

The liver is exposed to portal venous bacteria on a regular basis and usually clears this bacterial load by the action of the Kupffer cells. Abscesses occur when normal hepatic clearance mechanisms fail, the system is overwhelmed, or when an inoculum of bacteria, regardless of the route of exposure, exceeds the liver's ability to clear it, resulting in tissue invasion, neutrophil infiltration, and the formation of an organized abscess. Amebic and pyogenic are the commonest types of liver abscesses. Rarer forms include tuberculosis and fungal abscesses. Amebic abscess is usually solitary while pyogenic abscesses can be multiple. The potential routes of spread of infection to the liver include the biliary tree, portal vein, hepatic artery, or direct extension from a nearby source of infection and trauma. In recent decades, the predominant etiology of pyogenic liver abscess has changed from pylephlebitis to a biliary origin.

Biliary obstruction results in bile stasis with the potential for subsequent bacterial colonization, infection, and ascending infection into the liver. Bilioenteric anastomoses (by virtue of causing ascending cholangitis), trauma, and biliary instrumentation (percutaneous or endoscopic) biliary procedures can lead to pyogenic liver abscesses. In Asia, intrahepatic biliary stones and cholangitis are common causes while in the West, malignant obstruction is the predominant cause. Any infectious disease of the gastrointestinal tract can result in liver abscess. The most common causes of pylephlebitis are diverticulitis, appendicitis, pancreatitis, inflammatory bowel disease, pelvic inflammatory disease, perforated viscus, and omphalitis in newborn. Systemic infections such as infective endocarditis, pneumonia, or osteomyelitis may also lead to bacteremia and seeding of infection into the liver via the hepatic artery. Direct extension includes suppurative cholecystitis, subphrenic abscess, perinephric abscess, and perforation of the bowel directly into the liver [1].

Fungal liver abscesses are uncommon. They are usually diagnosed in immunocompromised patients and are due to *Candida albicans* infection. Liver abscesses may follow radiofrequency ablation as a result of thermal injury to the bile duct with resultant bacterial contamination and growth in the zone of coagulation necrosis.

HIV/AIDS and organ transplant have led to a new patient population at risk for liver infections [1].

The most common organisms cultured are *Escherichia coli* and *Klebsiella pneumoniae*. Other organisms encountered are *Staphylococcus aureus, Enterococcus* sp., *Streptococci viridans,* and *Bacteroides* [2].

## CLINICAL PRESENTATION

The patient with a pyogenic liver abscess can present with fever and abdominal pain, although symptoms can include a broad range of complaints ranging from nausea and vomiting to malaise and weight loss.

Jaundice may be the first and only clinical manifestation of the disease. Apart from jaundice, physical examination may show tender hepatomegaly in about 50% of cases. Less commonly, patients may present with cough, hiccups, or referred right shoulder tip pain due to diaphragmatic irritation.

Comorbid conditions associated with pyogenic abscess are cirrhosis, diabetes, chronic renal failure, and a history of malignant disease. Appropriate treatment of these conditions is necessary.

Up to 40% of patients develop complications from pyogenic liver abscesses which include generalized sepsis, pleural effusions, empyema, and pneumonia. Rarely, abscesses may rupture intraperitoneally, which may result in fatality. More commonly, the abscess does not rupture but develops a controlled leak, resulting in a perihepatic abscess. Pyogenic abscesses may also cause hemobilia and hepatic vein thrombosis. Rarely, liver abscess can rupture into the thoracic cavity and even lead to the formation of hepatobronchial fistulae.

The unique characteristic of *Klebsiella pneumoniae* liver abscess is its potential for septic metastatic infection, which may present as endophthalmitis, pulmonary septic emboli, meningitis, or septic arthritis [2].

## INVESTIGATIONS
### Blood tests

Leucocytosis is present in 70–90% of patients along with normocytic anemia. Abnormalities in liver function tests include hypoalbuminemia, coagulopathy, and elevated transaminase with or without an elevation in the alkaline phosphatase and even serum bilirubin levels [3].

### Imaging

A chest X-ray may show an elevated hemidiaphragm, pleural effusion, atelectasis, or right lobar consolidation. However, it is normal in over 50% of patients (as was seen in our patient).

Abdominal ultrasound and CT scan are the mainstay in terms of diagnostic modalities, and tend to complement each other. On an ultrasound, a pyogenic liver abscess appears as a round or oval cavity that is hypoechoic in comparison to the surrounding liver parenchyma. The sensitivity of ultrasound in diagnosing liver abscesses approaches 80–95% [1]. An abdominal CECT scan (Figure 32.1) helps with diagnosis in determining the size of the abscess, and guides management. It also helps to rule out other differential diagnoses. In patients with monomicrobial *Klebsiella pneumoniae* abscesses, the lesion may appear solid and mimic a hepatic tumor [2].

In patients with a liver abscess and jaundice (supported with deranged liver function tests), additional imaging such as magnetic resonance cholangiopancreatography (MRCP) may help confirm, or rule out, a communication between the abscess cavity and the biliary tree.

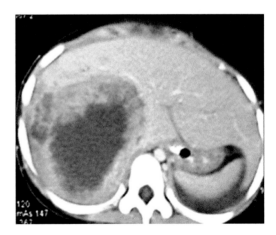

**Figure 32.1**  Axial CECT scan of the abdomen showing a large hypoattenuated lesion with rim enhancement in the right lobe of liver.

The differentiation of a pyogenic from an amebic abscess is assisted by amebic serology (indirect hemagglutination and gel diffusion precipitin) being negative and blood culture being positive in a pyogenic abscess. Performance of Gram staining on the percutaneous aspirate (see below) from the abscess cavity will demonstrate polymorphonuclear leucocytes and bacteria in pyogenic abscess, unlike in amebic abscess where the pus is sterile.

## TREATMENT

Survival from pyogenic liver abscess was rare before the turn of the century, with open drainage being the main stay of therapy. Improvement in therapeutic modalities over the years has helped reduce the case-fatality rate for this disease to 5–30% [3].

Treatment of most hepatic abscesses involves a combination of pharmacotherapy and percutaneous image-guided drainage (Figure 32.2).

Broad-spectrum intravenous antibiotics should be started immediately to control ongoing bacteremia and its associated complications. Blood samples and specimens of the abscess from aspiration should be sent for aerobic and anaerobic cultures. The optimal duration of antibiotic treatment is not well defined and must be individualized, depending on the success of the drainage procedure. Recommendations include parenteral therapy for two to three weeks or until there is a favorable clinical response, followed by an oral regimen for two to six weeks. Active liaising with the infectious disease unit is warranted to avoid the risk of development of antibiotic resistance. The antibiotic therapy should consist of a combination of a third generation of cephalosporin or an aminoglycoside with either metronidazole or clindamycin [3]. Antibiotic therapy alone, may be adequate in patients who are systemically well and who have a

solitary, or micro abscesses smaller than 2 cm in diameter.

Percutaneous drainage along with targeted antimicrobial therapy is the accepted treatment modality in most patients. Criteria for percutaneous drainage includes abscess size >4 cm, ongoing pyrexia despite 48–72 hours of appropriate medical therapy and clinical, or imaging features suggestive of impending rupture. Continuous percutaneous catheter drainage is more efficient than intermittent percutaneous needle aspiration. Intermittent percutaneous needle aspiration is reserved for small abscesses. Endoscopic drainage by endoscopic retrograde cholangiopancreatography can cure pyogenic liver abscess in selected patients with abscesses due to bile duct stones or strictures, by facilitating biliary drainage.

Indications for surgery (open or laparoscopy) includes abscess rupture, uncorrected primary pathology (e.g. pylephlebitis due to an unresolved enteric infection), abscesses that are inaccessible to percutaneous drainage, multiloculated abscesses, and inadequate clinical response after four to seven days of percutaneous drainage where the diagnosis is in doubt (Figure 32.3).

In case of non-responders, one must consider alternative diagnoses, such as a hepatic malignancy or chronic granulomatous diseases like tuberculosis or sarcoidosis, and an attempt should be made to further investigate the patient and obtain a tissue diagnosis.

## LIVER ABSCESS IN SPECIAL CLINICAL SITUATIONS

### *Klebsiella pneumoniae* liver abscess

It has been reported as the leading cause of pyogenic liver abscess in Southeast Asia and is described as a globally emerging infectious disease. Monomicrobial cryptogenic invasive *Klebsiella pneumoniae*-associated liver abscess syndrome typically affects diabetic patients and alcoholics along with healthy individuals and is complicated by involvement of other organs such as the eyes, lungs, brain, and joints. The outcome is good but requires prolonged hospitalization, and after successful treatment the recurrence rate is reported to be low. After successful treatment, the recurrence rate of *Klebsiella pneumoniae* liver abscesses is reported to be low [2].

## PYOGENIC LIVER ABSCESS FOLLOWING TRANSARTERIAL CHEMOEMBOLIZATION OR RADIOFREQUENCY ABLATION

Abscess formation is a serious complication of transarterial chemoembolization and

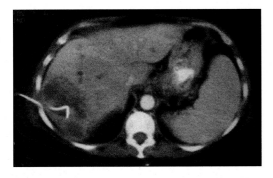

**Figure 32.2** Axial section of a CT scan of the abdomen demonstrating a pigtail in situ placed for the drainage of a liver abscess.

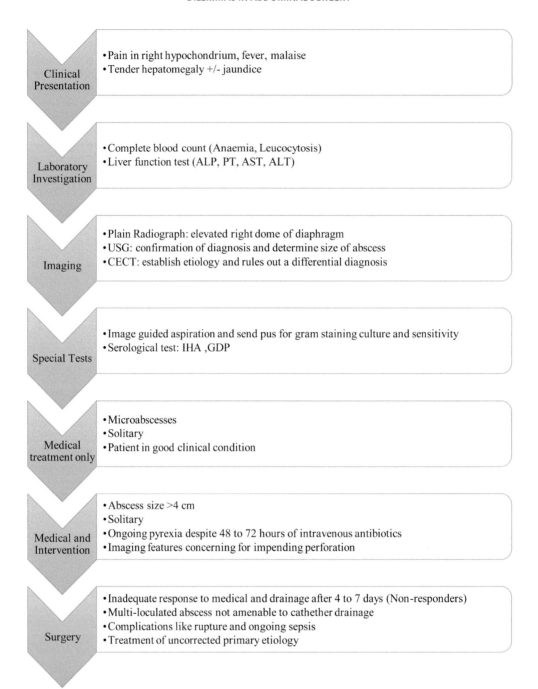

**Clinical Presentation**
- Pain in right hypochondrium, fever, malaise
- Tender hepatomegaly +/- jaundice

**Laboratory Investigation**
- Complete blood count (Anaemia, Leucocytosis)
- Liver function test (ALP, PT, AST, ALT)

**Imaging**
- Plain Radiograph: elevated right dome of diaphragm
- USG: confirmation of diagnosis and determine size of abscess
- CECT: establish etiology and rules out a differential diagnosis

**Special Tests**
- Image guided aspiration and send pus for gram staining culture and sensitivity
- Serological test: IHA ,GDP

**Medical treatment only**
- Microabscesses
- Solitary
- Patient in good clinical condition

**Medical and Intervention**
- Abscess size >4 cm
- Solitary
- Ongoing pyrexia despite 48 to 72 hours of intravenous antibiotics
- Imaging features concerning for impending perforation

**Surgery**
- Inadequate response to medical and drainage after 4 to 7 days (Non-responders)
- Multi-loculated abscess not amenable to cathether drainage
- Complications like rupture and ongoing sepsis
- Treatment of uncorrected primary etiology

**Figure 32.3** Algorithm of the management of a pyogenic liver abscess. (*Abbreviations:* ALP – alkaline phosphatase, PT – prothrombin time, AST – aspartate transaminase, ALT – alanine transaminase, USG – ultrasonography, CECT – contrast-enhanced computed tomography, IHA – indirect hemagglutination assay, GDP – gel diffusion precipitin assay.)

radiofrequency ablation. Reported incidence of liver abscess following transarterial chemoembolization is 0.3–2.7%, and following radiofrequency ablation is 0.6–2.4% [4]. Incidence is high in metastatic neuroendocrine tumors and sarcomas. Time to abscess formation varies from within the first few days to up to eight weeks after transarterial chemoembolization or after radiofrequency ablation. The diagnosis may be challenging because fever can be a confounding factor – more often due to post-ablation syndrome. Percutaneous aspiration or drainage remains the treatment of choice. Prophylactic use of antibiotics, including prolonged use in high-risk patients, is recommended [4].

## LIVER ABSCESS AND LIVER TRANSPLANT

Infections occurring during the first month post-liver transplant are usually nosocomial, donor-derived infections, or the result of systemic immunosuppression or perioperative complications (hepatic artery thrombosis). During the highly intense period of immunosuppression (one to six months) opportunistic infections such as Aspergillus, cytomegalovirus, and reactivation of latent infections such as *Mycobacterium tuberculosis* are more frequent [5]. The diagnosis may be delayed since immunosuppressive therapy diminishes inflammatory responses and so clinical signs of infection may be blunted or absent. Preventive strategies are awareness of potential transmissions in donor evaluation process, comprehensive workup for pretransplant infectious diseases, and immunizations.

## PROGNOSIS

With modern treatment approaches, the prognosis depends more on the underlying etiology and comorbidities rather than the pyogenic liver abscess itself, although delay in presentation and diagnosis contribute to a poor outcome. Risk factors for an adverse outcome are presence of acute respiratory failure on the first day of ICU admission, septic shock, raised bilirubin levels (> 3.5 mg/dL), coagulopathy, encephalopathy, hepatobiliary malignancy, and immunocompromised status. Complications like multiple abscesses or large volume abscess cavity and intraperitoneal rupture add to the morbidity and mortality rates.

## KEY MESSAGES

- Most liver abscesses are bacterial (80–90%), other causes are amebic, fungal, and tuberculosis.
- Portal bacteremia was a common cause up until 50–60 years ago. Biliary causes have since dominated with a rising trend in iatrogenic abscesses.
- There is a high mortality (10–15%) in patients with high-risk factors. However, the overall prognosis is good due to appropriate treatment modalities.
- Percutaneous drainage and pharmacotherapy are the mainstay of treatment. Surgery is only indicated in complicated cases and in patients who do not respond to the more conservative options.

## REFERENCES

1. Johannsen EC, Sifri CD, Madoff LC. Pyogenic liver abscesses. *Infec Dis Clinics North Am* 2000 Sep 1;14(3):547–563.
2. J Tsai FC, Huang YT, Chang LY et al. Pyogenic liver abscess as endemic disease, Taiwan. *Emerging Infect Dis* 2008 Oct;14(10):1592.
3. Heneghan HM, Healy NA, Martin ST et al. Modern management of pyogenic hepatic abscess: A case series and review of the literature. *BMC Res Notes* 2011 Dec;4(1):80.
4. Su XF, Li N, Chen XF et al. Incidence and risk factors for liver abscess after thermal ablation of liver neoplasm. *Hepatitis Monthly* 2016 Jul;16(7):e34588.
5. Justo I, Jiménez-Romero C, Manrique A et al. Management and outcome of liver abscesses after liver transplantation. *World J Surgery* 2018 Oct 1;42(10):3341–3349.

# 33 Hepatocellular Carcinoma

## 10 cm Lesion in a Child-Pugh Class A Cirrhotic Patient

*Masakazu Yamamoto and Shun-ichi Ariizumi*

## CONTENTS

## CASE SCENARIO

An 83-year-old man presented with a 10 cm hepatocellular carcinoma in the right liver. He underwent right partial resection of the lung for lung cancer in 1999 and transurethral resection of a bladder tumor (TUR-Bt) in 2013. He was followed-up for alcoholic liver cirrhosis at a department of gastroenterology. In 2015, he underwent radiofrequency ablation therapy for hepatocellular carcinoma 2 cm in diameter in segment 6. A local recurrence 3.7 cm in diameter was detected in August 2018. He underwent transarterial chemoembolization in October 2018 because he had concomitant aortic valve stenosis, renal dysfunction, and chronic obstructive pulmonary disease, and was therefore given an assessment of the American Society of Anesthesiologists (ASA) classification of 3 by anesthesiologists. However, the tumor increased in size, and he underwent transarterial chemoembolization again in March 2019. Tumor markers increased after the second transarterial chemoembolization and the patient was referred to our surgical department.

## BACKGROUND

Most hepatocellular carcinomas develop in persons with liver cirrhosis; therefore, liver function has to be considered in planning treatments for patients with hepatocellular carcinoma. The Barcelona Clinic Liver Cancer treatment algorithm recommends that surgery is the most suitable treatment for very early and early hepatocellular carcinoma patients with Child-Pugh A/B; however, liver transplantation is recommended for patients with Child-Pugh C and Milan criteria of one lesion ≤5 cm or two to three lesions not exceeding 3 cm [1]. Indocyanine green retention rate at 15 minutes (ICG-R15) has been used for evaluating liver function in Japan for over 30 years. ICG-R15 is applied in the Japanese Clinical Guidelines for hepatocellular carcinoma by the Japanese Society of Hepatology.

Makuuchi proposed that normal serum bilirubin levels and normal ICG-R15 are required for major hepatectomy by his criteria. However, abnormal ICG-R15 is often noted in patients with hepatocellular carcinoma and liver cirrhosis. This constitutes a dilemma for major hepatectomy when a patient has a large hepatocellular carcinoma in a cirrhotic liver. Makuuchi's criteria guarantee definite safety after hepatectomy; therefore, the criteria sometimes do not match the actual clinical setting. Takasaki reported on the prediction of the remnant liver function using ICG-R15 [2]. Takasaki's log table made it possible to calculate the allowable hepatic resection volume using ICG-R15.

Figure 33.1 shows a logarithmic graph for the allowable hepatic resection based on the ICG-R15. In cases with clinical cirrhosis, a postoperative ICG-R15 of 40% has to be preserved to avoid liver failure because ICG-R15 of 40% indicates severe liver dysfunction. The ICG-R15 12% point on the X vertical axis is connected by a solid line to the 100% point on the Y vertical axis. The line drawn vertically from the intersection of the solid line and the 40% point of the Y vertical axis indicate that the maximum allowable hepatic resection is 58%. Likewise, in cases without clinical cirrhosis and preoperative ICG-R15 of 10%, the allowable hepatic resection is 70%. We have performed over 5,000 hepatectomies with Takasaki's remnant liver function prediction, resulting in postoperative liver failure in less than 1% of cases. Takasaki's prediction of future remnant liver function using ICG-R15 is more attractive and practical in liver surgery [2]. A new 3D software program (Synapse Vincent, Fujifilm Co., Japan)

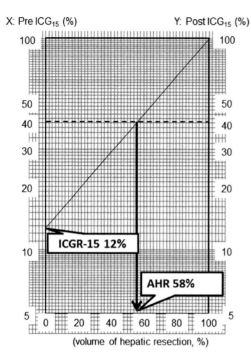

X: Pre ICG$_{15}$ (%)   Y: Post ICG$_{15}$ (%)

(volume of hepatic resection, %)

ICGR-15 12%

AHR 58%

**Figure 33.1** The allowable hepatic resection volume was 58% by Takasaki's log table if the future ICG-R15 in the remnant liver was predicted to be less than 40%.

with multidetector computed tomography (MDCT) provides not only the hepatic anatomy but also precise evaluation of the liver resection volume for hepatectomy [3]. ICG-R15 and volumetry by the new software program are mandatory for precise evaluation of the predicted remnant liver.

Oncological aspects should also be considered. The incidence of portal vein invasion and intrahepatic metastasis of hepatocellular carcinoma increases with increasing tumor size. Therefore, surgery is sometimes avoided for patients with huge hepatocellular carcinoma with portal vein invasion and multiple intrahepatic metastases. However, favorable outcomes have been reported in patients with hepatocellular carcinoma over 10 cm in diameter without portal vein invasion nor intrahepatic metastasis. The five-year survival after surgery for single hepatocellular carcinoma over 10 cm in diameter was reported to be 79% [4]. Therefore, surgery should be considered even if the tumor size is larger than 10 cm in diameter if the patient's condition is suitable for surgery.

## APPROACH TO MANAGEMENT
The patient's general condition, blood chemistry tests, Child-Pugh grade, and ICG-R15 are assessed before surgery. ICG-R15 is the most

valuable test for evaluating liver function; however, there is some discrepancy between ICG-R15 and other blood chemistry tests which reflect liver function. If patients have abnormal ICG-R15 levels exceeding 70–80%, and normal serum albumin levels and coagulation tests, we have to consider the possibility of constitutional ICG excretory defect. Therefore, we should always check ICG-R15 and other blood chemistry tests and coagulation tests which reflect liver function. Tumor markers such as alpha fetoprotein and protein induced by vitamin K absence or antagonists-II (PIVKA-II) should be checked before surgery to consider oncological aspects. MDCT is performed to construct 3D images of the vessels in the liver. Magnetic resonance imaging (MRI) is performed to check for intrahepatic metastasis and portal vein invasion. The allowable hepatic resection is determined with a logarithmic graph based on ICG-R15. The hepatic resection volume excluding volume of tumors is measured using 3D-CT. Perioperative risks are predicted according to the novel National Clinical Database risk calculator. Anesthetists always check the patient's preoperative condition and assess the ASA class. High-risk control meetings and cancer board meetings are held before surgery.

## CLINICAL FINDINGS
The patient was older than 80 years with comorbidities. Therefore, previous gastroenterologists did not recommend surgery. However, treatment of hepatocellular carcinoma with radiofrequency ablation and transarterial chemoembolization failed, and the size of the tumor and the tumor marker levels increased after treatment. Fortunately, the tumor did not have intrahepatic metastasis or portal vein invasion at the time of referral to our department. The patient was therefore investigated further. Blood chemistry test results were: hepatitis B antigen negative, hepatitis C virus antibody negative, hemoglobin level 12 mg/dL, platelet 14.3 10⁻4/μL, prothrombin time 76.9%, total bilirubin level 0.9 mg/dL, albumin level 3.3 g/dL, AST 31 U/L, ALT 59 U/L, creatinine 1.06 mg/dL, alpha fetoprotein 26067 ng/dl, PIVKA-II 1367 mAU/ml. Child-Pugh class was evaluated as A (point 6) and ICG-R15 12%. MDCT showed a 10 cm hepatocellular carcinoma in the right liver. The tumor was attached to the right hepatic vein and the right anterior portal vein (Figure 33.2). There was neither intrahepatic metastases nor portal vein tumor thrombus. According to 3D-CT, the right liver volume without the tumor was 434 ml and the remnant left liver volume was 333 ml. The hepatic resection volume

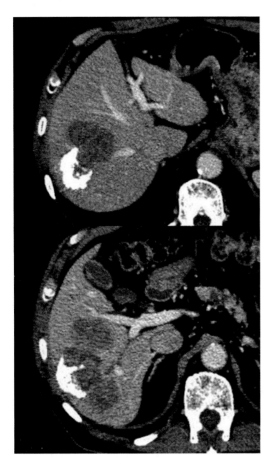

**Figure 33.2** CT showed a 10 cm hepatocellular carcinoma attached to the right hepatic vein and the right anterior portal vein.

was 57% (Figure 33.3). The allowable hepatic resection was 58% by Takasaki's log table if the future ICG-R15 in the remnant liver was predicted to be less than 40% (Figure 33.1). Portal vein embolization before surgery does therefore not need to be considered. The patient underwent right hepatectomy in April 2019 (Figure 33.4) and he was discharged from the hospital on the 14th day after surgery without complications. The macroscopic findings showed a 10 cm hepatocellular carcinoma (Figure 33.5) and the pathological findings yielded a diagnosis of poorly differentiated hepatocellular carcinoma with liver cirrhosis.

## FACTORS TO BE CONSIDERED WITH LARGE TUMORS

Liver function is a very important factor in considering the operative procedure. However, if a tumor in the liver exceeds 10 cm in diameter, major hepatectomy can be considered in most cases. Makuuchi's criteria do not recommend major hepatectomy for the patient presented in our clinical scenario because the ICG-R15 was over 10%. However, Makuuchi's criteria do not consider the resected liver volume. If a large hepatocellular carcinoma is present in the whole resected liver, major hepatectomy can be performed with ICG-R15 over 10%. Therefore, we should assess the volume of the liver considering the tumor volume when the tumor is large. This is a very important message regarding major hepatectomy.

The incidence of portal vein invasion and intrahepatic metastasis increases with

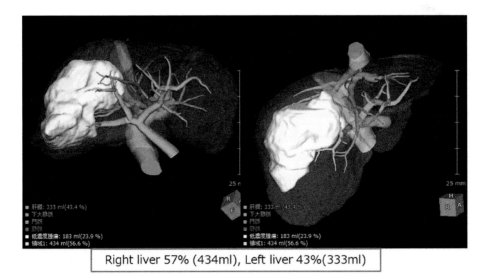

Right liver 57% (434ml), Left liver 43%(333ml)

**Figure 33.3** 3D-CT scan showed the volume of the right liver without the tumor to be 434 mL or 57% of the whole liver.

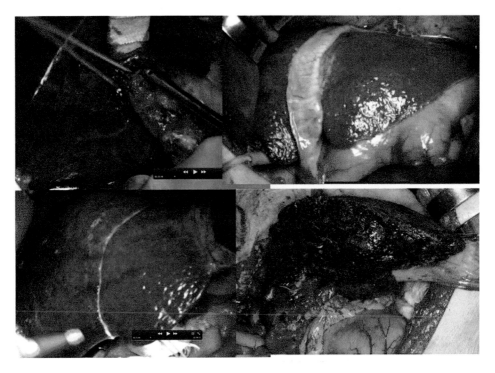

**Figure 33.4**  Right hepatectomy was performed with the extrahepatic Glissonean pedicle approach. The operation time was 2 hours and 30 minutes and the blood loss was 900 g.

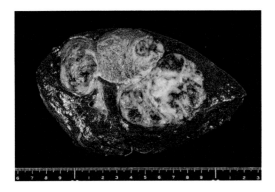

**Figure 33.5**  The cut surface of the specimen showed a 10 cm hepatocellular carcinoma with liver cirrhosis.

increasing tumor size. However, several articles reported favorable surgical outcomes in patients with solitary hepatocellular carcinoma even if the tumor size exceeds 10 cm in diameter [4]. Macroscopic findings of a solitary tumor without portal vein invasion may reflect a good tumor progression like that of a benign tumor. These are some other reasons why surgery need not be abandoned even if the tumor size exceeds 10 cm in diameter.

## TREATMENT OPTIONS

The Barcelona Clinic Liver Cancer treatment algorithm recommends treatments in consideration of performance status, Child-Pugh class, tumor number, portal vein invasion, and tumor size. Surgery is the first option for a single hepatocellular carcinoma with good liver function without considering tumor size. The algorithm does not consider the patient's age, comorbidity, or future remnant liver function after surgery [1]. If surgery is not suitable, transarterial chemoembolization, radiofrequency ablation, and liver transplantation should be considered. However, radiofrequency ablation and transarterial chemoembolization were not effective for this patient, and liver transplantation could not be selected due to the patient's age and the Milan criteria; therefore, external beam radiation therapy and systemic therapy should be considered. Median survival has improved by several months by systemic therapy with Sorafenib and other multikinase inhibitors. However, systemic therapy sometimes cannot be used because of severe side effects and its expensive cost. If hepatocellular carcinomais localized without metastasis, radiation therapy should be considered as another option. There is a lack of evidence of radiation therapy for large hepatocellular carcinoma; however, stereotactic body radiation therapy and proton beam therapy have been reported in patients unsuitable for other established local therapies [5].

ICG-R15. ICG-R15 and liver volumetry on 3-dimensional computed tomography are keys for success when planning major liver surgery even if the liver is cirrhotic.

## KEY MESSAGES

■ There is a dilemma when patients present with large hepatocellular carcinoma and liver cirrhosis. However, liver resection is the most suitable treatment for patients with single hepatocellular carcinoma even if the tumor size is over 10 cm in diameter. Makuuchi proposed that normal serum bilirubin levels and normal indocyanine green retention rate at 15 minutes (ICG R-15) are required for major hepatectomy by his criteria. However, abnormal ICG-R15 is often noted in patients with hepatocellular carcinoma and liver cirrhosis. This chapter shows an attractive and practical procedure which could predict future remnant liver function. The allowable liver resection volume could be predicted by Takasaki's log table with

## REFERENCES

1. Marrero JA, Kulik LM, Sirlin CB et al. Diagnosis, staging, and management of hepatocellular carcinoma: 2018 Practice guidance by the American Association for the Study of Liver Diseases. *Hepatology* 2018;68(2):723–750.
2. Takasaki K, Kobayashi S, Suzuki S et al. Predetermining postoperative hepatic function for hepatectomies. *Int Surg* 1980;65(4):309–313.
3. Ariizumi S, Takahashi Y, Kotera Y et al. Novel virtual hepatectomy is useful for evaluation of the portal territory for anatomical sectionectomy, segmentectomy, and hemihepatectomy. *J Hepatobiliary Pancreat Sci* 2013;20:396–402.
4. Ariizumi S, Kotera Y, Takahashi Y et al. Impact of hepatectomy for huge solitary hepatocellular carcinoma. *J Surg Oncol* 2013;107(4):408–413.
5. Klein J, Dawson LA. Hepatocellular carcinoma radiation therapy: Review of evidence and future opportunities. *Int J Radiat Oncol Biol Phys* 2013;87(1):22–32.

# 34 Metastatic Colorectal Cancer

## Three Discrete 2 cm Lesions in the Right Lobe with a 1 cm Central Lesion in the Segment 2/3

*Ganesh Nagarajan and Kaushal Kundalia*

## CONTENTS

## CASE SCENARIO

A 55-year-old man who had been operated for a rectal cancer two years prior was referred with imaging (done on follow-up) suggestive of liver metastases. There were three lesions in the right lobe and a solitary central lesion in the left lobe. The patient also had an elevated serum carcinoembryonic antigen level and was otherwise fit and healthy. The liver was the only site of metastases on further imaging.

## BACKGROUND OF THE PATHOLOGY

The last decade has witnessed rapid advances in the treatment of colorectal liver metastases. Colorectal cancer is the third most common cancer worldwide [1]. More than 50% of patients with colorectal cancer will develop metastatic disease to their liver in their lifetime, which ultimately results in death in more than two-thirds of these patients. Currently, hepatic resection of the metastasis in patients with isolated liver disease remains the only option for potential cure. The aim of surgery is to resect all metastases with negative histological margins and to preserve an adequate residual liver volume.

However, only about 20–25% of patients with colorectal liver metastases are amenable to surgical resection [2]. Colorectal liver metastases is usually quite a challenge to treat and requires a multimodality approach by a multidisciplinary team.

## WORKUP AND INVESTIGATION

The aim of the initial imaging is to assess the status of the primary tumor and the metastatic lesions. It helps stage the disease accurately, assess response to chemotherapy, and plan surgery.

Multidetector helical contrast-enhanced computed tomography (CECT) scans have increased the sensitivity of detecting colorectal liver metastases to 70%–90%[3]. They possess the ability to measure the expected resection and residual functional liver volumes. This is achieved by tracing the liver regions on transverse CT images and by liver resection simulation using a dedicated 3D image analysis software.

Contrast-enhanced magnetic resonance imaging (MRI) offers no further advantage when compared with CT scans in most situations, however, it is useful to identify lesions that cannot be characterized on CT scan. Moreover, MRI is superior to CT scan in severe steatohepatitis resulting from chemotherapy, as well as for identification of disappearing liver metastases.

For detection of extrahepatic disease, preoperative staging techniques, such as 18F-fluorodeoxyglucose positron emission tomography (FDG-PET) scanning and/or laparoscopic staging, have been shown to be effective. The sensitivity has been shown to increase from 75% to 89% when CT and FDG-PET are combined, and is considered the gold standard [3].

After obtaining all the desired clinical, biochemical, and radiological information, patients with colorectal liver metastases must be discussed in a multidisciplinary team meeting to plan the appropriate management.

## NEOADJUVANT CHEMOTHERAPY

Neoadjuvant chemotherapy has a number of potential benefits, such as increasing resectability (conversion rates up to 60% have been reported), limiting the extent of hepatectomy, treating micrometastases, and enabling the evaluation of chemosensitivity of the disease, which helps identify patients who are likely to benefit from surgical resection and whether chemotherapy should be given after the resection of metastases. Some of the common regiments include capecitabine and oxaliplatin; Folinic acid, 5-fluorouracil, and oxaliplatin; and 5-fluorouracil, leucovorin, irinotecan, and oxaliplatin, with or without targeted agents like bevacizumab or cetuximab.

The duration of chemotherapy administration has shown to be an important factor affecting morbidity rates after liver resection. Chemotherapy-associated steatohepatitis also referred to as the yellow liver syndrome is seen following treatment with irinotecan. "Blue liver" syndrome due to sinusoidal dilation may follow treatment with oxaliplatin. In these patients, one must be mindful that when planning a liver resection, a larger future remnant (>30%) needs to be taken into consideration.

## PREOPERATIVE HEPATIC ARTERY EMBOLIZATION

If a major hepatic resection is planned, one should ensure that in a healthy liver, about 25–30% of liver volume is spared and in a compromised liver due to multiple chemotherapy cycles, at least 40% of liver is left behind. If not, it could result in postoperative hepatic insufficiency. A good way to optimize and increase the liver volume is to embolize the portal vein branch on the side to be resected using glue or coils. The preferential blood flow diversion to the remnant side increases the volume over the subsequent four to six weeks [4]. This hypertrophy of liver volume reduces the incidence of liver failure postoperatively.

## PRINCIPLES OF SURGICAL RESECTION

The only contraindications to liver resection for colorectal liver metastases (occurring after treatment of the primary cancer) in addition to a patient being unfit or unwilling for surgery include uncontrollable/untreatable extrahepatic disease, extensive nodal disease (retroperitoneal or mediastinal) and bone or central nervous system metastases.

A diagnostic laparoscopy is first performed to rule out peritoneal disease. A good exposure and complete mobilization of both lobes of the liver is essential to have a good assessment of all segments. An intraoperative ultrasound is then performed to map out the liver lesions. This is correlated with the findings of the preoperative imaging.

The general principle of hepatic resection is to preserve as much of parenchyma as possible. Non-anatomical resections have similar outcomes to anatomical resections. A 0.5 cm margin is acceptable and in cases where the lesion is adherent to the major vessels, a negative margin is all that one looks for [5]. In a non-anatomical resection, especially deep in the parenchyma, one should be wary of bile leaks. Meticulous use of clips and ligatures and patient underrunning of any biliary tracts is recommended to reduce morbidity.

In patients who were otherwise considered unresectable, a two-stage hepatectomy procedure, with or without portal vein occlusion, has been shown to allow a curative resection in up to 20% of patients. However, approximately 20–30% of these patients will not complete the second-stage resection because of disease progression [4].

The associating liver partition and portal vein ligation for staged hepatectomy (ALPPS) technique is gaining popularity in some units for otherwise unresectable liver metastasis with low residual liver volume. However, its role in the routine management of patients who would otherwise need a second-stage hepatectomy has not yet been defined.

## ABLATIVE TECHNIQUES

While a complete surgical resection is always the most desirable treatment for colorectal liver metastases, often ablative procedures are used as a standalone treatment, or in combination with surgery. This is usually preferred for lesions which are deep seated in the parenchyma which would otherwise need a lot of parenchymal sacrifice (large/formal anatomical resections for relatively small lesions). Previously, the only modality was radiofrequency ablation. The main drawback of this technique is a heat-sink effect which would result in inadequate and incomplete ablation of the lesions in close proximity of major blood vessels. Over the last few years, microwave ablation is being more commonly used in many centers. Electromagnetic waves agitate water molecules in tissue producing heat and friction and thus cell death. This technique is faster than radiofrequency ablation, has a wider zone of ablation, and has a lesser heat sink effect. One needs to be cautious regarding thermal damage along the tract if the technique is improper. Some centers have recently tried irreversible electroporation as an ablative modality with promising results but the costs are presently prohibitive.

## CASE SCENARIO DISCUSSION

When we approach any case of colorectal liver metastases, it is important to ascertain if the liver metastases are potentially resectable or not. More than 80% of colorectal liver metastases are unresectable on presentation. The above scenario is a case of bilobar metastasis but can be potentially resectable. Before starting any treatment, a multidisciplinary oncology team along with the radiologist need to see the imaging and provide a road map for the patient's care.

Usually, if three or more segments of liver are free of disease there is a likelihood colorectal liver metastases will eventually be resectable. If all segments of the liver have metastatic lesions, it is unlikely that the patient would ever come up for a curative resection. This decision of potential resectablility must be taken before the treatment is started. It helps plan the intent of chemotherapy, use of targeted therapy and helps prognosticate the long-term outcomes to the patient and care givers.

The entire line of management of bilobar colorectal liver metastases is determined by three important factors, namely the size of the tumor, its location in the liver, and response to chemotherapy.

To understand this better we can look at the same clinical picture of three lesions on the right lobe and one central lesion in the left lateral lobe as two different scenarios. The approach to both these scenarios will be discussed.

## SCENARIO 1

In this scenario, the right lobe lesions are about 2 cm in size each, peripherally located close to the liver surface with a central left lobe lesion (Figure 34.1). If the primary tumor has been resected earlier, this scenario can be approached in two ways.

Upfront resection is an option which will involve resection of the tumors with a sufficient margin. While the right lobe lesions can be excised with a 0.5 cm margin, the left lobe lesion can have a wide local excision or, a left lateral hepatectomy can be performed if the portal pedicle is involved. Alternatively, these patients may be treated with neoadjuvant chemotherapy prior to resection. The only difficulty in neoadjuvant chemotherapy is that if too many cycles of chemotherapy are given, some of the metastasis may disappear on further imaging. As discussed earlier, most patients with a disappearing lesion on

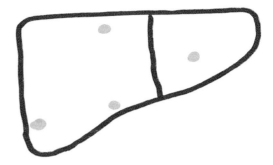

**Figure 34.1** Schematic representation of the liver with metastases. The lesions in the right lobe of liver are about 2 cm in size each, peripherally located close to the liver surface with a central left lobe lesion.

CT or PET scan will still harbor viable disease and this will manifest as a recurrence in the near future. Hence, it is important to keep the patient under surveillance while on chemotherapy with serial scans after every two to three cycles. In case of small lesions, if one plans to administer neoadjuvant chemotherapy, ultrasound-guided fiducial markers may be placed. These help locate the lesion after neoadjuvant chemotherapy during the surgery.

For the left lobe, if the lesion is small and centrally located and the liver is unhealthy, one can consider an ablative procedure (radiofrequency ablation or microwave) instead of a formal liver resection.

## SCENARIO 2

This is a scenario where the size of the lesions is relatively small (similar to Scenario 1) and the number of lesions is the same. The location of the lesions, however, is not as conducive to upfront surgery as in Scenario 1. These lesions are located deep in the parenchyma and in close proximity to the hepatic veins (Figure 34.2). An upfront resection without chemotherapy will involve resecting a large volume of the liver. It may hence be prudent to administer two to four cycles of neoadjuvant chemotherapy to the patient and then assess the response. Such a strategy will also enable sterilization of the margins especially where the lesions are adherent to the veins. This will ensure a negative margin during the resection of the lesion while dissecting it off the right and middle hepatic veins and the right portal pedicle as seen in the figure above. This will be an appropriate case for ultrasound-guided liver surgery, and one may not need to sacrifice too much of liver parenchyma to get the lesions out even if they are deep in the parenchyma or close to the pedicles.

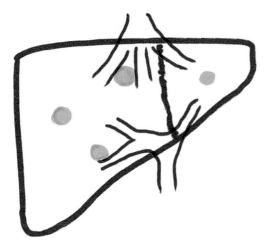

**Figure 34.2** Schematic representation of the liver with metastases. The lesions are located deep in the parenchyma of the right and left lobes of liver with an additional lesion between the right and middle hepatic veins.

The other option for this situation is to combine surgical resection for some of the more superficial lesions and a suitable ablative technique for the deep-seated lesions. This will help preserve liver parenchyma especially in patients with severe chemotherapy-associated steatohepatitis.

### KEY MESSAGES

- A multidisciplinary team comprising of colorectal and hepatobiliary surgeon, medical and radiation oncologist, radiologist, and pathologist should see every such patient and chart out the plan.
- Frequent imaging after every two to three cycles is important to minimize the chances of disappearing liver metastasis.

- Newer chemotherapeutic regimens and targeted molecular level drugs hold the key in increasing resectablility.
- A complete R0 resection offers the best chance of cure and every effort should be made to achieve this. Compared to most other cancers, colorectal liver metastases has reasonably good outcomes, even in bilobar disease.
- Advances in ablative measures may hold promise in targeting deep-seated lesions thereby saving liver parenchyma.
- It is critical to understand molecular mechanisms of tumorigenesis underlying new therapeutic strategies that specifically target tumors. This will lead to the evolution of personalized therapies for patients with colorectal liver metastases.

### REFERENCES

1. Ferlay J, Soerjomataram I, Dikshit R et al. Cancer incidence and mortality worldwide: Sources, methods and major patterns in GLOBOCAN 2012. *Int J Cancer* 2015;136(5):E359–E386.
2. Tomlinson JS, Jarnagin WR, DeMatteo RP et al. Actual 10-year survival after resection of colorectal liver metastases defines cure. *J Clin Oncol* 2007;25(29):4575–4580.
3. Bipat S, van Leeuwen MS, Comans EF et al. Colorectal liver metastases: CT, MR imaging, and PET for diagnosis – Meta-analysis. *Radiology* 2005;237(1):123–131.
4. Nordlinger B, Benoist S. Benefits and risks of neoadjuvant therapy for liver metastases. *J Clin Oncol* 2006;24(31):4954–4955.
5. Jaeck D, Oussoultzoglou E, Rosso E et al. A two-stage hepatectomy procedure combined with portal vein embolization to achieve curative resection for initially unresectable multiple and bilobar colorectal liver metastases. *Ann Surg* 2004;240(6):1037–1049; discussion 49–51.

# 35 Metastatic Colorectal Cancer Bilobar Metastatic Disease That Has Completely Disappeared Following Systemic Chemotherapy

*Yuki Kitano and René Adam*

## CONTENTS

## CASE SCENARIO

A 59-year-old man had a sigmoid colon adenocarcinoma with multiple unresectable synchronous bilobar liver metastases and had already undergone the sigmoidectomy. The therapy that was administered was 5-fluorouracil, l-leucovorin, and oxaliplatin. After seven cycles of chemotherapy, a partial response by response evaluation criteria in solid tumors was observed. Some tumors had a complete radiological response on contrast-enhanced CT (Figure 35.1). Also, carcinoembryonic antigen sharply decreased from 8.0 ng/ml to normal value. After multidisciplinary discussion, this patient was proposed for surgical resection. At operation, six lesions were detected, and the patient underwent partial hepatectomy for two lesions which were detected by palpation, and radiofrequency ablation for four lesions which were detected by intraoperative ultrasound. A pathological examination revealed that the two resected lesions were completely necrotic with a thick capsule. After the hepatectomy, the patient was treated with six cycles of 5-fluorouracil, l-leucovorin, and oxaliplatin as adjuvant chemotherapy and did not present any sign of recurrence after 1ten years of follow-up.

## APPROACH TO MANAGEMENT

### Definition of "missing" liver metastases

Thanks to the improvement of systemic treatment modalities, an increasing number of patients with initially unresectable colorectal liver metastases could be converted to resectability with a survival benefit. However, such an excellent response to preoperative systemic therapy sometimes causes complete radiological disappearance of liver metastases. This is the phenomenon of missing liver metastases. From previous reports, the percentage of patients with one or more missing liver metastases ranged widely from 7–37%, but the incidence of total disappearance of all liver metastases is very low (0–6%) [1]. On the other hand, we showed that although a complete pathological response was observed in 4% of patients with colorectal liver metastases treated by preoperative chemotherapy and such patients was associated with better survival than patients without complete pathological response (five-year overall survival rate; 76% versus 45%; P=0.004), a complete pathological response correlated poorly with a complete complete radiological response [2]. Therefore, complete pathological response and complete radiological response correspond to two different entities. When missing liver metastases were resected, microscopically residual tumor cells were found in up to 80% of the specimens, and a conservative management for missing liver metastases resulted in 19–74% local recurrence, mostly within two years [1]. This means that most of missing liver metastases are still viable and require an aggressive surgical treatment. However, the accurate resection of missing liver metastases is very difficult when the metastases cannot be detected during preoperative and intraoperative setting.

### How to detect "missing" liver metastases for surgical treatment

Although several studies described the phenomenon of missing liver metastases, they showed a wide range of preoperative and intraoperative imaging modalities for restaging colorectal liver metastases after preoperative chemotherapy. The most common restaging imaging regimes include a CT scan and intraoperative ultrasound. Recent advances of imaging technology have provided a higher sensitivity to detect colorectal liver

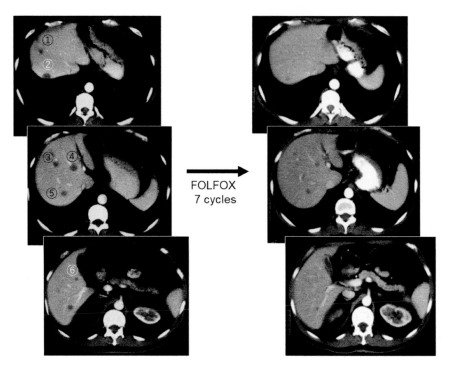

**Figure 35.1** CT assessment before and after seven cycles of chemotherapy. Tumors with white number were treated by hepatectomy and tumors with black number were treated by radiofrequency ablation.

metastases than conventional modalities. Van Kessel et al. performed a systematic review and meta-analysis to identify the optimal imaging modality for preoperative evaluation of patients with colorectal liver metastases treated with systemic therapy. In this study, the pooled sensitivities of magnetic resonance imaging (MRI), CT, fluorodeoxyglucose positron emission tomography (FDG-PET), and FDG-PET/ CT were 85.7%, 69.9%, 54.5%, and 51.7%, respectively [3]. Recently, various up-to-date contrast agents have been introduced to provide a much better sensitivity than conventional contrast enhanced MRI. For the intraoperative setting, although most lesions on the surface of the liver are usually detectable intraoperatively as a scar by inspection or palpation of the liver capsule, it is difficult to find lesions deeply located in the liver. Intraoperative ultrasound has been used as a key tool for this purpose, but only 10–30 % of missing liver metastases are reportedly identified using intraoperative ultrasound. Arita et al. showed that contrast-enhanced intraoperative ultrasound identified 79% of missing liver metastases which were not able to be detected by using all the following imaging modalities: gadolinium ethoxybenzyl diethylenetriamine pentaacetic acid enhanced MRI (EOB-MRI), contrast-enhanced CT, and contrase-enhanced ultrasound preoperatively. And, in fact, the sensitivity of contrast-enhanced intraoperative ultrasound for tumors 1 cm or less reached 100 %, which was notably higher than the sensitivities of other modalities [4]. Furthermore, the sequential use of EOB-MRI and contrast-enhanced intraoperative ultrasound offers 93% sensitivity and 77% positive predictive value to identify viable missing liver metastases. These results suggest that missing liver metastases should be resected when detected by sequential inspection that visualize missing liver metastases containing residual tumors [5]. Novel techniques are being developed to detect small metastases which are likely to disappear after systemic therapy. One study described a new technique to mark small lesions with coils before chemotherapy. They used this marking technique in patients with deep small lesions likely to disappear following systemic chemotherapy. In this study, five patients underwent coil placement and three patients had a complete radiological response to chemotherapy on preoperative CT, and two of them were not detectable with intraoperative ultrasound [6]. To overcome such a difficult situation of liver surgery, further research will be needed, and the combination of various preoperative and intraoperative modalities with expertise can minimize the chance of missing metastases, consequently.

### Prognostic impact of untreated "missing" liver metastases

Fortunately, thanks to the development of the imaging technology, there is only a small proportion of patients who demonstrate complete radiological response even after an assessment that combines the various modalities. As previously stated, although the prognosis of patients with complete pathological response was associated with better survival, the correlation between complete pathological and radiological response was not so good. However, one study showed that in patients with missing liver metastases, factors like the use of hepatic arterial infusion chemotherapy, the inability to detect the missing liver metastases on MRI, and normalization of the carcinoembryonic antigen level were associated independently with complete pathological response [7]. Another study showed, in patients with preoperative systemic chemotherapy, overall survival rate was not significantly different for patients with missing liver metastases left in situ when compared to patients with a radiological response in whom all original metastatic sites were surgically treated (three-year overall survival rate; 63.5% versus 70.8%; P=0.66), although the intrahepatic recurrence rate was higher for patients with missing liver metastases left in situ (three-year intrahepatic recurrence-free survival rate; 16.1% versus 35.1%; P=0.04) [8].

### Practical policy for patients with "missing" liver metastases

Because untreated missing liver metastases have a high risk of in situ recurrence, surgical resection should be considered for those in whom all the original sites can be treated. But if the remnant disease cannot be detected preoperatively or intraoperatively, even after the combination of various modalities, how should we manage such missing liver metastases? The first policy to treat such missing liver metastases is to perform systematic resection of the previous metastatic sites according to CT images prior to preoperative chemotherapy. However, in such a case, the lesion sometimes cannot be resected easily without anatomic resection of the liver. The second policy is to "wait and see", which means to leave them in situ. However, it can be considered only when a majority of metastatic sites cannot be detected or the incorporation of undetected original sites in a resection is unsafe. However, by performing surgery when lesions reappear

means that surgery will be done in progression and surgery should be avoided in case of progression since the survival benefit of patients who underwent hepatic resection in progression is much more limited than that of patients with partial response or stability. So, we have to consider how to treat each patient with missing liver metastases in a multidisciplinary discussion. However, the most important thing is to avoid such situation and to perform hepatic resection as soon as the resectability is obtained after systemic chemotherapy. This means that preoperative treatment to induce resectability should be as short as possible because of not only for missing liver metastases but also liver toxicity. The more cycles we do before surgery, the more toxicity the liver may suffer, and the less cycles we can deliver after surgery. We know that prolonged chemotherapy gives a "blue liver" related to the administration of oxaliplatin or the "yellow (steatotic) liver" related to the prolonged administration of irinotecan, and these livers are exposed to a higher risk of morbidity and mortality. The aim of conversion strategy is just to achieve resectability but not a complete response. The number of cycles until disappearance of the liver metastases varies widely between 5 and 25 cycles in the studies that describe missing liver metastases. And we recommend that the optimal timing for assessment of response to chemotherapy to be every two months to reduce the risk of missing liver metastases.

### CONCLUSION

Thanks to the improvement of systemic treatment modalities, an excellent response of systemic therapy sometimes causes missing liver metastases. However, in most cases, complete radiological response does not mean complete pathological response, and untreated missing liver metastases have a high risk of in situ recurrence. Therefore, the combination of various preoperative and intraoperative modalities should be used to minimize the risk of missing liver metastases and an aggressive surgical approach toward missing liver metastases should be considered.

### REFERENCES

1. Kuhlmann K, van Hilst J, Fisher S et al. Management of disappearing colorectal liver metastases. *Eur J Surg Oncol* 2016;42(12):1798–1805.
2. Adam R, Wicherts DA, de Haas RJ et al. Complete pathologic response after preoperative chemotherapy for colorectal liver

metastases: Myth or reality? *J Clin Oncol* 2008;26(10):1635–1641.

3. van Kessel CS, Buckens CF, van den Bosch MA et al. Preoperative imaging of colorectal liver metastases after neoadjuvant chemotherapy: A meta-analysis. *Ann Surg Oncol* 2012;19(9):2805–2813.

4. Arita J, Ono Y, Takahashi M et al. Usefulness of contrast-enhanced intraoperative ultrasound in identifying disappearing liver metastases from colorectal carcinoma after chemotherapy. *Ann Surg Oncol* 2014;21:S390–S397.

5. Oba A, Mise Y, Ito H et al. Clinical implications of disappearing colorectal liver metastases have changed in the era of hepatocyte-specific MRI and contrast-enhanced intraoperative ultrasonography. *HPB (Oxf)* 2018;20(8):708–714.

6. Zalinski S, Abdalla EK, Mahvash A et al. A marking technique for intraoperative localization of small liver metastases before systemic chemotherapy. *Ann Surg Oncol* 2009;16(5):1208–1211.

7. Auer RC, White RR, Kemeny NE et al. Predictors of a true complete response among disappearing liver metastases from colorectal cancer after chemotherapy. *Cancer* 2010;116(6):1502–1509.

8. van Vledder MG, de Jong MC, Pawlik TM et al. Disappearing colorectal liver metastases after chemotherapy: Should we be concerned? *J Gastrointest Surg* 2010;14(11):1691–1700.

# PART 8
# PANCREAS

# 36 Pyrexia Two Weeks after an Attack of Alcohol-Induced Acute Pancreatitis

*John A. Windsor*

## CONTENTS

## CASE SCENARIO

A 45-year-old man presented with a history of five previous admissions in the last 12 months for acute pancreatitis related to excess alcoholic consumption. He is a heavy smoker, his "binge" drinking pattern is largely confined to the weekends and he is struggling to hold down his job as an IT consultant. His wife and two young daughters have left him. With the most recent episode, he had been admitted when he was found heavily intoxicated and lying on the sidewalk. In the emergency department he was found to be intoxicated, had a scalp laceration, a distal radial fracture, abdominal pain, and an elevated serum lipase level (6× upper limit of normal). He self-discharged after five days in hospital after the acute pain had settled. He was readmitted ten days later with abdominal pain, elevated serum lipase (4× upper limit of normal), elevated blood alcohol level, and a fever of 38.5°C.

## BACKGROUND OF THE PATHOLOGY

The gross pathology of acute pancreatitis is remarkably similar across the different aetiologies. It is customary to distinguish interstitial edematous acute pancreatitis (which is usually associated with milder acute pancreatitis), from necrotizing pancreatitis. The latter is also associated with edema and is a hallmark of more severe disease. The necrosis can be patchy and minimal, confluent, and extensive and/or involving the peripancreatic tissue in the retroperitoneum. The extent of necrosis appears to be related to disease severity [1,2].

The morphological classification of local complications has been an important diagnostic advance [1]. It is based on cross sectional imaging and takes into account whether the local complication has become encapsulated or "walled off" (*walled-off necrosis*). This tends to occur after three to four weeks. Prior to that, the local complications are considered to include *acute fluid collections* (in the absence of necrosis) or *acute necrotic collections* (when necrosis is present). The term *"pseudocyst"* is now a more restricted definition and is only applied after four weeks, and if the content of the collection is only fluid. Any of these local complications can become infected, and this is more common if necrosis is present. It can become infected from enteric or extra-pancreatic sources and at any time, although infection is most is common between two and six weeks [3].

When severe, and in common with other acute and critical diseases, acute pancreatitis is associated with two syndromes: systemic inflammatory response syndrome and multiple organ dysfunction syndrome. The organ systems most often affected are the respiratory, cardiovascular, and renal. Early organ failure appears to be cytokine mediated, while organ failure after three to four weeks is infection mediated.

The main determinants of clinical outcome from pancreatitis have been infected pancreatic necrosis and organ failure that lasts for more than 48 hours (persistent organ failure). Notable progress has been made with the treatment of infected local pancreatic necrosis. Thus, it is no longer considered an important determinant of severity and mortality. In contrast persistent organ failure, in the absence of specific treatments that target the drivers of persistent organ failure, is the leading cause of mortality, and its management remains intensive care support. Over one-third of those with recurrent acute pancreatitis develop chronic pancreatitis, and this is more likely in men who smoke and drink [4].

## CLINICAL FINDINGS

This man was examined by the emergency physician on readmission. He was inebriated and dishevelled. On examination he was a thin man with nicotine staining but no clinical signs of anemia or liver disease. He had cool peripheries but a normal capillary refill time, was sweating, had a fever (38.5°C), tachycardia (heart rate 106/min), and tachypnea (respiratory rate 26/min) but was normotensive (blood pressure 124/68). Oximetry revealed an oxygen saturation of 86% while on 2 litres of oxygen by nasal prongs. His abdomen was tender in the epigastrium with mild rebound. There was an ill-defined fullness in the left upper quadrant. There was no Grey Turner's sign, Cullen's sign, or erythema ab igne. There was evidence of urinary incontinence. There was superficial bruising over the left skull, associated with a 5 cm flap laceration that was sutured and healing, bruising over the left shoulder, and a swollen, tender but not displaced left wrist.

## INVESTIGATIONS

Routine bloods were sent on readmission and this confirmed that serum lipase was elevated at > 4× upper limit of normal, now two weeks after initial admission. He also had a blood alcohol level of 280 mg/dL. Hematology revealed a hemoglobin of 132 g/L, total white blood count of $15.2 \times 10^{-9}$/L, and a platelet count of $224 \times 10^{-9}$/L. The hematocrit was 0.45. Electrolytes were normal but his renal function was impaired, with a blood urea nitrogen of 11 mmol/L (Normal range = 2.5–7.1). Liver function tests were normal other than a mildly elevated gamma glutamyl transferase. Random blood glucose was 11.2 mmol/L. An arterial blood gas confirmed hypoxemia and respiratory acidosis (pH 7.32, bicarbonate 30 mEq/L, partial pressure of carbon dioxide of 49 mmHg).

A chest X-ray revealed bilateral pleural effusions, more on the left than the right. Although subtle, there were also signs of early adult respiratory distress syndrome (diffuse bilateral opacities partly obscuring the vascular markings). Because of the tender mass in the left upper quadrant, a computed tomography (CT) scan of the abdomen was done in the emergency department and this revealed signs of acute on chronic pancreatitis. There was evidence of parenchymal calcification, pancreatic duct irregularity, and a maximum duct diameter of 6 mm in the body of the pancreas. There was significant peripancreatic "stranding", indicative of extensive pancreatic and retroperitoneal inflammation. As a result, it was unclear whether there was any underlying pancreatic atrophy. In addition, there was a complex collection centered on the body of the pancreas, with what appeared to have both fluid and solid contents, but without any evident gas. The mass measuring 8 cm in maximum diameter was indenting the posterior stomach and showed early signs of encapsulation. The arterial enhanced phase failed to reveal normal perfusion of the pancreas, with patchy hypoperfusion, particularly in the body and tail of the pancreas. The radiologist correctly reported an acute necrotic collection.

## APPROACH TO MANAGEMENT

There are different phases to the management of acute pancreatitis and these apply irrespective of the aetiology. At the time of admission several important questions need to be addressed:

1) Is it acute pancreatitis? In this patient, a confident diagnosis of acute pancreatitis can be made on the basis of typical abdominal pain, pancreatic enzyme elevation (>3× upper limit of normal), and CT evidence of pancreatitis [1].

2) What is the duration of acute pancreatitis? While most patients present within 24 hours of the onset of abdominal pain, this is not always the case. In this patient, it was not possible to determine the duration of symptoms prior to the first admission, given the alcohol intoxication. And with the second readmission, it is not known whether this was new attack of pancreatitis, an exacerbation, continuation, or complication of the first attack. What was clear is that the symptoms must have been present for at least 15 days.

3) What is the aetiology? The aetiology was not in question in this case, given the pattern of drinking, multiple admissions to hospital following binge drinking, the markedly elevated blood alcohol concentration, and the absence of other causes. Gallstones had been excluded on previous admissions with an abdominal ultrasound.

4) How severe will this attack be? On readmission there were four positive systemic inflammatory response syndrome criteria (elevated temperature, heart rate, respiratory rate, and white blood count) which predict severe acute pancreatitis [1, 2]. Also, of prognostic value was the mildly elevated hematocrit, blood urea nitrogen, and evidence of respiratory dysfunction.

During the first hour after admission, these investigations should be completed and the initial steps in management initiated. This involves the following:

### Pain relief

Acute pancreatitis is a very painful condition and prompt analgesia is indicated. It is usual to provide intravenous narcotic analgesia (e.g. morphine sulphate) to achieve relief. Careful monitoring of the patient is required for early detection of a suppressed respiratory drive [2].

### Fluid resuscitation

This is widely acknowledged to be the cornerstone of treatment, but in this patient should the same approach be taken with the readmission as was taken at the time of the first admission? The answer to this is "probably not", although there is a serious lack of high quality evidence to guide the choice of fluid, the rate of intravenous fluids, and the goal for resuscitation [2]. There is some recent evidence indicating that aggressive fluid replacement is beneficial in the first six hours, but if it is continued beyond that period, it can be harmful. The generalized capillary leak syndrome means that there will be an increase in edema which can exacerbate organ dysfunction and cause abdominal compartment syndrome and sequelae. In this patient, there is also the need for caution with fluid resuscitation because of the incipient acute respiratory distress syndrome. It would be reasonable to provide a litre of Ringer's lactate over four hours and then review the patient's fluid balance status. The elevated hematocrit and blood urea nitrogen suggests the need for some volume repletion, which might correct a degree of prerenal failure, and these tests should be repeated at the four hour review. Note that urine output is misleading as a guide to the need for volume repletion, since oliguria is a normal physiological response to acute illness.

### Locus of management

On the basis of predicted severe acute pancreatitis, respiratory and renal dysfunction, and the large acute necrotic collection, urgent transfer to a regional center should be arranged and management should be in a high dependency unit [2].

### Respiratory care

The respiratory dysfunction could be made worse with excess fluid resuscitation and the early signs of acute respiratory distress syndrome indicate the need for careful management. Although no specific therapy exists for acute respiratory distress syndrome, treatment is initially non-invasive ventilation (i.e. high flow oxygen, humidification, and positive pressure) and later mechanical ventilation using low tidal volumes (to minimize lung injury), if required. And conservative "maintenance" fluid management is indicated rather than resuscitation. Cardiovascular support with vasopressors should be considered early to avoid excess fluid administration. The judicious use of diuretics might help improve lung function, but should not be given until normal renal function is confirmed.

### Sepsis screen

This patient has been readmitted with a fever and elevated white blood count. Given the interval from the first admission (15 days), the fever is unlikely to be part of an acute systemic inflammatory response syndrome to acute pancreatitis. The key question is whether this is due to infection of the acute necrotic collection or not. A thorough search for other causes should be undertaken and not just assume it is due to infection of the acute necrotic collection. There are several other possibilities, including a nosocomial chest, urinary or intravenous cannula site infection from the recent admission, or an aspiration pneumonia with intoxication. A concomitant appendicitis or cholecystitis is unlikely.

The timing of the fever is worthy of comment. It has been commonly accepted that infection of pancreatic necrosis is something that occurs after four weeks. Previously it was shown that half of all infections in patients with acute pancreatitis occur in the first week of admission, including pneumonia and bacteremia [3]. Bacteremia is an independent predictor of death and is associated with an increased risk of infected pancreatic necrosis, and this almost certainly reflects gut barrier dysfunction which is a common feature of acute pancreatitis [3]. A fever at 15 days could therefore be from the acute necrotic collection in this patient.

## Antibiotics

The evidence is now very clear that prophylactic antibiotics are not indicated in acute pancreatitis, but there should be a low threshold for treatment antibiotics if there is a high suspicion of infections, as in this patient. Blood cultures should be taken prior to commencement of broad spectrum antibiotics (e.g. meropenem) and there should be a commitment to treatment for a limited period (e.g. five to seven days) and then review. Adequate drainage should facilitate earlier cessation of antibiotic treatment.

## Nutritional support

Acute pancreatitis is a highly catabolic disease and alcoholics are often malnourished. The presence of respiratory dysfunction means that he will be encouraged to have oral nutrition drinks and, if tolerated, allowed to eat so long as the pain is not significantly exacerbated by doing so. If after 72 hours he is unable to tolerate at least 80% of his calorie and protein requirements, and if the respiratory function has not deteriorated, it would be appropriate to consider nasogastric feeding. The tube can be advanced for nasojejunal feeding if required due to feeding intolerance (nausea and vomiting). Occasionally, supplementary parenteral feeding is required.

## Monitoring the response to initial treatment

This is an important principle of management, as exacerbation of organ dysfunction will exhaust physiological reserves and result in clinical deterioration. This is more likely in older patients with comorbidities. A formal reassessment of this patient at four hours is recommended, because a lack of response is a grave prognostic indicator, and a deterioration will warrant admission to an intensive care unit. The cornerstone of monitoring is covered by the three Cs: regular clinical assessment to determine the patient's trajectory, daily C-reactive protein estimation, and CT scanning when there are concerns. Recently the Pancreatitis Activity Scoring System (PASS) has been introduced for this purpose and may prove helpful in indicating response to initial therapy (or lack of it) and for the early detection of deterioration [5]. It considers organ failure (100 points per system), intolerance to solid diet (40 points), systemic inflammatory response syndrome (25 points per criteria), abdominal pain (up to 10 points), and intravenous morphine equivalent dose (up to 5 points).

## The management of uninfected acute necrotic collection

The *dilemma in this case is the cause of the patient's temperature.* There are several possibilities, including a cytokine-mediated systemic inflammatory response syndrome response, bacteremia secondary to gut translocation, extra-pancreatic infection, and/or infected local complication the pancreas. It is most likely, in the absence of any other infections, that this patient was readmitted because of bacteremia secondary to bacterial translocation or early infection of the acute necrotic fluid collection. Either way, a full set of blood cultures should be collected, and antibiotics commenced. If the patient is stable (or improves) then continued conservative management is indicated. It has been shown that occasionally some patients have required no more than antibiotic treatment. On careful monitoring, and with clinical evidence of deterioration, drainage of the collection will be required. Drainage can be done either endoscopically (with endosonographic guidance) or percutaneously (with fluoroscopic or ultrasound guidance). The choice is primarily based on the location of the collection. Centrally located collections are suitable for endoscopic transgastric drainage (with the added advantage including dilatation, insertion of metal stents, and endoscopic debridement). Collections that extend into the paracolic gutters are suitable for percutaneous drainage. On this basis, this patient would have been referred for endoscopic drainage. However, owing to the immaturity of the wall with the attendant risk of leakage into the lesser sac and peritonitis, a percutaneous approach was preferred. If endoscopic and radiological expertise are not available, then this patient should be transferred to a referral center. Early drainage (less than three weeks) not only permits the ability to obtain a specimen for bacteriology, but it also helps to "buy time", allowing patients to improve, the necrosum to sequester, and walls of the collection to become more defined. This makes it safer for subsequent debridement should that be required (enabling insertion of a guidewire for dilatation, insertion of a metal stent, and debridement). Drainage alone can suffice in up to 50% of patients. If drainage is not available, a cystojejunostomy or cystogastrostomy (open or laparoscopic) can be considered in large or symptomatic mature cysts a few weeks down the track [6].

## Management of alcohol problems

This patient clearly requires support with regard to his alcohol abuse. In the acute setting, regular review for signs of alcohol withdrawal, and the administration of thiamine for potential alcohol withdrawal are indicated. A social worker should be engaged to explore what measures have been taken and what options are available to assist him, should he be willing. Further education should be offered about recurrent acute and chronic pancreatitis and their long-term sequelae. He should be offered smoking cessation programs. It is also important to screen the patient in the future for pancreatic endocrine (HBA1c) and exocrine insufficiency (fecal elastase). This is best done at the time of a subsequent clinic appointment.

## Excluding a malignancy

Another consideration is whether the pancreatic mass harbors a malignancy. In this context and given his age, this is less likely. Nevertheless, he should have a baseline serum carbohydrate antigen 19-9 (CA 19-9) and this should be repeated since patients with chronic pancreatitis are at an increased risk of pancreatic cancer. Interval cross section imaging at three and six months should also be performed to demonstrate resolution of this acute problem and establish interval baseline imaging of the pancreas.

## KEY MESSAGES

- This patient illustrates the challenge that clinicians are faced with when a patient has signs of infection before the three-to-four week threshold for full intervention.
- Early drainage without debridement allows confirmation of infection and it often allows the patient to improve sufficiently to allow the maturation of the acute necrotic collection to walled-off necrosis (or to resolve).
- A step-up approach can help avoid overtreatment, by allowing some patients to be managed with antibiotics and/or drainage alone.
- Drainage can be performed by endoscopy or radiology, depending on the topography of the collection and local expertise. The initial goal is adequate drainage and not removal of necrotic tissue.

## REFERENCES

1. Banks PA, Bollen TL, Dervenis C et al. Classification of acute pancreatitis—2012: Revision of the Atlanta classification and definitions by international consensus. *Gut* 2013;62(1):102–111.
2. Working Group IAPAPAAPG. IAP/APA evidence-based guidelines for the management of acute pancreatitis. *Pancreatology* 2013;13(4):e1–e15.
3. Besselink MG, van Santvoort HC, Boermeester MA et al. Dutch acute pancreatitis study G. Timing and impact of infections in acute pancreatitis. *Br J Surg* 2009;96(3):267–273.
4. Sankaran SJ, Xiao AY, Wu LM et al. Frequency of progression from acute to chronic pancreatitis and risk factors: A meta-analysis. *Gastroenterology* 2015;149(6):1490–1500 e1.
5. Buxbaum J, Quezada M, Chong B et al. The pancreatitis activity scoring system predicts clinical outcomes in acute pancreatitis: Findings from a prospective cohort study. *Am J Gastroenterol* 2018 May;113(5):755–764.
6. van Dijk SM, Hallensleben NDL, van Santvoort HC et al. Acute pancreatitis: Recent advances through randomised trials. *Gut* 2017;66(11):2024–2032.

# 37 Ten-Year History of Chronic Pancreatitis Presents with Pancreatic Head Mass

*Courtney E. Barrows and Tara S. Kent*

## CONTENTS

## CASE SCENARIO

A 64-year-old woman with a ten-year history of chronic pancreatitis was referred for intractable abdominal pain and a new pancreatic head mass. She endorses intermittent epigastric pain and nausea over the past 18 months, resulting in worsened quality of life and several hospitalizations for pain control, a 12-pound weight loss, but no steatorrhea or diabetes. Serum CA 19-9 was normal.

A pancreas protocol computed tomography (CT) revealed stable main pancreatic duct dilation, but with new abrupt narrowing at the pancreatic head, and an ill-defined low-density mass in the pancreatic head and uncinate process (Figure 37.1A), with attenuation and stranding of the portal-superior mesenteric vein confluence (Figure 37.1B). She underwent several endoscopic ultrasounds and endoscopic retrograde cholangiopancreatography over the preceding 18 months, demonstrating main pancreatic duct dilation in the head with abrupt cutoff at the neck (Figure 37.2A) and a hypoechoic 1.5 cm pancreatic head/uncinate mass (Figure 37.2B). Despite multiple negative fine-needle biopsies/aspirations, malignancy could not be ruled out because of her pain, weight loss, and concerning CT findings. She thus underwent a staging laparoscopy (negative) followed by pylorus-preserving pancreatoduodectomy with an uneventful postoperative course. Her final histopathology revealed chronic pancreatitis and pancreatic intraepithelial neoplasm, but no malignancy.

## BACKGROUND OF THE PATHOLOGY

Chronic pancreatitis is itself a risk factor for the development of pancreatic ductal adenocarcinoma. In this disease process, chronic inflammation and duct obstruction cause atrophy of the normal pancreatic parenchyma, which is subsequently replaced with fibrotic tissue. This is not a symmetric process and can occasionally present as a local heterogeneous inflammatory mass in approximately 15–30% of chronic pancreatitis patients. This has been referred to as "mass-forming pancreatitis" or "pseudotumor", and can easily be mistaken for pancreatic ductal adenocarcinoma or other pancreatic neoplasms [1,2].

The ability to discriminate between mass-forming pancreatitis and pancreatic malignancy is critical in order to avoid an inappropriate resection for inflammatory disease, or conversely a delay in curative resection/treatment for pancreatic neoplasms. Despite improvements in diagnostic modalities, differentiating these two disease processes remains a challenge, and such patients require a multidisciplinary approach to both diagnosis and management.

## CLINICAL SYMPTOMS/SIGNS

Recurrent or chronic abdominal pain is the most common presenting symptom of chronic pancreatitis and the most common indication for surgical intervention. The classic constellation of symptoms include repeated bouts of epigastric abdominal pain radiating to the mid to upper back, nausea, and inability to tolerate

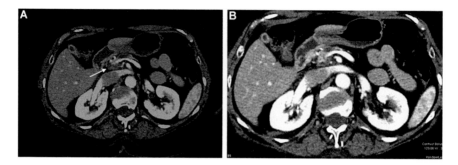

**Figure 37.1**  Preoperative computed tomography angiogram pancreas protocol demonstrating: (A) a new ill-defined low-density area (arrows) along the superior aspect of the pancreatic head and uncinate process with increased stranding and slight nodularity extending posteriorly toward the inferior vena cava and left renal vein, encasing the inferior pancreaticoduodenal artery, with associated pancreatic duct dilation, (B) low density area causing attenuation (arrow) and stranding along the portal/ superior mesenteric vein confluence raises concern for potential malignancy with vascular invasion.

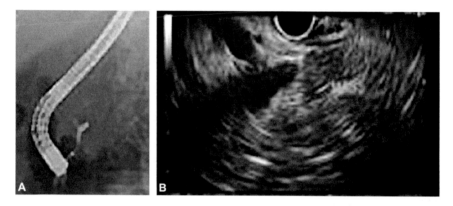

**Figure 37.2**  (A) Endoscopic retrograde cholangiopancreatography demonstrating a pancreatic duct partially filled with contrast, dilated to 3 mm in the pancreatic head, with an abrupt cut off between the pancreatic head and neck. (B) Endoscopic ultrasound demonstrating a 1.5 cm hypoechoic mass with ill-defined borders in the pancreatic head/uncinate. Fine-needle aspirate and biopsies were negative for malignancy.

oral intake with resultant weight loss. In this context, patients may present with ongoing opioid requirements and/or the inability to work. Additionally, due to destruction of normal pancreatic parenchyma and resultant glandular dysfunction, patients often present with exocrine and/or endocrine pancreatic insufficiency, such as fat malabsorption, diarrhea or steatorrhea, weight loss, and diabetes mellitus. Biliary obstruction may occur due to either benign biliary stricture from repeated bouts of inflammation (which occurs in approximately 25% of chronic pancreatitis patients [3]) or extrinsic compression from an inflammatory mass, the latter of which can also result in gastric outlet obstruction. While these symptoms are also common to pancreatic cancer, the onset or timing may assist with delineating the underlying etiology.

### DIAGNOSTIC STUDIES

Chronic pancreatitis is diagnosed clinically based on the patient's constellation of recurrent symptoms as described above. Unlike with acute pancreatitis, elevation in serum amylase and/or lipase levels is uncommonly noted due to the progressive destruction of the exocrine portion of the gland over time. However, cross-sectional imaging is often helpful to delineate chronic pancreatitis from other pathologies when the diagnosis is uncertain, or to evaluate for complications of pancreatitis such as the formation of a pseudocyst or mass. A multimodality approach affords the best opportunity at distinguishing mass-forming pancreatitis from malignant neoplasm.

### Computed tomography (CT)

A triple-phase, pancreatic protocol contrast-enhanced CT is often the initial study of choice for evaluating a pancreatic head mass. A hypodense mass is characteristic of both pancreatic ductal adenocarcinoma and mass-forming pancreatitis, but delayed washout is more prominent with the former. Secondary findings more commonly associated with pancreatic ductal adenocarcinoma include upstream segmental pancreatic parenchymal atrophy and a "double duct" sign [2] (dilated common bile ducts and main pancreatic duct, with abrupt cutoff at the mass). While mass-forming pancreatitis can result in pancreatic duct dilation, it is typically less prominent than that associated with pancreatic ductal adenocarcinoma, and often the main duct and/or side branches are still visualized within the lesion itself (also known as "duct penetrating sign"), a key distinguishing feature between the two entities [4]. Despite some of these distinguishing features, there is still considerable overlap in parameters between the two disease entities. Furthermore, CT is also limited in detecting lesions smaller than 2 cm.

### Magnetic resonance imaging (MRI) and magnetic resonance cholangiopancreatography (MRCP)

MRCP allows for better visualization of ductal anatomy to assess for the "duct penetrating sign". The addition of diffusion-weighted imaging technology is particularly useful, which evaluates the free movement of water molecules within the pancreatic tissue, quantified by the apparent diffusion coefficient. Compared to chronic pancreatitis/inflammatory masses, pancreatic ductal adenocarcinoma is characterized by high signal and lower apparent diffusion coefficients [1].

### Endoscopic modalities

endoscopic ultrasound and endoscopic retrograde cholangiopancreatography have pivotal roles in the diagnosis of chronic pancreatitis associated with a pancreatic head mass. Endoscopic retrograde cholangiopancreatography allows access to the major and minor papillae, through which brushings can be obtained for cytology of any ductal strictures. Standard endoscopic ultrasound is able to evaluate the echotexture of the lesion and surrounding pancreatic parenchyma, lesion boundaries, duct properties, surrounding lymph nodes, and vascular involvement.

It is also superior to CT for detecting smaller lesions (<2 cm). Features suggestive of a mass-forming pancreatitis lesion on conventional endoscopic ultrasound include intralesional Doppler signal, hyperechoic septa, and multilobularity. Endoscopic ultrasound-mediated fine-needle aspiration has demonstrated 90% sensitivity for detecting pancreatic ductal adenocarcinoma in the background of normal pancreatic parenchyma, however only 50–75% when performed in the setting of chronic pancreatitis. With improved techniques such as core needle biopsy and increasing the number of passes, the sensitivity and specificity has been reported as high as 90% [2,4].

Endoscopic ultrasound-based adjunct techniques improve the diagnostic accuracy and provide more objective/quantifiable information. Endoscopic ultrasound-elastography measures the tissue stiffness of solid lesions, which can be quantitatively represented by the "strain ratio". Stiffness tends to be higher in malignant masses compared to inflammatory masses, and when quantified using the strain ratio is >90% sensitive and 66–93% specific for pancreatic ductal adenocarcinoma.

Contrast-enhanced endoscopic ultrasound exploits the principle that pancreatic ductal adenocarcinoma tends to be hypovascular, injecting air-filled albumin-coated microspheres that cannot diffuse out of blood vessels, allowing for a longer period to evaluate vascular structures. In order to minimize inter-observer variability, this can also be quantitatively measured using the "contrast uptake ratio index" which is significantly lower in pancreatic ductal adenocarcinoma compared to chronic pancreatitis with >90% sensitivity and specificity using a cutoff of 0.17 [2].

Endoscopic retrograde cholangiopancreatography is useful for the diagnosis and management of both chronic pancreatitis and pancreatic head masses.

In our practice, these patients with long-standing chronic pancreatitis are often found to have a mass on the CT scan or MRI performed for the evaluation of worsening symptoms, or for resolution following an acute exacerbation of pain. For those who undergo either an MRI or non-pancreas protocol CT detecting a suspicious mass, we perform CT pancreas protocol to evaluate for vessel involvement. Patients with a suspicious pancreatic head mass, or symptoms but no discrete mass on cross-sectional imaging are referred for endoscopic ultrasound, with fine-needle aspirate and core needle biopsy to obtain a tissue diagnosis. An endoscopic retrograde cholangiopancreatography will also be performed at that time with possible stenting for those with biliary obstruction.

## TREATMENT OPTIONS

In this section, we will focus on the treatment options for chronic pancreatitis associated with a pancreatic head mass, while the management of other neoplasms including pancreatic ductal adenocarcinoma will be covered elsewhere. It should be emphasized that patients with chronic pancreatitis, mass-forming pancreatitis, and pancreatic malignancy should be managed at high-volume centers experienced at managing patients with these disease processes, which requires cooperative multidisciplinary involvement of gastroenterology/advanced endoscopy, diagnostic and interventional radiology, surgery, oncology, nutritional specialists, and social work.

In general, chronic pancreatitis is managed medically, with surgery reserved for those with refractory disease (to be covered later). Nonoperative management consists of the following principles:

1) *Analgesia:* Minimizing the use of narcotic pain medications when possible through multimodality pain management strategies.

2) *Risk factor mitigation:* Minimizing further gland damage, slow progressive inflammatory changes, and potentially decrease the risk of malignant transformation. Patients are advised to pursue both alcohol and smoking cessation.

3) *Oral pancreatic enzyme replacement therapy:* Pancreatic enzymes inhibit cholecystokinin release, theoretically decreasing the frequency of acute inflammatory attacks. While this is somewhat controversial, we advocate for oral enzyme replacement therapy for patients with symptoms of fat malabsorption, such as steatorrhea and/or postprandial diarrhea and/or abnormal fecal elastase measurements. We recommend a starting dose of 30,000 units of lipase per meal, which can be titrated according to symptom relief. An acid-suppressing medication such as proton pump inhibitors (omeprazole, pantoprazole, lansoprazole, etc.) or histamine 2 receptor blockers (ranitidine, famotidine, etc.) should be coadministered in order to prevent the denaturation of pancreatic enzymes by gastric acid.

4) *Endoscopic therapy:* Endoscopic retrograde cholangiopancreatography can be an effective therapy to treat patients with biliary and/or pancreatic duct strictures, as well as pancreatic duct stones through the use of

balloon dilation or stent placement. Larger duct stones may require extracorporeal shockwave lithotripsy. In general, while endoscopic therapies provide good initial symptom relief, more than half of patients with chronic pancreatitis will ultimately require surgical intervention. In addition, endoscopic ultrasound and/or endoscopic retrograde cholangiopancreatography can also help to distinguish chronic pancreatitis from malignancy in some cases through biopsy and/or brushings. Particularly in the setting of mass-forming pancreatitis, we advocate for early surgical intervention for patients with an acceptable performance status without prohibitive comorbidities.

### Surgical management

Surgery for chronic pancreatitis may be indicated in the following circumstances:

1) Pain interfering with quality of life

2) Biliary obstruction not amenable to endoscopic intervention

3) Duodenal or gastric outlet obstruction

4) Concern for malignancy and inability to establish definitive tissue diagnosis

There are several different surgical options for chronic pancreatitis, further categorized into drainage or combined drainage/resection procedures:

1) Lateral pancreaticojejunostoy (Puestow procedure)

2) Pancreaticoduodenectomy (Whipple procedure)

3) Duodenum-preserving pancreatic head resection (Beger procedure)

4) Duodenum-preserving pancreatic head resection with lateral pancreaticojejunostomy (Frey procedure)

5) Duodenum-preserving pancreatic head resection (Berne procedure)

Of note, drainage procedures are inadequate for mass-forming chronic pancreatitis, therefore the remainder of this section will focus on the combined drainage/resection techniques, summarized in Table 37.1. If there is suspicion for underlying malignancy or irreversible duodenal/gastric outlet obstruction, classic or pylorus-preserving pancreaticoduodenectomy should be performed. In the setting of chronic pancreatitis with a background of inflammation, it may be difficult to disprove a malignancy. In these cases, a partial pancreatic

**Table 37.1 Comparison of Surgical Techniques for Chronic Pancreatitis Presenting with Pancreatic Head Mass**

| Procedure | Description | Indication | Benefits | Risks |
|---|---|---|---|---|
| Pancreatoduodenectomy (PD) | Pylorus preserving or classic | Inflammatory HOP mass for which PDAC cannot be ruled out, and/or causing irreversible duodenal/gastric outlet obstruction | | • Pancreatic insufficiency (exocrine 25-50%; endocrine 12-48%)<br>• Longer operative time, LOS<br>• Pancreatic fistula (less common w/CP)<br>• Delayed gastric emptying |
| **Duodenum-Preserving Pancreatic Head Resections** | | | | |
| Frey Procedure | • Central pancreatic head resection ("cored out"), no neck transection<br>• Longitudinal RNY PJ | Inflammatory HOP mass with main pancreatic duct dilation | Complete pancreatic parenchymal drainage<br>Single anastomosis<br>Less bleeding risk than Beger<br>Retains more HOP parenchyma, less risk of pancreatic insufficiency (theoretical) | Incomplete resection, disease recurrence (theoretical) |
| Beger Procedure | Subtotal pancreatic head resection, transected at neck, rim of head tissue along medial duodenum<br>2 PJ anastomoses to same RNY loop of jejunum (side-to-side head, end-to-side body/tail) | Inflamed pancreatic head mass, secondary portal hypertension, biliary stenosis | • More complete resection for larger masses<br>• Can modify to include choledochojejunostomy if concomitant biliary stenosis | • Increased bleeding risk<br>• Technically challenging<br>• At least 2 anastomoses – longer operative time, increased risk of leak (theoretical) |
| Berne Procedure | • Subtotal pancreatic head resection similar to Beger but without neck transection<br>• Side-to-side RNY PJ | • Inflammatory HOP mass without pancreatic duct dilation/stricture<br>• Concern for significant inflammation/portal hypertension, high bleeding risk | • Avoids pancreatic neck dissection, decreased bleeding risk<br>• Shorter operative and recovery time (vs Beger) | Limited PD drainage |

**Abbreviations:** PJ – pancreaticojejunostomy, PD – pancreatoduodenectomy, LOS – length of stay, HOP – head of pancreas, RNY – Roux-en-Y.

233

head resection is contraindicated on oncologic grounds, and a pancreaticoduodenectomy should be performed.

In the absence of these situations, we recommend considering one of the duodenum-preserving pancreatic head resections for pancreatic head mass-forming chronic pancreatitis, as these have demonstrated similar efficacy with regards to pain relief, but with improved perioperative morbidity, quality of life, shorter hospital stay, and less postoperative exocrine insufficiency compared to pancreaticoduodenectomy [3, 5].

The Frey's procedure combines a limited pancreatic head resection with a complete pancreatic duct drainage procedure, and is indicated for a clearly inflammatory pancreatic head mass with a dilated main pancreatic duct without biliary dilation. The central portion of the pancreatic head is cored out anteriorly. The main pancreatic duct is opened anteriorly along the head, body, and tail and anastomosed to a Roux-en-Y limb of jejunum.

The Beger procedure involves a more radical pancreatic head resection than the Frey, with complete resection of the pancreatic neck at the confluence of the splenic and mesenteric veins, leaving only a small rim of pancreatic head tissue along the medial border of the duodenum. The pancreatic reconstruction requires two anastomoses, with a Roux-en-Y loop of jejunum sewn to both the preserved head tissue (side-to-side) and the transected neck (end-to-side). The procedure can be modified to include a choledochojejunostomy to the same Roux limb in the setting of a biliary stricture, which is required in approximately 25% of cases [3]. This is often the most technically challenging of the three procedures.

The Berne procedure combines elements of both the Frey and Beger procedures. The extent of pancreatic head resection is similar to Beger, leaving only a small rim of head left on the medial duodenum, but differs in that a small amount of tissue is also left anterior to the superior mesenteric and/or portal vein. This obviates the need for pancreatic neck transection and is particularly advantageous in situations with extensive inflammation or portal hypertension with collaterals, due to the increased risk of major bleeding during the posterior pancreatic neck dissection. Reconstruction consists of a single Roux-en-Y side-to-side pancreaticojejunostomy, which, similar to the Beger, can be modified to include a cholechoje-junostomy when indicated. A notable limitation is that unlike the Frey, it does not decompress

the entire length of the main pancreatic duct, therefore would not be the procedure of choice in patients with multiple ductal obstructions or strictures.

Despite an extensive body of literature comparing outcomes between duodenum-preserving pancreatic head resection and pancreaticoduodenectomy, there is insufficient data at this time to recommend one type of duodenum-preserving resection over another. The preferred operative approaches vary according to patient presentation and imaging findings, concern for malignancy, and as per unit-specific protocols.

While data are limited, no differences have been observed in postoperative pain relief or quality of life. We therefore recommend a tailored approach to each patient based on the individual clinical setting and anatomy, as well as the individual surgeon and institution's experience.

Surveillance consists of monitoring for abatement of symptoms and return to normal life activities. We do not have a specific time interval that imaging is performed.

## KEY MESSAGES

- Approximately 15–30% of cases of chronic pancreatitis present as a mass, also known as mass-forming pancreatitis or "pseudotumor", which can appear similar to a pancreatic neoplasm.
- Distinguishing mass-forming pancreatitis from pancreatic cancer and other neoplasms is challenging and requires a multimodality approach including CT, MRCP, endoscopic retrograde cholangiopancreatography, and/or endoscopic ultrasonography. These patients should be evaluated at high-volume centers with expertise in managing pancreatic diseases utilizing a multidisciplinary approach.
- While medical management remains the mainstay of treatment, surgery is indicated if there is suspicion for underlying malignancy, intractable pain interfering with quality of life or ability to function at work, biliary obstruction not amenable to endoscopic therapy, or duodenal/gastric outlet obstruction.
- Duodenum-preserving pancreatic head resections (Frey, Berne, or Beger) are similarly efficacious as

pancreaticoduodenectomy in providing long-term pain relief, with improved outcomes such as quality of life, morbidity, length of stay, and lower rates of exocrine insufficiency.

■ Pancreaticoduodenectomy is the gold-standard treatment for mass-forming pancreatitis of the head/uncinate if malignancy cannot be ruled out, or in cases of irreversible duodenal/gastric outlet obstruction.

## REFERENCES

1. Ruan Z, Jiao J, Min D et al. Multi-modality imaging features distinguish pancreatic carcinoma from mass-forming chronic pancreatitis of the pancreatic head. *Oncol Lett* 2018;15(6):9735–9744. doi:10.3892/ol.2018.8545.

2. Dutta AK. Head mass in chronic pancreatitis: Inflammatory or malignant. *World J Gastrointest Endosc* 2015;7(3):258. doi:10.4253/wjge.v7.i3.258.

3. Tillou JD, Tatum JA, Jolissaint JS et al. Operative management of chronic pancreatitis: A review. *Am J Surg* 2017;214(2):347–357. doi:10.1016/j.amjsurg.2017.03.004.

4. Narkhede RA, Desai GS, Prasad PP et al. Diagnosis and management of pancreatic adenocarcinoma in the background of chronic pancreatitis: Core issues. *Dig Dis* 2019;37(4):315–324. doi:10.1159/000496507.

5. Diener MK, Rahbari NN, Fischer L et al. Duodenum-preserving pancreatic head resection versus pancreatoduodenectomy for surgical treatment of chronic pancreatitis: A systematic review and meta-analysis. *Ann Surg* 2008;247(6):950–961. doi:10.1097/SLA.0b013e3181724ee7.

# 38 Chronic Pancreatitis: Small Duct Disease with Uncontrolled Pain

*Michael F. Nentwich and Jakob R. Izbicki*

## CONTENTS

## CASE SCENARIO

A 43-year-old woman presented with a history of dull aching abdominal pain for about 16 months. The pain was felt to lie deep in the upper part of the abdominal cavity and radiated into the back from time to time. The pain gradually increased in frequency and severity and was associated with food intake. Prior to presentation, the pain had become constant necessitating regular opioid analgesics and was associated with about 15% loss of her body weight in the last six months. Investigations by her general practitioner did not reveal any reasons for her symptoms. The pain had prompted the patient to become agitated warranting a reactivation of her old smoking habit (she had quit several years prior).

## BACKGROUND OF THE PATHOLOGY

Though being in the focus of clinicians and scientific research for decades, the pathogenesis leading to a chronic pancreatitis is not fully understood. Several risk factors such as toxic, metabolic, obstructive, autoimmune, genetic, and idiopathic are well known. The premature activation of pancreatic enzymes (mainly trypsin) within the acinar cells and the pancreas leads to a local inflammation. Recurrent inflammation induces the proliferation of connective tissue resulting in a fibrosis of pancreatic tissue and a stenosis of small pancreatic ducts. Further fibrotic changes to the pancreas lead to main duct irregularities and usually end up in a dilation of the main duct.

Though chronic alcohol abuse is one of the main risk factors for the development of chronic pancreatitis, other additional factors, especially genetic factors, seem to play at least an equally relevant role, considering chronic alcohol abuse does not regularly result in the development of a chronic pancreatitis.

One of the additional independent factors in the development of a chronic pancreatitis is smoking. Though often associated with alcohol abuse, the negative effect of smoking on disease progression has been noted in patients with non-alcoholic, idiopathic chronic pancreatitis. Therefore, smoking cessation seem to slow down the disease progression of chronic pancreatitis.

The structural changes to the pancreas usually include a main pancreatic duct dilation with atrophy of the rest of the glandular tissue over time. However, there is a small subgroup of patients who present with the classic symptoms of a chronic pancreatitis without a dilation of the main pancreatic duct (<3.5 mm). The reason for this is unclear. As with classic large duct pancreatitis, one of the leading symptoms of the small duct entity is the recurrent, and often hardly controllable, pain. Potential reasons for pain development consist of pancreatic fibrosis-associated inflammation and neural interaction, necrosis, increased pressure in the pancreatic ducts and tissue, and local nerval dysfunction [1–3].

## APPROACH TO MANAGEMENT
### Clinical findings

The diagnostic workup in chronic pancreatitis is commonly initiated when patients complain of recurrent upper abdominal pain, often radiating to the back, associated with food intake, nausea, and vomiting. These symptoms may be accompanied by signs of exocrine (lack of digestive enzymes leading to malabsorption) and endocrine (reduced glycemic control due to lack of insulin production) pancreatic dysfunction, yet exocrine and endocrine insufficiency may also appear without recurrent episodes of pain. Malabsorption leads to steatorrhea (stool is voluminous and hard to flush in toilet because of the high fat content), diarrhea, and results in weight loss that may be accompanied by deficiencies of fat soluble vitamins (vitamin A, D, E, and K) and cobalamin (vitamin B12). As the clinical presentation is variable, one needs to consider the diagnosis of chronic pancreatitis as one of the differential diagnoses of recurrent abdominal pain and weight loss.

Features and symptoms of a "classic" chronic pancreatitis may differ from those in small duct pancreatitis. Small duct pancreatitis seems to be more common in females and the development of a manifest steatorrhea is uncommon [1–3].

## INVESTIGATIONS

The diagnostic workup of a chronic pancreatitis usually consists of assessing structural changes of the pancreas on the one hand as well as losses in exocrine and endocrine function on the other hand. Commonly, the structural changes that develop in the pancreas, such as calcifications and duct dilation can be seen on most image modalities. Though being the gold standard of diagnosis, obtaining a pancreas biopsy is often not possible.

### Image modalities

*Sonography:* Easily available and performable without effort and patient preparation. The pancreatic assessment, especially in the body and tail areas, is difficult and is investigator dependent but warning signs such as bile duct dilation, hepatic lesions, and free abdominal fluid can be ruled out.

*Computed tomography (CT) scan:* Mostly easy, available, and performable with low effort. A CT-scan offers a good depiction of the upper abdominal organs including the pancreas and changes in the pancreatic gland structure such as calcifications and large dilations of the main pancreatic duct. Additionally, a CT scan can detect signs and pathologies such as hepatic lesions, intrahepatic and extrahepatic bile duct dilation, and tumorous masses. Yet, assessment of the pancreatic duct and its side branches is not detailed enough.

*Magnetic resonance cholangiopancreatography:* Oftentimes not as quickly available as a CT scan. Magnetic resonance cholangiopancreatography offers a good depiction of pancreatic gland and duct morphology without the necessity of an invasive procedure that can be further enhanced by performing a secretin magnetic resonance cholangiopancreatography. Figure 38.1 shows a narrowed pancreatic duct on magnetic resonance cholangiopancreatography.

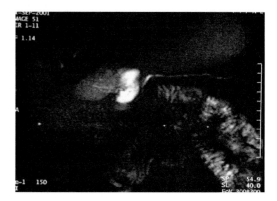

**Figure 38.1** Magnetic resonance cholangiopancreatography depicting a narrowed duct seen in small duct chronic pancreatitis. (Reproduced with permission from Yekebas EF, Bogoevski D, Honarpisheh H, et al. Long-term follow-up in small duct chronic pancreatitis: A plea for extended drainage by V-shaped excision of the anterior aspect of the pancreas. *Ann Surg.* 2006;244(6):940–6; discussion 6–8.)

*Endoscopic retrograde cholangiopancreatography:* Requires planning and patient preparation plus sedation. Endoscopic retrograde cholangiopancreatography gives a good depiction of pancreatic duct anatomy and pathology, additionally the visual and chemical assessment of duct fluid (e.g. mucinous in intraductal mucinous neoplasms) can add to the process of diagnosis. Yet, being an invasive procedure, endoscopic retrograde cholangiopancreatography harbors a risk of procedure related complications such as post-endoscopic retrograde cholangiopancreatography pancreatitis, and a rare chance of (especially duodenal) bowel perforation.

*Endoscopic ultrasound:* Requires planning and patient preparation. In endoscopic ultrasound, pancreatic changes are detectable earlier than with endoscopic retrograde cholangiopancreatography (and possibly magnetic resonance cholangiopancreatography). With endoscopic ultrasound, the parenchymal as well as ductal changes can be visualized and classified using the "Rosemont criteria" to assess for a chronic pancreatitis. It additionally offers the option of endoscopic ultrasound-guided puncture of areas of interest, such as fluid aspiration of cystic lesions. Endoscopic ultrasound harbors the risks of any endoscopic examination with rare incidences of severe complications, unless invasive procedures such as punctures are performed.

Due to its peculiarity, a small duct pancreatitis is not as obvious on imaging studies as a large duct pancreatitis is. Calcifications of the pancreas are infrequent and the modalities depicting mainly the main duct such as endoscopic retrograde cholangiopancreatography or magnetic resonance cholangiopancreatography might only show minimal or no abnormalities at all.

Therefore, functional tests can help to diagnose a small duct pancreatitis. One of the seldom used, but very sensitive and specific, tests is the secretin stimulation test.

*Secretin stimulation test:* Requires planning and patient preparation. An endoscopically placed duodenal tube is aspirated after injection of secretin and the aspirate is assessed for bicarbonate and pancreatic enzyme activity (e.g. lipase). By that, almost one-third of patients with only minimal changes of side branch duct morphology on imaging studies or those with no changes at all can be detected having an abnormal test. Not uncommonly, patients with clear signs of chronic pancreatitis on imaging may have a normal secretin stimulation test.

*Fecal elastase:* Easy to perform. Measuring fecal elastase is a very sensitive and specific test of pancreatic function especially in early phases of pancreatic insufficiency. Only one stool sample is needed and results are not obscured by oral pancreatic enzyme supplementation. It has superseded the 72-hour quantitative fecal fat determination due to its easy application.

*Serum trypsinogen:* Widely available. Serum trypsinogen levels correlate with pancreatic acinar mass and has a high sensitivity in advanced pancreatic insufficiency. In earlier stages of pancreatic insufficiency, the test is not as sensitive and serum trypsinogen levels rise in abdominal pain of non-pancreatic origin as well as in acute pancreatitis.

Serum Immunogolbulin G4 (IgG4): Widely available. Serum IgG4-levels are increased in autoimmune pancreatitis, a condition to be ruled out especially in suspected small duct pancreatitis.

In the Case Scenario, the patient underwent a sonography (with no "red flags") as well as a CT scan ruling out abdominal masses. Taking the patient history into account, a fecal elastase test was performed showing pathologically low elastase-levels. Therefore, a magnetic resonance cholangiopancreatography was done, revealing a slightly narrowed pancreatic main duct, serum IgG4-levels were normal.

## TREATMENT OPTIONS WITH BENEFITS AND RISKS

*The goals of treatment* of a small duct pancreatitis are equal to those of a classic large duct chronic pancreatitis. The treatment revolves around improving the daily quality of life – which is severely compromised by recurrent devastating pain and may be accompanied by symptoms of malabsorption and endocrine insufficiency – just like the patient had reported. These goals can be addressed by combining a variety of treatment options, ranging from lifestyle changes to surgical procedures.

*Lifestyle changes* include a cessation of smoking and alcohol consumption, dietary changes such as a low fat and higher protein diet, and regular sports activity. Additionally, some patients may benefit from relaxation and meditation practices to better cope with disease related stress and pain.

*Exocrine insufficiency* leading to steatorrhea, diarrhea, and malabsorption due to the lack pancreatic enzymes can be treated by oral pancreatic enzyme supplementation. The dose of supplementation can be easily calculated by checking the fat content of the food, as approximately 1 g of fat needs 2,000 units of lipase. For example, a meal containing about 20 g of fat would need a 40.000 unit supplementation, a small snack with 8.5 g fat would need 17.000 units of lipase. Online, several pages exist helping to estimate the fat content of a meal and to find the right amount of enzyme supplement. Several formulations of pancreatic enzyme supplementation exist, some are enteric coated while some are not (to avoid acid inactivation of enzymes, H2-antagonists or proton pump inhibitors should be taken additionally). The enzyme supplement is usually taken right before the meals (best with room temperature water) and should not be chewed.

Though steatorrhea is not fully stopped by lipase substitution, it is reduced to a level where sufficient fat absorption can be achieved and body weight can be gained. Pancreatic enzyme substitution is not only helpful in treating malabsorption, but it also plays a role in pain relief especially in small duct pancreatitis. The effect of pain reduction with pancreatic enzyme substitution is thought to be derived by a negative feedback mechanism. Usually, the pancreatic exocrine secretion is inhibited by intraduodenal serine proteases. As protease activity is reduced in patients with chronic pancreatitis, the feedback mechanism fails and continues to stimulate pancreatic secretion and by supplementing enzyme preparations (that should already be released in the duodenum), constant pancreatic stimulation is thought to be reduced.

*Pain control* is one of the main goals in the treatment of a chronic pancreatitis, and often is difficult to achieve. The conservative therapy consists of analgesics (nonsteroidal anti-inflammatory drugs up to combination therapies with opiates), co-analgesics (e.g. gabapentin and antidepressants), pancreatic secretion suppression (octreotide), and interventional attempts of pain control via celiac plexus neurolysis. As the treatment options are numerous yet the understanding of pancreatic pain pathophysiology is incomplete, a thorough review on therapeutic strategies as well as insights on experimental findings is given in [4].

*The indication for surgery* in small duct disease is a severe, continuous uncontrollable pain that affects daily life and leads to repeated hospital admissions. During the course of disease, pain usually will not spontaneously decrease ("burnout") with vanishing pancreatic tissue. This can result in an addiction to pain medication; yet without adequate pain relief, the pain can have a severe effect on the patient's life. The ongoing destruction of pancreatic tissue is unpredictable and surgery does not cure a chronic pancreatitis, but it can offer sufficient pain relief. As surgery for chronic pancreatitis can be performed with acceptable morbidity and mortality rates (in specialized centers), it offers a durable and good therapeutic option for pain control as well as for management of chronic pancreatitis complications (strictures, pseudocysts, pseudo tumors, etc.) and surgery is favored by randomized controlled trials over endoscopic therapies.

Surgical procedures can be divided in both drainage or resection procedures, combination procedures, and denervation procedures. Thereby, the aim of surgery is to achieve a good drainage of the ductal system including the side ducts, to remove an inflammatory (or potentially malignant mass) and to preserve a maximum of pancreatic functionality. A larger number of procedures for drainage, resection, drainage, and resection, as well as for denervation exist (Table 38.1) and are beyond the scope of this chapter to be described in detail. Reference [2] gives a good figured overview on these techniques.

In case of a dominant head mass in small duct pancreatitis, a pancreatoduodenectomy was initially the preferred approach. However, nowadays, the duodenum-preserving pancreatic head resection and its modifications are more commonly performed. Distal pancreatectomy seems to be beneficial only in a small subset of patients with disease limited to the body and tail of the pancreas. Near-total pancreatectomies failed to achieve a satisfactory pain relief along with severe pancreatic functional loss and should therefore be considered last.

For small duct pancreatitis, the operation of choice in the authors' view is a combination of resection and drainage of the pancreas, the "Hamburg V-shaped excision". The Izbicki modification to the Partington-Rochelle procedure, as well as the Frey and Amikura procedures, includes an excision of the pancreatic head as well as a V-shaped longitudinal excision of the ventral pancreas to not only achieve drainage of the main pancreatic duct but also of the secondary and tertiary ducts in the periphery of the gland, the sought to be place of the small duct pancreatitis origin. This surgical technique, as reported in the long-term follow-up study after introduction of this technique, led to an increase of the global quality-of-life index in median by 54%, the median pain score decreased by 95%, and 73% of patients had a complete pain relief. Forty-three percent of patients developed diabetes, the exocrine function was well-preserved in 78% of patients, with 0% mortality and a morbidity of 19.6%. [1–3,5]. Figure 38.2 shows the hollowing of the pancreatic head, followed by pancreatic duct-incision and V-shape resection resulting in a V-shaped cut-out throughout the pancreatic body and tail. The reconstruction is done by a side-to-side pancreaticoojejunostomy using continuous sutures.

The patient in this Case Scenario had an exocrine, but no endocrine, pancreatic insufficiency. IgG4-levels were normal and magnetic resonance cholangiopancreatography showed subtle changes to the main pancreatic duct. CT

## Table 38.1 Overview of Surgical Procedures

**Surgical Procedures**

| *Drainage* | *Resection* | *Drainage plus resection* | *Denervation* |
|---|---|---|---|
| • Duval<br>• Puestow and Gillespie<br>• Partington and Rochelle | • Duodenum preserving pancreatectomy<br>• Kausch-Whipple pancreatoduodenectomy<br>• Pylorus preserving pancreatoduodenectomy<br>• Subtotal pancreatectomy<br>• Distal pancreatectomy | • Beger<br>• Frey<br>• Berne procedure<br>• Hamburg V-shape (Izbicki procedure) | • Splanchniectomy<br>• Coeliac ganglionectomy<br>• Denervated pancreatic flap surgery |

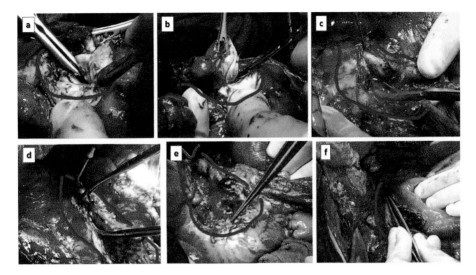

**Figure 38.2** Intraoperative photographs demonstrating a duodenum-preserving pancreatic head resection with V-shape excision (blue lines indicate pancreas borders). (a and b) Pancreatic head incision and "hollowing" of the pancreatic head. (c) Incision of the pancreatic duct toward the pancreatic tail. (d) Increasing the cut-out toward the pancreatic borders to achieve a V-shape resection. (e) Final resection status (red lines depict the V-shaped cut-out). (f) Reconstruction by side-to-side pancreatojejunostomy using running sutures (forceps pointing toward pancreatic tail).

scans did not reveal other suspicious findings such as abdominal masses or metastases. A pancreatic enzyme supplementation was begun, leading to a moderate improvement of steatorrhea and weight loss, but did not improve pain control. After discussing the therapeutic options interdisciplinary and with the patient, she opted for a surgical approach instead of a coeliac plexus blockade or an endoscopic intervention in hope of best pain relief. The patient underwent a Hamburg V-shape resection, had an uneventful postsurgical course, and a substantial decrease of pain post-surgically. Unfortunately, she was lost to a long term follow-up to especially ask for persistent pain decrease. Though being anecdotal, this case demonstrates the severity of pancreatitis and pancreatitis-associated life affections.

### KEY MESSAGES

- Small duct pancreatitis is a rare form of chronic pancreatitis without clear dilation of the main duct and difficult to depict dilation of the pancreatic side branches. As the classic large duct chronic pancreatitis, it can result in uncontrollable pain as well as malabsorption.
- In case of recurrent abdominal pain, the possibility of a small duct pancreatitis has to be considered.

- Diagnostic workup includes imaging studies (endoscopic ultrasound, secretin-MCRP, endoscopic retrograde cholangiopancreatography, etc.) as well as functional tests.
- The therapeutic approach consists of supplementation and substitution of exocrine (pancreatic enzymes) and endocrine (diabetes control) function as well as pain control.
- Pain control can be hard to achieve via conservative methods and surgery can offer a substantial pain improvement. Thereby, the authors prefer a combination of resectional and drainage techniques resulting in a local pancreatic head excision with a V-shaped longitudinal excision of the pancreas not only draining the pancreatic main duct but also reaching the ducts of second and tertiary order.
- Though surgery does not cure chronic pancreatitis, it can substantially increase the quality of life by pain reduction.

### REFERENCES

1. Gupta V, Toskes PP. Diagnosis and management of chronic pancreatitis. *Postgrad Med J* 2005;81(958):491–497.

2. Pujahari AK. Chronic pancreatitis: A review. *Indian J Surg* 2015;77(Suppl 3):1348–1358.

3. Shrikhande SV, Kleeff J, Friess H et al. Management of pain in small duct chronic pancreatitis. *J Gastrointest Surg* 2006;10(2):227–233.

4. Barreto SG, Saccone GT. Pancreatic nociception – Revisiting the physiology and pathophysiology. *Pancreatology* 2012;12(2):104–112.

5. Yekebas EF, Bogoevski D, Honarpisheh H et al. Long-term follow-up in small duct chronic pancreatitis: A plea for extended drainage by 'V-shaped excision" of the anterior aspect of the pancreas. *Ann Surg* 2006;244(6):940–946; discussion 6–8.

# 39 Multifocal Branch Duct Intraductal Papillary Mucinous Neoplasm with 3 cm Lesion in Head of Pancreas

*Atsushi Oba, Robert J. Torphy, Richard D. Schulick, and Marco Del Chiaro*

## CONTENTS

## CASE SCENARIO

A 55-year-old woman presented to a local hospital with abdominal pain. An abdominal ultrasound was advised that revealed a 3 cm cystic mass in the head of pancreas. Abdominal computed tomography (CT) and magnetic resonance imaging (MRI) scans were performed which showed three cystic lesions in the pancreatic head (34 mm), body (5 mm), and tail (8 mm) with a maximal main pancreatic duct diameter of 2.4 mm (Figure 39.1). The serum carbohydrate antigen (CA) 19-9 level was 15.4 U/mL and carcinoembryonic antigen was 2.2 mg/dL. The patient had no significant personal or family history neither for pancreatic, nor other malignancies. Her abdominal pain was treated with simple analgesia. An endoscopic ultrasound was performed which confirmed the findings noted on cross-sectional imaging. No solid components were identified in the cyst. A fine-needle aspiration was performed. Cystic fluid carcinoembryonic antigen was 400 ng/mL. Based on all the investiagtions, the patient was diagnosed as a case of multifocal branch duct type intraductal papillary mucinous neoplasm for which a total pancreatectomy was recommended. She was referred to our hospital for a second opinion regarding the management of her lesions.

## BACKGROUND OF THE PATHOLOGY

Intraductal papillary mucinous neoplasm is a type of pancreatic cystic neoplasm which is increasingly being identified on cross-sectional imaging. Of all the pancreatic cystic neoplasms, the ones with malignant potential, namely main duct intraductal papillary mucinous neoplasm, branch duct type intraductal papillary mucinous neoplasm, and

mucinous cystic neoplasm should be clearly identified [1].

On pathology, intraductal papillary mucinous neoplasms are grossly visible (generally >1 cm in diameter) neoplasms arising from the main pancreatic duct or branch ducts, with varying degrees of duct dilatation. On microscopy, they are noninvasive, mucin-producing, predominantly papillary, or rarely flat epithelial lesions and include a variety of cell types with a spectrum of cytologic and architectural atypia.

Main duct intraductal papillary mucinous neoplasm is characterized by a segmental or diffuse dilation of the main pancreatic duct to ≥5 mm in the absence of other causes of obstruction. Considering its ability for cancer transformation, surgery is recommended even in cases with a relatively small maximal main pancreatic duct dilatation (between 5–9.9 mm) [2]. Branch duct type intraductal papillary mucinous neoplasm is generally believed to have the lowest malignant potential among the mucinous pancreatic cystic neoplasms. As a result, these lesions need to be accurately diagnosed and characterized so that the appropriate treatment can be advised. For intraductal papillary mucinous neoplasm, all pancreatic ductal epithelial cells could be at risk of dysplastic change, as most typically shown in patients with multifocal branch duct type intraductal papillary mucinous neoplasms. Currently, most international guidelines propose radiological and clinical criteria to assess the risk of high-grade dysplasia or cancer in patients with intraductal papillary mucinous neoplasms. Their management should be evidence based. The European Guidelines on Cystic Tumors of the Pancreas is one of the preferred evidence-based

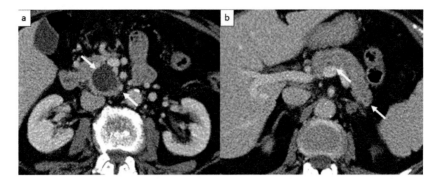

**Figure 39.1** Axial CT scan images in venous contrast phase demonstrating multifocal cystic lesions (white arrows) in the pancreas with a main pancreatic duct diameter of 2.4 mm. (a) 34 × 24 mm cystic lesion in pancreatic head. (b) 5 × 5 mm cystic lesion in pancreatic body and 8 × 4 mm cystic lesion in pancreatic tail.

guidelines for the management of pancreatic cystic neoplasms [2].

## APPROACH TO MANAGEMENT

### Cross-sectional imaging

A dedicated pancreatic-protocol CT and pancreatic MRI/magnetic resonance cholangiopancreatography (MRCP) are reported to have a similar accuracy for the characterization of pancreatic cystic neoplasms. MRI/MRCP is more sensitive than CT for identifying a communication between the pancreatic cystic neoplasm and pancreatic ductal system, as well as the presence of a mural nodule or internal septations [2]. In addition, it is very sensitive for identifying whether a patient has a single or multiple pancreatic cystic neoplasms, with the latter favoring a diagnosis of multifocal branch-duct type intraductal papillary mucinous neoplasm. Patients with pancreatic cystic neoplasm may require lifelong imaging follow-up. This is important, as studies have shown that repeated exposure to ionizing radiation following CT increases the risk of malignancy. For this reason, MRI is also considered the best method for surveillance of patients affected by pancreatic cystic neoplasms [2]. Otherwise, multimodality imaging should be considered in cases where the identification of calcifications is important for tumor staging or for diagnosing postoperative recurrent disease. The use of CT should be restricted to the following clinical situations:

a) For the detection of parenchymal, mural, or central calcification, and especially when differentiating pseudocysts associated with chronic pancreatitis from pancreatic cystic neoplasm.

b) When there is a suspicion of a malignant pancreatic cystic neoplasm or concomitant

pancreatic cancer, and when assessment of vascular involvement, peritoneal, or metastatic disease is required.

c) When there is suspicion of postoperative recurrence of pancreatic cancer.

d) In patients who are unable to undergo an MRI.

### Endoscopic ultrasound/endoscopic ultrasound with fine-needle aspiration

Endoscopic ultrasound is a useful adjunct to other imaging modalities. Endoscopic ultrasound is helpful for identifying pancreatic cystic neoplasms with features that should be considered for surgical resection. Similar to MRI and CT, endoscopic ultrasound is imperfect at identifying the exact type of pancreatic cystic neoplasm. Endoscopic ultrasound is recommended if the pancreatic cystic neoplasm has either clinical or radiological features of concern identified during the initial investigation or follow-up. Data for endoscopic ultrasound-based differentiation between benign and malignant pancreatic cystic neoplasms are conflicting. In addition, there is considerable inter-observer variation in endoscopic ultrasound-based diagnoses.

Contrast-enhanced harmonic endoscopic ultrasound should be considered for further evaluation of mural nodules. Contrast-enhanced harmonic endoscopic ultrasound is also helpful in assessing vascularity within the cyst as well as septations. The presence of hyperenhancement of a mural nodule, solid mass, or septations on contrast-enhanced harmonic endoscopic ultrasound raises concern for malignant transformation, and endoscopic ultrasound with fine-needle aspiration of the lesion should be considered. Contrast-enhanced harmonic endoscopic ultrasound seems superior to standard endoscopic ultrasound and CT for the identification of mural nodules. Interobserver agreement is excellent for contrast-enhanced harmonic endoscopic ultrasound using Sonazoid (perflubutane), and moderate for SonoVue (sulfur hexafluoride).

While endoscopic ultrasound is used for the diagnosis and follow-up of intraductal papillary mucinous neoplasms and pancreatic cystic neoplasms, there is no evidence supporting its superiority in diagnostic accuracy. The main drawback of endoscopic ultrasound it its invasiveness (especially when associated with fine-needle aspiration and biopsy) with the attendant risk of complications. The Euroepan guidelines recommend the use of endoscopic ultrasound (and endoscopic ultrasound with fine-needle aspiration) only if it will provide additional information that will alter the clinical strategy [2]. For example, it is very unlikely that endoscopic ultrasound can change a clinical decision regarding a 2 cm branch duct type intraductal papillary mucinous neoplasm without any radiological sign of high-grade dysplasia or cancer. In contrast, in a 4 cm suspected branch duct type intraductal papillary mucinous neoplasm, an endoscopic ultrasound with fine-needle aspiration can help differentiate between a branch duct type intraductal papillary mucinous neoplasm and an oligocystic serous adenoma. Consequently, it could help to decide if surgical resection is indicated. A combined analysis of cyst fluid carcinoembryonic antigen, lipase levels, and cytology provides the highest accuracy for differentiating mucinous from non-mucinous pancreatic cystic neoplasms. An endoscopic ultrasound with fine-needle aspiration should not be performed if the diagnosis is already established by cross-sectional imaging, or where there is a clear indication for surgery. The role of endoscopic ultrasound with fine-needle aspiration in the diagnosis of pancreatic cystic neoplasm is still a matter of debate, and consensus in the literature is lacking.

## Surgery

Surgical resection is the only treatment option for patients with intraductal papillary mucinous neoplasms with risk of high-grade dysplasia or cancer. According to the European Guidelines, there are absolute and relative criteria for resection. The absolute criteria are associated with a high risk for cancer; therefore every patient fit for surgery, with one of these absolute criteria, should be offered a resection. Relative criteria are aimed at detecting high-grade dysplasia and lesions with an increased

risk for cancer. In these patients the aim is to resect pre-cancerous lesions. Patients fit for surgery and with a long life expectancy should be offered resection when relative criteria are met.

- *Absolute Criteria for Resection*
  - The presence of (tumor-related) jaundice
  - Cytology positive for high-grade dysplasia or cancer
  - The presence of a contrast-enhancing mural nodule ($\geq$5 mm), solid mass, or a maximal main pancreatic duct measuring $\geq$10 mm
- *Relative Criteria for Resection*
  - Maximal main pancreatic duct dilatation between 5–9.9 mm
  - Cyst growth rate $\geq$5 mm/year
  - Increased level of serum CA 19.9 (>37 U/mL)
  - Clinical symptoms
  - Enhancing mural nodules (<5 mm)
  - New-onset diabetes mellitus
  - Acute pancreatitis (caused by intraductal papillary mucinous neoplasm)
  - Cyst diameter $\geq$40 mm

Interestingly, cyst size is becoming less important as a criterion for resection. According to the European Guidelines, a cyst size of 40 mm in diameter, in the absence of other features concerning for malignancy or high-grade dysplasia, is considered a relative indication for surgery. Several studies that have include-surgically resected and observed intraductal papillary mucinous neoplasms, have reported an increased risk of malignancy ranging from 12–47% in cases of a cyst $\geq$30 mm. In some of these studies [3], the impact of cyst size on the risk of malignancy was analyzed using stratification based on the presence of other features for malignancy. The studies confirmed what we now know about the lack of importance of cyst size on the risk of malignancy in the absence of other features. This was even confirmed in a large series of patients with branch duct type intraductal papillary mucinous neoplasms [4].

The surgical approach for main duct intraductal papillary mucinous neoplasm and most branch duct type intraductal papillary mucinous neoplasm is an oncological resection with standard lymphadenectomy. Parenchyma-sparing pancreatectomy is a non-oncological procedure, which is suitable only for lesions with a very low probability of malignancy including patients without risk factors who have a strong desire to be operated on. The indications for parenchyma-sparing pancreatectomy are very limited considering that surgery is rarely indicated for benign cysts and the morbidity of parenchyma-sparing pancreatectomy is the same as that of conventional pancreatectomies.

### Multifocal branch duct type intraductal papillary mucinous neoplasm

In multifocal branch duct type intraductal papillary mucinous neoplasm, each cyst should be evaluated individually for the presence of features associated with malignancy in order to determine their need for surgical extirpation. Once this appraisal is performed, a tailored surgical approach can be planned. An intraoperative analysis of the surgical margins may help to determine the need for expanded resection [3]. Cysts without concerning features can undergo surveillance.

### Case scenario (continued) and follow-up

In the patient presented at the beginning of the chapter, none of the individual cysts met absolute or relative criteria for resection, which meant that they were amenable to follow-up. Follow-up of branch duct type intraductal papillary mucinous neoplasm is required as progression of disease is expected in about 10–15% of patients in the ensuing three to five years. Surveillance should also include the entire pancreatic gland because of an increased risk of new-onset cancer [5]. In patients with main duct intraductal papillary mucinous neoplasm and those with mixed-type intraductal papillary mucinous neoplasm several factors may predict progression during surveillance (e.g. diffuse maximal main pancreatic duct dilatation, serum CA 19-9, serum alkaline phosphatase, and absence of extra pancreatic cysts).

MRI is the preferred imaging modality for the follow-up of intraductal papillary mucinous neoplasm. Endoscopic ultrasound can be used in selected cases. A six-month follow-up in the first year, and yearly follow-ups thereafter is adequate when no risk factors are present that establish an indication for surgery. In contrast to the American Guidelines, the progression risk in branch duct type intraductal papillary mucinous neoplasms increases over time, as demonstrated by several studies [2,4]. Changes in clinical symptoms should trigger investigations. For patients with a relative indication for surgery who do not immediately proceed to surgical resection given age or comorbidities, a six-month follow-up is recommended.

### KEY MESSAGES

- In multifocal branch duct type intraductal papillary mucinous neoplasm, each cyst should be evaluated individually for the presence of features associated with malignancy.
- The absolute criteria (jaundice, cytology positive, a contrast-enhancing mural nodule, solid mass, or a maximal main pancreatic duct measuring ≥10 mm) are associated with a high risk for cancer and therefore surgery must be considered in the management of patients fit for surgery.
- There has been a recent trend toward a reduced focus on cyst size as an indication for surgical resection. A cyst size of ≥40 mm in diameter, in the absence of other risk factors for malignancy, is only considered a relative indication for resection according to the European Guidelines.
- MRI is the preferred imaging modality for the follow-up of intraductal papillary mucinous neoplasm and a six-month follow-up in the first year, and yearly follow-up thereafter, is adequate when no risk factors are present.

### REFERENCES

1. Hruban RH, Takaori K, Klimstra DS et al. An illustrated consensus on the classification of pancreatic intraepithelial neoplasia and intraductal papillary mucinous neoplasms. *Am J Surg Pathol* 2004;28(8):977–987.
2. European Study Group on Cystic Tumours of the P. European evidence-based guidelines on pancreatic cystic neoplasms. *Gut* 2018;67(5):789–804.
3. Del Chiaro M, Beckman R, Ateeb Z et al. Main duct dilatation is the best predictor of high-grade dysplasia or invasion in intraductal papillary mucinous neoplasms of the pancreas. *Ann Surg* 2019.
4. Del Chiaro M, Segersvard R, Pozzi Mucelli R et al. Comparison of preoperative conference-based diagnosis with histology of cystic tumors of the pancreas. *Ann Surg Oncol* 2014;21(5):1539–1544.
5. Han Y, Lee H, Kang JS et al. Progression of pancreatic branch Duct intraductal papillary mucinous neoplasm associates with cyst size. *Gastroenterology* 2018;154(3):576–584.

# 40 Resectable Pancreatic Cancer Post Roux-en-Y Gastric Bypass for Obesity

*Sarah Bormann and Savio George Barreto*

## CONTENTS

## CASE SCENARIO

A 60-year-old obese woman presented with pyrexia of unknown origin to her general practitioner. The patient reported abdominal pain and so a computed tomography (CT) scan of the abdomen was performed. The scan revealed an obstructed common bile duct secondary to a periampullary mass. She was referred for further management of this likely malignancy. Her only significant past surgical history was that four years prior she had undergone bariatric surgery (a Roux-en-Y gastric bypass) that was complicated postoperatively by a collection that needed a repeat laparoscopy and drain placement. The details of this intervention were unclear, but the patient volunteered that no further intervention was required.

## BACKGROUND OF THE PATHOLOGY

The global incidence of obesity has steadily increased over the last few decades. Obesity and increased body mass index (BMI) have been linked to an increased risk of pancreatic cancer while sarcopenic obesity has been shown to be result in an increased postoperative complication rates and shorter overall survival. The underlying pathophysiologic mechanisms postulated for this observed phenomenon include lower insulin sensitivity, cross talk between tumor cells and surrounding adipocytes, obesity-induced hypoxia, oxidative stress, and chronic inflammation, migrating adipose stromal cells, functional defeat of the immune function, aberrations in fatty acid metabolism and shared genetic susceptibility [1]. While bariatric surgery, with likely attendant weight reduction, may offer the hope of reducing the risk of developing cancer, this has not been conclusively demonstrated in pancreatic and periampullary cancer. Regardless, there has been an exponential increase in the number of bariatric surgeries performed around the world. Thus, pancreatic surgeons and surgical oncologists are going to be treating a substantial number of patients with pancreatic cancer who have undergone prior bariatric surgery. It is thus important to understand what options are possible in terms of reconstruction, especially after a Roux-en-Y gastric bypass and the altered anatomy resulting therefrom. In the case of a prior adjustable gastric band or a sleeve gastrectomy, the anatomical alterations are not as significant to impact on the ensuing pancreatic surgery.

## APPROACH TO MANAGEMENT

The approach to a patient with suspected pancreatic head or periampullary cancer follows a standard algorithm. Most patients present with jaundice, as was the case in the patient referred, and so the initial workup consists of blood investigations and an ultrasound. The various blood investigations performed are as follows:

a) *Complete blood counts*: An elevated white cell count may be seen in cholangitis secondary to biliary obstruction and may help the clinician consider biliary drainage first. In our patient, with a prior Roux-en-Y gastric bypass, an endoscopic retrograde cholangiopancreatography was not feasible at the time and so if she had been cholangitic necessitating biliary drainage, we would have had to resort to a percutaneous transhepatic approach. Patients with periampullary tumors may present with anemia as these tumors tend to slough off and cause occult bleeding.

b) *Liver function tests*: Alterations in serum bilirubin, gamma glutamyl transpeptidase, and alkaline phosphatase are encountered in patients with surgical obstructive jaundice.

c) *Renal function tests*: It is important to check renal functions before embarking on contrast-enhanced CT scans.

d) *Prothrombin time and international normalized ratio*: Being aware of the coagulation status in a patient with surgical obstructive jaundice is imperative prior to preoperative biliary drainage, surgery, or in the event that the anesthetist is considering the placement of an epidural catheter.

e) *Blood sugar levels*: In patients with obesity and suspected pancreatic cancer, in general, it is important to measure the blood glucose levels.

f) *Other tests to be done in a patient after bariatric surgery*: Metabolic profile, thyroid function tests, iron studies, Vitamin B12, and fat-soluble vitamins.

### Abdominal ultrasound

This is the first investigation performed in a patient with a suspected pancreatobiliary pathology. While its use may be limited by body habitus in obese patients, it still should be performed as it may provide useful preliminary information that may help guide the next important test. Findings may vary from a dilated biliary tree to liver metastases and ascites. The visualisation of gallstones and a dilated common bile duct without a clear cause for the biliary dilation should prompt further investigations such as a magnetic resonance cholangiopancreatography (MRCP), in the least.

If these initial investigations raise the suspicion of a pancreatic head or periampullary malignant process, then the next useful investigations include:

### Tumor marker

Serum carbohydrate antigen 19-9 (CA 19-9): This is useful as a complementary test to support the diagnosis of pancreatic or periampullary cancer. Caution must be advised in interpreting a mildly elevated result in a patient with biliary dilation as this may be an erroneous value. The flip side is also pertinent for patients who are unable to secrete CA 19-9 due to being Lewis blood group antigen negative.

### Radiological investigations

a) Pancreas protocol multidetector computed tomography (MDCT) scan of the abdomen and pelvis with multiplanar reconstruction: This modality comprises a pre-contrast scan and three post-contrast phases with axial section thickness ≤5 mm. It also uses water or mannitol as negative contrast to distend the stomach and duodenum. It is regarded as the best investigation not only for assessing the primary tumor, but also its locoregional and distant intra-abdominal spread. It also provides valuable preoperative delineation of the vascular anatomy which is essential for preoperative surgical planning. Figure 40.1 demonstrates the CT findings in the patient discussed in this chapter.

b) Magnetic resonance imaging (MRI) of the abdomen and pelvis, and MRCP: These are useful alternatives to MDCT if patients have contrast allergies or if the facilities for performing, or the expertise needed to report a CT scan, are unavailable. MRIs may also be of value in the assessment of isoattenuating cancers.

c) Chest X-ray or CT of the chest: Used to rule out lung metastases.

Other tests in the preoperative workup of obese patients:

- Cardiovascular evaluation including an electrocardiogram and possible stress test to detect occult coronary artery disease

- Respiratory evaluation: Arterial blood gas, and pulmonary function tests

- Doppler ultrasound: To rule out deep venous thrombosis

It is important to note that both CT and MRI have their limitations in determining the presence of, or delineating, smaller lesions <2 cm, in the accurate characterisation of venous involvement, as well as in the diagnosis of small liver metastases, especially on its surface, and peritoneal disease. In this situation, if there is a strong suspicion of advanced disease or vascular invasion, complementary investigations include endoscopic ultrasound, positron emission tomography CT (PET-CT), venography, or staging laparoscopy.

### Endoscopy

a) Side-viewing endoscopy may be performed to visualize the ampulla and obtain biopsies of ampullary and duodenal carcinomas.

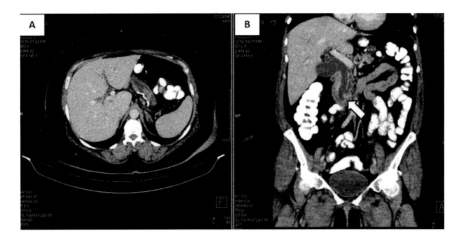

**Figure 40.1** Contrast-enhanced CT scan of sections of the abdomen. (A) Axial post-contrast CT section showing staple line of the pouch post Roux-en-Y gastric bypass. (B) Coronal section of the abdomen with a dilated common bile duct down to the level of a mass in the ampulla reformation showing common bile duct and pancreatic duct dilation due to suspicion of a periampullary tumor (*white arrow*). (Reproduced with permission from Malhotra S, Barreto SG. Surgery for Cancer after previous Bariatric Surgery. In: *Surgical Emergencies in the Cancer Patient.* Edited by Fong Y, Kauffmann RM, Marcinkowski E, Singh G, Schoelhammer H. Pp 371–382.)

b) Endoscopic retrograde cholangiopancreatography is useful in patients with pancreatic head and periampullary cancer to obtain biliary cytology for diagnosis, but more importantly to relieve biliary obstruction (with the placement of stents) in patients who have cholangitis, or in those who are debilitated by severe jaundice or other comorbidities as these patients need optimisation prior to surgery. Endobiliary drainage with self-expanding metal stents offers useful palliation of obstructive jaundice in patients with advanced disease.

c) Endoscopic ultrasound plays a complementary role by aiding in the delineation of periampullary lesions (suspected on imaging) or lesions <2 cm. It is also useful in providing an access for the performance of fine-needle aspiration cytology to confirm the diagnosis of malignancy prior to commencing neoadjuvant (in borderline resectable or locally advanced disease) or palliative (metastatic disease) chemotherapy or radiotherapy, and in the assessment of vascular involvement suspected on CT or MRI.

Endoscopic procedures are feasible in patients who have undergone prior adjustable gastric band or a sleeve gastrectomy. However, in the patient presented above (with a prior Roux-en-Y gastric bypass), the altered gastric anatomy precludes the performance of these procedures. The options to biliary drainage (if absolutely indicated) include the percutaneous transhepatic approach or a laparoscopic (endoscopic) transgastric approach performed via the gastric remnant of the Roux-en-Y gastric bypass. For pancreatic head and periampullary cancers, obtaining a preoperative histological diagnosis is not an absolute necessity prior to surgical resection.

### Complementary investigations

a) *PET-CT*: This scan is recommended by most national guidelines for the routine staging of resectable pancreatic cancer.

b) *Staging laparoscopy and laparoscopic ultrasonography*: The main indication for these modalities include the assessment of non-metastatic, unresectable, or borderline resectable disease on conventional imaging to rule out peritoneal disease as their presence will alter the intent of treatment from curative to palliative.

### SURGICAL MANAGEMENT

A patient who has been fully and adequately worked up must be discussed in a multidisciplinary team meeting comprising of surgeons, medical and radiation oncologists, pathologists, and radiologists.

A complete surgical resection with negative microscopic margins and a standard lymphadenectomy offers the best chance of cure in patients with pancreatic and periampullary cancer. In patients with a pancreatic head or periampullary cancer, the appropriate operation is a pancreatoduodenectomy while patients with cancers of the body and tail would require a distal pancreatectomy with splenectomy.

In patients who have had an adjustable gastric band or a sleeve gastrectomy, the ensuing pancreatic cancer surgery follows the standard principles. The possibility of adhesions from the previous surgery presents the only additional challenge to the operation. In patients who have had a prior adjustable gastric band, the removal of the band at the time of pancreatic cancer surgery must be considered. In the case of patient with a previous sleeve gastrectomy, a pylorus-preserving pancreatoduodenectomy with preservation of the right gastric artery should be performed [2] (Figure 40.2).

In patients who have undergone a previous Roux-en-Y gastric bypass, the following considerations need to be made during pancreatic surgery.

### Distal pancreatectomy and splenectomy

a) Careful adhesiolysis: Specific attention needs to be given to obtaining a safe access into the lesser sac behind the Roux limb, creation of a safe plane behind the Roux limb, and dissecting the gastric remnant off the gastric pouch without compromising the pouch and the gastroenterostomy.

b) The division of the short gastric vessels presents a theoretical concern of affecting the blood supply of the remnant (excluded portion of) stomach. In the case of damage to the remnant stomach during dissection, or if the blood supply is compromised during splenectomy, the surgeon must consider

a resection of the remnant and stapling off the pylorus.

### Pancreatoduodenectomy

a) Careful adhesiolysis.

b) The resection portion of the pancreato-duodenectomy proceeds as in the case of a standard pancreatoduodenectomy with care taken to perform [3] a supracolic division of duodenum to ensure a sufficient length of the biliopancreatic limb. Specific attention needs to be given to the mobilization of the safe duodenojejunal flexure which can be impeded by the pre-existing Roux-limb.

c) A complete resection of the remnant stomach *in toto* with the pancreatoduodenectomy should be performed so long as it can be safely carried out without injuring the Roux limb and the gastroenterostomy. In the patient presented above, the complication following the Roux-en-Y gastric bypass had caused significant scarring which precluded a safe resection of the remnant. Thus, an additional gastroenterostomy had to be performed between the Roux limb and the remnant stomach to help drain the remnant.

d) Reconstruction depends on the length of the remaining biliopancreatic limb. If there is sufficient length to permit a safe pancreaticojejunostomy [4] and hepaticojejunostomy

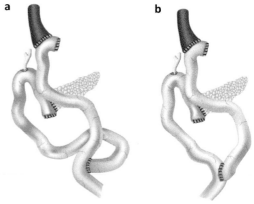

**Figure 40.3** Diagrammatic representation of the reconstruction following a pancreato-duodenectomy in a patient who has undergone a previous Roux-en-Y gastric bypass. (a) Sufficient length of the biliopancreatic limb. (b) Insufficient length of the biliopancreatic limb. In this case, a new Roux limb downstream needs to be created for anastomosis to the pancreatic and hepatic ducts with an enteroenterostomy between the two Roux limbs.

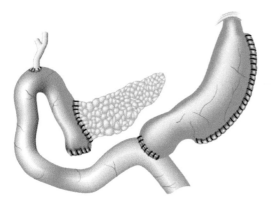

**Figure 40.2** Diagrammatic representation of the reconstruction following a pylorus-preserving pancreatoduodenectomy in a patient who has undergone a previous sleeve gastrectomy.

without tension, then this can be carried out by delivering the limb to the supracolic compartment behind the Roux limb (Figure 40.3a). In this scenario, no further enteroenterostomy is warranted. This type of reconstruction was performed in the patient presented in this chapter. However, if the biliopancreatic limb is not of adequate length to enable a safe anastomosis without tension, then a new "Roux limb" should be fashioned (for anastomosis to the pancreatic stump and cut end of the common hepatic duct) from the jejunum downstream of the previous enteroenterostomy. A new enteroenterostomy between the two Roux limbs should be created at a distance of >40 cm downstream from the hepaticojejunostomy (Figure 40.3b).

The postoperative course and the risks are no different from a routine pancreatic resectional surgery.

Patients should be considered for adjuvant therapy based on the pathological staging of their cancer after discussion within a multidisciplinary team meeting taking into account the patient's performance status and comorbidities [5].

### KEY MESSAGES

- Obesity presents an increased risk for most solid organ cancers, including pancreatic cancer.
- The altered anatomy must be considered when planning preoperative endoscopic interventions in these patients.
- Prior bariatric surgery does not preclude a safe pancreatic resection and every attempt must be made to offer the patient the best chance of cure.
- Obese patients tend to be malnourished and preoperative nutritional (micronutrient) optimization is imperative before surgery.

- In patients who have undergone previous Roux-en-Y gastric bypass, the gastric remnant (excluded portion of stomach) should be resected in toto with the pancreatoduodenectomy specimen, if feasible. If the remnant is not resected, an additional gastroenterostomy must be performed between it and the Roux limb.
- The pancreaticojejunostomy and hepaticojejunostomy reconstruction must be tailored to the length of available biliopancreatic limb. The principles of pancreatic surgery, namely, a well vascularized duct-to-mucosa anastomosis with fine sutures and "no tension" on the anastomosis is absolutely essential.

### REFERENCES

1. Malhotra S, Barreto S. Surgery for cancer after previous bariatric surgery. In: Fong Y, Kauffmann R, Marcinkowski E, Singh G, Schoelhammer H, editors. *Surgical Emergencies in the Cancer Patient*. Cham, Switzerland: Springer; 2016. p. 371–382.
2. Hatzaras I, Sachs TE, Weiss M et al. Pancreaticoduodenectomy after bariatric surgery: Challenges and available techniques for reconstruction. *J Gastrointest Surg* 2014 Apr;18(4):869–877.
3. Shukla PJ, Barreto G, Pandey D et al. Modification in the technique of pancreaticoduodenectomy: Supracolic division of jejunum to facilitate uncinate process dissection. *Hepatogastroenterology* 2007 Sep;54(78):1728–1730.
4. Barreto SG, Shukla PJ. Different types of pancreatico-enteric anastomosis. *Transl Gastroenterol Hepatol* 2017;2:89.
5. Shrikhande S, Barreto S, Sirohi B et al. Indian Council of Medical Research consensus document for the management of pancreatic cancer. *Indian J Med Paediatr Oncol* 2019;40(1):9–14.

# 41 Managing a Grade C Pancreatic Fistula after Pancreatoduodenectomy

*Maxwell T. Trudeau and Charles M. Vollmer*

## CONTENTS

## CASE SCENARIO

A 76-year-old man undergoes a pylorus-preserving pancreatoduodenectomy for a 3 cm ampullary adenocarcinoma causing jaundice from biliary obstruction. The pancreatic gland is of soft texture, with an observed duct diameter of 3 mm, and an estimated blood loss of 750 cc. The fistula risk score is 7 (high-risk zone). The pancreaticojejunostomy is constructed with two interrupted layers and a bulb-suction drain is left next to the pancreaticojejunostomy anastomosis. On the first postoperative day, the drain fluid amylase is 3,560 U/L and the drain is removed on postoperative day three. The patient is discharged to home on day seven but presents to the hospital on postoperative day nine with respiratory distress, tachypnea, and a white cell count of 21,000/μl. Subsequently, he is intubated. A computed tomography (CT) scan (Figure 41.1) of the abdomen reveals complete dehiscence of the pancreaticojejunostomy (ISGPF Grade C). Given profound sepsis with need for pressor support and progressive clinical deterioration, what is the optimal management?

## BACKGROUND OF THE PATHOLOGY

At high volume centers, the mortality rate for pancreatoduodenectomy has improved significantly in recent decades and hovers around 2%. Despite this advancement, postoperative pancreatic fistula incidence is still reported between 10–30%. Postoperative pancreatic fistula remains the greatest contributor to morbidity in pancreatoduodenectomy as it can lead to sepsis, delayed gastric emptying, and even hemorrhage due to a gastroduodenal artery stump blowout.

Pancreatic fistula entails a leak from the pancreatic anastomosis and was definitively defined by the International Study Group on Pancreatic Fistula (ISGPS) in 2005, which broadly includes an increased drain fluid amylase level, as well as any clinically relevant sequelae that necessitates change in regular management. This grading system classified postoperative pancreatic fistula as grade A, B, or C based on the clinical severity and impact on patient outcomes. Since 2005, the ISGPS definition and grading of postoperative pancreatic fistula has been accepted universally. Due to postoperative pancreatic fistula remaining as one of the most relevant and harmful complications following pancreatoduodenectomy, in 2016 the ISGPS updated and refined the definition and grading of postoperative pancreatic fistula [1]. New guidelines redefined grade A postoperative pancreatic fistula as having a drain fluid amylase greater than three times the institutional normal serum amylase value, and is now termed as a "biochemical leak", because it has no clinical relevance and requires no change in management. Grade B postoperative pancreatic fistula is now defined by changes in the postoperative management requiring either drains left in place for longer than three weeks, pharmacologic treatments, or the use of endoscopic or percutaneous procedures. Grade C postoperative pancreatic fistula is the most infrequent (2% of all pancreatoduodenectomies performed) but severe and is defined by management requiring reoperation (one-third of cases), or any postoperative pancreatic fistula that leads to single or multiple organ failure (one-third of cases), or mortality (one-third of cases). Thus, grade B and C postoperative

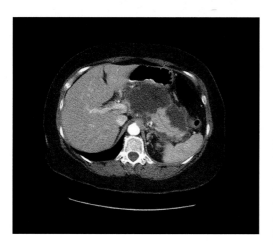

**Figure 41.1** Axial CT scan image of a dehisced pancreaticojejunostomy with evidence of a perianastomotic collection.

pancreatic fistula are commonly referred to as clinically relevant pancreatic fistula.

In a series of 4,301 pancreatic resections, McMillan et al. characterized the 79 (1.9%) grade C postoperative pancreatic fistulas that occurred [2]. The 90-day mortality rate was 35%, with reoperations occurring 72.2% of the time. Rates of single- and multi-system organ failure were 28.2 and 39.7%, respectively. The median length of stay was 32 days (interquartile range: 21–54), with a median number of four complications incurred per patient (interquartile range: 2–5). Using this data, predictive models for occurrence of grade C postoperative pancreatic fistula were created with preoperative and intraoperative variables. The following predictors were identified: alcohol consumption, previous cardiac event, high-risk disease pathology, and operative time in minutes.

In accordance with the evolution of the definition and characterization of postoperative pancreatic fistula, the management of postoperative pancreatic fistula has improved starting with the ability to predict its occurrence. In 2013, Callery et al. developed the fistula risk score, which has been externally validated as a highly predictive tool for the occurrence of clinically relevant postoperative pancreatic fistula [3]. The fistula risk score (0 to 10 points) can be calculated at the time of pancreatic anastomotic reconstruction (Table 41.1). The weighted risk score incorporates four independent factors: (1) soft pancreatic parenchyma, (2) high-risk disease pathology, (3) pancreatic duct diameter (in mm), and (4) estimated intraoperative blood loss. Discrete risk zones with escalating propensity for clinically relevant postoperative pancreatic fistula have been identified;

negligible (fistula risk score 0), low (fistula risk score 1–2), moderate (fistula risk score 3–6), and high (fistula risk score 7–10).

The cases of the high-risk zone have been reported to account for just a tenth of all pancreatoduodenectomies, but demonstrate a clinically relevant postoperative pancreatic fistula rate of approximately 30%. While these high-risk fistula risk score scenarios present challenging anastomotic reconstructions, best practice mitigation strategies have been established to reduce the occurrence of clinically relevant postoperative pancreatic fistula. Specifically, externalized stents and omission of prophylactic octreotide, in the setting of intraperitoneal drainage and pancreaticojejunostomy reconstruction, has been associated with optimal outcomes [4]. Considering the increased risk for clinically relevant postoperative pancreatic fistula, a high-risk patient may be managed more specifically. Thus, prevention of clinically relevant postoperative pancreatic fistula development from the outset may indeed be the best management.

## APPROACH TO MANAGEMENT

The infrequent scenario of a grade C postoperative pancreatic fistula presents challenges, and the optimal management is highly debated. The major controversy originates from the fine line of successfully utilizing conservative management, while opting for a necessary relaparotomy when the patient clinically deteriorates. This dilemma can be best navigated using Smits et al. step-up approach, based on primary catheter drainage being associated with better clinical outcomes as the first intervention when compared to relaparotomy [5].

### Percutaneous drainage

In their series of 309 patients, the first intervention for postoperative pancreatic fistula was either catheter drainage or relaparotomy. Primary catheter drainage alone was successfully completed in 77.1% of patients. Furthermore, propensity score matching was used to compare patients undergoing primary catheter drainage versus initial relaparotomy in a 1:1 manner (N = 64). Employing the first intervention of primary catheter drainage proved to be the optimal first step, yielding lower mortality rates (14.1 vs 35.9%; P = 0.007), new-onset single organ failure (4.7% vs 20.3%; P = 0.007), and multiorgan failure (15.6% vs 39.1%; P = 0.008). The authors ultimately conclude that catheter drainage should be the primary step in management of severe pancreatic fistula. Relaparotomy should be reserved for patients who are not candidates for a minimally

## Table 41.1 Fistula Risk Score for Prediction of Clinically Relevant Pancreatic Fistula after Pancreatoduodenectomy

| Risk Factor | Parameter | Points |
|---|---|---|
| Gland texture | Firm | 0 |
| | Soft | 2 |
| Pathology | Pancreatic adenocarcinoma or pancreatitis | 0 |
| | Ampullary, duodenal, cystic, islet cell | 1 |
| Pancreatic duct diameter (mm) | ≥5 | 0 |
| | 4 | 1 |
| | 3 | 2 |
| | 2 | 3 |
| | ≤1 | 4 |
| Intraoperative blood loss (ml) | ≤400 | 0 |
| | 401–700 | 1 |
| | 701–1,000 | 2 |
| | >1,000 | 3 |

| Fistula Risk Zones | Points |
|---|---|
| Negligible | 0 |
| Low | 1–2 |
| Moderate | 3–6 |
| High | 7–10 |

Total 0–10 points

invasive intervention or whose condition is progressively worsening despite catheter drainage.

### Operative interventions

When approaching surgical intervention, it is recommended that only highly experienced surgeons should perform this procedure, perhaps in tandem, as, due to rarity and severity, it is possibly the most challenging operation a pancreatic surgeon has to face. With that being said, a deteriorating clinical status associated with grade C postoperative pancreatic fistula may mandate re-exploration to prevent continued sepsis and organ failure. During re-exploration, surgeons are faced with three basic options: completion pancreatectomy, wide external peripancreatic drainage with an attempt to better control the leak, or conversion to an alternative pancreaticoenteric anastomosis (either pancreaticojejunostomy or pancreaticogastrostomy). The sparse literature on this topic provides a glimpse as to how management may proceed.

### Completion pancreatectomy

Historically, completion pancreatectomy was considered the only plausible treatment. In a multi-institutional study in 2008, Fuks et al. [6] analyzed 680 pancreatoduodenectomy cases, consisting of half the original reconstructions performed in pancreaticojejunostomy fashion

(50.4%) and an overall fistula rate of 16.3% [6]. Grade C postoperative pancreatic fistula was observed in 36 patients, 47% suffered from sepsis due to an abdominal collection, 44% had postoperative bleeding, 28% had bleeding associated with abdominal collection, and 9% had multiorgan failure due to other causes. Grade C postoperative pancreatic fistula resulted in an increased length of stay in comparison to grade A and B postoperative pancreatic fistula (46 vs 29 days; $P<0.001$). While no risk factors for grade C postoperative pancreatic fistula were identified in a multivariate analysis, univariate analysis showed soft gland texture ($P = 0.011$), perioperative blood transfusion ($P = 0.003$), and postoperative bleeding were risk factors ($P = 0.001$).

Of the patients suffering from Grade C postoperative pancreatic fistula, 97% underwent reoperation. In patients who presented with sepsis secondary to intrabdominal collections ($N = 17$), ten patients went straight to surgery, while seven patients underwent percutaneous drainage which failed to be an effective therapy, and consequentially required reoperation. Operative management consisted of the following: surgical drainage was performed in nine patients, six of whom had their anastomoses reduced following necrosis and dehiscence, four patients underwent disconnection of the anastomosis with resection of the body and conservation of a small remnant, and two patients underwent a completion pancreatectomy [6]. While not fully discerning a best practice approach, this study concluded that completion pancreatectomy/splenectomy may be the best approach if major dehiscence of the anastomosis occurs.

More recently, utilization of a completion pancreatectomy has become viewed as a less favorable approach. The associated extensive dissection exposes the patient to a greater risk of short-term mortality as opposed to alternative options. Furthermore, removal of the remnant pancreas commits the patient, who survives, to lifelong total endocrine and exocrine insufficiency leading to a long-term risk of mortality due to the considerably elevated risk for severe hypoglycemia or hyperglycemia due to a brittle control.

### Wide external peripancreatic drainage

Another strategy to address a high-grade pancreaticojejunostomy leak is to utilize wide external peripancreatic drainage with an attempt to mitigate the leak. Wronski et al. recently published their data analyzing 616 patients [7]. The study compared three surgical approaches to manage grade C postoperative pancreatic fistula; simple drainage (N = 16), completion pancreatectomy (N = 17), and external wirsungostomy (N = 10). External wirsungostomy entailed taking down the pancreaticojejunostomy, closing the intestine with a linear stapler, inserting a small caliber catheter into the main pancreatic duct that could then be exteriorized in the epigastric region, and placement of two large-bore drains close to the pancreatic cut surface.

The mortality rate for simple drainage was 56%, compared with 47% for completion pancreatectomy (p = 0.598), and 50% for external wirsungostomy (p = 0.883). Simple drainage was associated with a higher rate of further reoperations for management of the fistula (56%) in comparison with completion pancreatectomy (24%; p = 0.055) and external wirsungostomy (0%; p = 0.003). Multivariate analysis showed the predictive factors of mortality after reoperation for grade C postoperative pancreatic fistula were organ failure on the day of reoperation (p = 0.001) and need for immediate surgical intervention (p = 0.007). Furthermore, patients managed by simple drainage had the highest rate of further interventions after reoperation, and more importantly, rescue completion pancreatectomy in these patients invariably resulted in mortality. Taking into account these observations, the authors suggested that simple drainage of the pancreatic

anastomosis should be avoided for the management of grade C postoperative pancreatic fistula, and other parenchyma-sparing techniques like the external wirsunostomy are recommended. However, it should be acknowledged that wirsunostomy does not provide definitive management, and the patient will most likely require a technically challenging elective operation months later to restore the continuity of the pancreatic duct if they survive the initial scenario.

### Conversion to an alternative pancreaticoenteric anastomosis

Building on this approach, our group has proposed a bridge stent technique to intraoperatively address a disrupted pancreaticojejunostomy [8]. We reviewed 357 pancreatoduodenectomies with a grade C fistula occurrence of 2%. The bridge stent technique was used for five patients who all had evidence of a dehisced pancreaticojejunostomy anastomosis. All patients survived this technique and were discharged from the hospital without any long-term external fistula, or any recognized pancreaticojejunostomy strictures or remnant atrophy.

To perform the bridge stent technique, it is recommended to proceed via the original incision tracing it back to the pancreaticojejunostomy anastomosis to observe the significance of the dehiscence. As opposed to utilizing a take down, the antecolic, isoperistaltic duodeno/gastrojejunostomy may be gently retracted laterally to the left. This maneuver should be performed meticulously to prevent any damage to the mesocolon or transverse colon. Once the anastomosis is located, it should be evaluated for: severity of surrounding inflammation, abscess or necrosis, extent of anastomotic dehiscence, distance between the pancreas and jejunal limb, and the quality of the pancreatic parenchyma and jejunal serosa. Debridement should be carefully utilized to reveal viable, well vascularized tissue, while avoiding damage to the critical vascular structures in the neighborhood.

Due to suboptimal conditions, a revised or "new" duct-to-mucosa anastomosis should be avoided, and the bridge stent technique is better advised (Figure 41.2). A 5-Fr or 8-Fr silastic feeding tube stent can be used to connect the pancreatic duct across the gap to the jejunal enterotomy, securing both ends with absorbable sutures. Stent size should be selected based on duct diameter. Given the 3 mm duct of this patient, an 8-Fr stent could be inserted establishing a larger caliber channel. It is imperative to ensure that the stent has been correctly

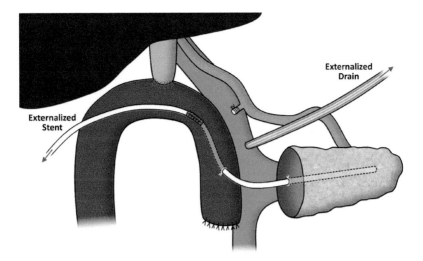

**Figure 41.2**   Bridge-stent technique with externalized stent and external drain adjacent to the gap.

inserted into the pancreatic duct, avoiding a false passage into the pancreatic parenchyma. It can be challenging to locate the pancreatic duct in these difficult situations.

Following successful placement of the stent, it must be anchored into place on the pancreatic side with absorbable sutures. Sutures should be placed carefully in the usually friable parenchyma and then attached to the stent. On the opposite side, the original bowel enterotomy could be used again with a purse-string closure around the stent if it is reasonably small and healthy. Alternatively, the bowel segment may be resected and a new enterotomy created proximally on the limb. Internalized stents, restricted to a short length (6–8cm), should be avoided. Instead, the stent should be externalized downstream on the bowel and passed through the abdominal wall. Drains are also placed in the operative bed and once there is decreased output, the stent can be capped to divert drainage into the bowel. While the stent remains open with exterior drainage, it is advised to supplement the patient's diet with pancreatic enzymes to counter exocrine insufficiency. Following the dissolution of the absorbable sutures (two to three months), the stent can be removed in the outpatient setting. A "neo-pancreatic duct" has been created with fibrotic scar around the stent tract, which usually displays long-term patency.

## CONCLUSION

Despite the best efforts at performing a safe and tension-free pancreatico-enteric anastomosis, a minority of patients will inevitably develop grade C postoperative pancreatic fistula after pancreatoduodenectomy. There are many surgical strategies to consider for managing this scenario. Although completion pancreatectomy definitively eliminates the pancreatic leak, this procedure is the most complex and traumatic to the patient. Resecting the remaining pancreas might be extremely challenging in the inflamed and hostile operative field. Similarly, the concept of reconstructing a pancreaticojejunostomy or pancreaticogastrostomy in this setting is unadvisable. Wide drainage or ductal externalization procedures, like the wirsunogostomy, typically prolong the hospital course and will require future reoperations and interventions. The bridge stent technique is our preferred approach as it allows for successful development of a "neo-anastomosis" to divert pancreatic secretions and restore the function of the original anastomosis.

### KEY MESSAGES

- Pancreatic fistula is a significant complication following pancreaticoduodenectomy, with grade C fistula presenting the greatest morbidity and mortality.
- Managing pancreaticojejunostomy anastomotic dehiscence following pancreatoduodenectomy is a rare and challenging complication – perhaps the hardest procedure a pancreatic surgeon has to perform.
- The preferred approach is the bridge stent technique as it requires minimal added dissection and allows for the creation of a new channel that can

successfully shunt pancreatic secretions internally.

- Wide external peripancreatic drainage can also be used at the outset, but is more difficult to manage over the longer term.
- Completion pancreatectomy should be avoided as it commits the patient to lifelong total endocrine and exocrine insufficiency with significant rate of both immediate and longer-term mortality.

## REFERENCES

1. Bassi C, Marchegiani G, Dervenis C et al. The 2016 update of the International Study Group (ISGPS) definition and grading of postoperative pancreatic fistula: 11 years after. *Surgery* 2017;161(3):584–591.
2. McMillan MT, Vollmer CV, Asbun H et al. The characterization and prediction of ISGPF Grade C fistulas following pancreatoduodenectomy. *J Gastrointest Surg* 2016;20(2):262–276.
3. Smits FJ, Santvoort HC, Besselink MG et al. Management of severe pancreatic fistula After pancreatoduodenectomy. *JAMA Surg* 2017;152(6):540–548.
4. Ecker BL, McMillan MT, Asbun HJ et al. Characterization and optimal management of high-risk pancreatic anastomoses during pancreatoduodenectomy. *Ann Surg* 2018;267(4):608–616.
5. Callery MP, Pratt WB, Kent TS et al. A prospectively validated clinical risk score accurately predicts pancreatic fistula after pancreatoduodenectomy. *J Am Coll Surg* 2013;216(1):1–14.
6. Fuks D, Piessen G, Huet E et al. Life-threatening postoperative pancreatic fistula (grade C) after pancreaticoduodenectomy: Incidence, prognosis, and risk factors. *Am J Surg* 2009;197(6):702–709.
7. Wronski M, Cebulski W, Witkowski B et al. Surgical management of the grade C pancreatic fistula after pancreatoduodenectomy. *HPB (Oxford)*. doi:10.1016/j.hpb.2019.01.006.
8. Kent TS, Callery MP, Vollmer CM, Jr. The bridge stent technique for salvage of pancreatojejunal anastomotic dehiscence. *HPB (Oxford)* 2010;12(8):577–582.

# 42 Acute Necrotizing Pancreatitis Post-Pancreatoduodenectomy

*Ibrahim Büdeyri, Onur Bayram, Christoph W. Michalski, and Jörg Kleeff*

## CONTENTS

## CASE SCENARIO

A 75-year-old man with periampullary (duodenal) adenocarcinoma (pT3N0M0) underwent a classical pancreatoduodenectomy. Intraoperatively, the pancreatic parenchyma was found to be soft and the main pancreatic duct was not dilated (2–3 mm in diameter). On postoperative day zero serum lipase was more than twice the upper limit of normal, which peaked at more than four times the upper limit of normal on postoperative day one and normalized on postoperative day three. On postoperative day six, a computed tomography (CT) scan showed a remnant pancreas with non-specific postoperative changes. On postoperative day 11, the patient's serum C-reactive protein peaked at 273 mg/L (normal <5 mg/L). The patient deteriorated clinically despite aggressive resuscitation and antibiotics and on postoperative day 17 an exploratory laparotomy was performed. At the time of exploration, resection of the pancreaticojejunostomy was performed due to partial pancreatic necrosis and the pancreatic duct was externalized using a 5 mm pediatric nasogastric tube. The patient recovered slowly and was discharged from the hospital on postoperative day 62.

## BACKGROUND OF THE PATHOLOGY

Post-pancreatectomy acute pancreatitis has a pathophysiological course similar to acute pancreatitis due to gallstones or heavy alcohol consumption. It is associated with pancreatic necrosis, cytokine release, increase in free radicals, systemic inflammatory response syndrome, and multiorgan dysfunction syndrome. The manifestation of post-pancreatoduodenectomy acute pancreatitis in the immediate postoperative period ranges from self-resolving inflammation to fulminant acute pancreatitis with multiorgan dysfunction syndrome and pancreatic necrosis.

The pathophysiology of postsurgical acute pancreatitis is multifactorial. Ischemia is believed to be one of the leading underlying factors. Blood flow to pancreatic acini is provided by singular end arteries. Temporary ischemia results in a transient rise in serum amylase or lipase, whereas prolonged ischemia can cause histological pancreatitis. Vasoconstriction leads to blood stasis and worsens tissue ischemia. This series of events starts 30 minutes after induction of acute pancreatitis and can cause capillary perfusion problems after three hours [1]. With progressive acute pancreatitis, tissue oxygenation is compromised due to increased pathological shunting of blood and thus capillary stasis, which is closely associated with the development of pancreatic necrosis. During pathological shunting, endothelial dysfunction develops and manifests itself as increased capillary permeability allowing fluid and activated proteolytic enzymes to leak into the pancreatic interstitium causing further local tissue damage. Systemically, increased capillary permeability leads to third space fluid losses as well as a dysfunction of the gut barrier giving rise to bacterial translocation.

Post-pancreatoduodenectomy acute pancreatitis may be caused by duct obstruction during placement of sutures for the pancreaticojejunal anastomosis and/or due to local pancreatic ischemia caused by factors related to anatomical features, vascularization, and intraoperative hemodynamics. A small main pancreatic duct is at significant risk of being completely occluded by one or more of the outer row stitches (may be avoided using intraoperative pancreatic duct stenting). This will lead to severe acute pancreatitis very early after the operation and needs to be avoided at all costs. Since the pancreas is extremely vulnerable to restrictions in both arterial supply and venous blood drainage, acute pancreatitis can be caused by transient hypoperfusion. In this case, a proper intraoperative fluid administration is crucial to avoid hypoperfusion and ensuing ischemia. In addition, surgical handling of the pancreas can also cause pancreatitis – thus, meticulous dissection of the remnant pancreas is warranted. Epidural analgesia may improve pancreatic perfusion and reduce severity of postoperative acute pancreatitis [2]. Patients with a soft pancreatic texture or with a non-dilated main pancreatic duct (diameter ≤3 mm) are at a high risk of developing postoperative acute pancreatitis [2], which again will lead in almost all cases to severe postoperative pancreatic fistula [3].

Postoperative pancreatic fistula and postoperative acute pancreatitis are two different entities. Postoperative acute pancreatitis mostly occurs in the first two postoperative days, whereas postoperative pancreatic fistula tends to form later than that, and is classically characterized by a drain amylase level more than thrice the upper limit of institutional normal serum amylase [1]. In addition, severe postoperative pancreatic fistula is usually one of the consequences of postoperative acute pancreatitis.

### INVESTIGATIONS

According to the Revised Atlanta Criteria in 2012 [4], two of the following three features must be present for the diagnosis of acute pancreatitis: epigastric pain radiating to back, serum amylase or lipase level at least three times the upper limit of normal, and confirmatory contrast-enhanced CT (CECT) or magnetic resonance imaging (MRI) or ultrasound findings. Yet, these criteria have not been widely applied in the setting of postoperative acute pancreatitis. To that end, Connor and colleagues [1] proposed a new definition of postoperative acute pancreatitis in which an elevation of serum amylase or lipase levels above the upper limit of normal on postoperative day zero or one is sufficient for the diagnosis of postoperative acute pancreatitis, irrespective of drain amylase/lipase levels.

Early diagnosis of postoperative acute pancreatitis is paramount to be able to mitigate its potentially life-threatening sequelae. In general, an increase of serum amylase/lipase on the first postoperative day to about 500 U/L is seen as a warning sign of a potentially severe postoperative acute pancreatitis. When there is an increase to about 1,000 U/L, particular attention needs to be paid. If there is additional clinical deterioration of the patient, as exemplified by features of a systemic inflammatory

response syndrome and significant increase in inflammatory markers such as serum C-reactive protein, diagnostic measures need to be undertaken to define the extent of postoperative acute pancreatitis. Drain amylase/lipase levels may or may not be helpful in decision making, mainly because these may also be elevated in patients with an uneventful postoperative course.

Morphological changes evident on CT imaging can only be detected 72 hours after the onset of postoperative acute pancreatitis. Therefore, recognizing the potential of a perioperative acute pancreatitis by observing intraoperative parenchymal changes such as edematous pancreatitis is essential for the surgeon to tailor postoperative hydration. Early diagnostic tests are needed to be developed to reduce morbidity and mortality from postoperative acute pancreatitis [2].

### MANAGEMENT

In post-pancreatoduodenectomy necrotizing pancreatitis, the treatment approach is guided by clinical signs and laboratory findings. Post-pancreatoduodenectomy necrotizing pancreatitis has been shown to be associated with prolonged intensive care unit or hospital stay, raised C-reactive protein, as well as acute physiology and chronic health evaluation (APACHE) II and sequential organ failure assessment (SOFA) scores [3]. Unlike acute pancreatitis due to other causes, in which the diagnosis can be made through biochemical evidence and clinical signs, postoperative acute pancreatitis is not easy to diagnose as a postoperative pancreatic fistula tends to be more commonly suspected. The clinical presentation is confounded by the radiological findings suggestive of fluid collections in the surgical bed [2]. There are no guidelines for the optimal treatment of postoperative acute pancreatitis, but it seems reasonable to follow the routine treatment strategies of acute pancreatitis due to other causes with fluid resuscitation and pain relief. If on imaging, the findings are suggestive of pancreatic necrosis with or without peripancreatic collections (Figure 42.1) which are highly suggestive of acute pancreatitis, then a step-up approach using percutaneous drainage to drain the collections first would be the way forward with surgery reserved only for clinical deterioration despite all these efforts.

If post-pancreatoduodenectomy acute pancreatitis is noted on imaging performed early in the postoperative course, and if the patient's status deteriorates with clinical signs and laboratory findings in line with superadded

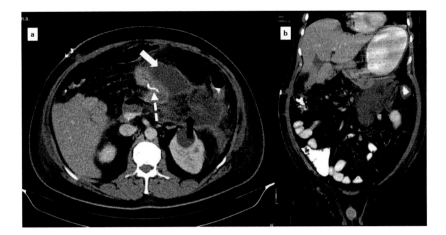

**Figure 42.1** Contraset-enhanced CT images of a patient who developed post-pancreatoduodenectomy acute necrotizing pancreatitis. (a) Axial section demonstrating necrosis of the remnant pancreas (black bold arrow) and peripancreatic collection (white bold arrow). The staple line of the jejunum used to fashion the pancreaticojejunostomy is also noted (dashed white arrow). (b) Coronal section demonstrating necrosis of the remnant pancreas (black bold arrow). The jejunal loop in the gallbladder fossa used to fashion the hepaticojejunostomy is also noted. (Images courtesy of Dr. Adarsh Chaudhary and Dr. Savio G. Barreto, HPB Surgeons, Medanta – The Medicity, India.)

sepsis, we advise a liberal consideration of re-exploration.

Generally speaking, there are two surgical approaches [5]. The first approach involves taking down the pancreatic anastomosis with externalization of the pancreatic duct. Alternatively, and if technically feasible, a completion pancreatectomy should be performed. Both are valid options and the final decision can often only be made intraoperatively. Factors in favor of a completion pancreatectomy include sepsis, organ failure, leakage, and bleeding from the pancreatico-enteric anastomosis [3]. Mortality after late revisions is higher than after early revisions due to destruction of the operating field by pancreatitis and necrosis and due to severe sepsis. Early diagnosis of postoperative acute pancreatitis is therefore a key to better outcomes, yet even after an early revision a prolonged recovery from disease must be expected [3]. It must be appreciated that completion pancreatectomy may be technically demanding, and rapid deterioration of the patient frequently requires damage control surgery. In such cases, disintegration of the pancreatic anastomosis and externalization of the pancreatic duct (e.g. using an infant nasogastric tube) may be warranted.

## RATIONALE FOR MANAGEMENT IN THE PATIENT PRESENTED

In the case of the patient presented in the Case Scenario, the remnant pancreas

post-pancreatoduodenectomy was soft. After an uneventful transection without using energy devices, a standard reconstruction was performed with a dual layer, interrupted 5-0 polydioxanone suture pancreaticojejunostomy. Serum lipase levels were checked in the immediate postoperative period, which were increased up to four times the upper limit of the normal. Due to postoperative analgesia the patient did not manifest any symptoms or signs. Based on the softness of the pancreas and the postoperative hyperlipasemia, the patient was kept nil per mouth and was generously hydrated. The patient was initially managed conservatively. During the postoperative course, the patient became unwell, developed fevers, and tachycardia on top of elevated systemic inflammatory markers, which warranted an abdominal CT scan. Although there was no strong suspicion of a necrotic pancreas based on the CT scan (which only revealed some free air and fluid within the operative field without contrast extravasation), we opted for re-exploration based on the clinical findings and laboratory values. The anastomosis was taken down due to pancreatic necrosis and accompanying anastomotic insufficiency, the necrotic parts of the remnant pancreas were debrided, and the remnant pancreatic duct was externalized. Given the age of the patient and the attendant risk of brittle diabetes in the aftermath of a completion pancreatectomy, a more conservative option was preferred.

## KEY MESSAGES

- Post-pancreatoduodenectomy acute necrotizing pancreatitis is an entity not widely discussed in the literature.
- Clinical symptoms and signs may be obscured by the postoperative course.
- In patients with a soft pancreas and a non-dilated pancreatic duct, there is a significant risk of post-pancreato-duodenectomy acute pancreatitis and sepsis. Thus, prevention is key with attention to detail and meticulous dissection of the remnant pancreas and care to avoid accidental closure of the main pancreatic duct during construction of the pancreatic anastomosis.
- Serum and drain amylase/lipase (on postoperative day one) are helpful in determining patients at risk and in guiding a decision for re-exploratory laparotomy versus conservative (sepsis) treatment.
- If a surgical procedure is required, an intraoperative decision must be made regarding whether to perform a completion pancreatectomy or merely dismantling of the anastomosis with externalization of the pancreatic duct.

## REFERENCES

1. Connor S. Defining post-operative pancreatitis as a new pancreatic specific complication following pancreatic resection. *HPB (Oxford)* 2016;18(8):642–651.
2. Bannone E, Andrianello S, Marchegiani G et al. Postoperative acute pancreatitis following pancreaticoduodenectomy: A determinant of fistula potentially driven by the intraoperative fluid management. *Ann Surg* 2018;268(5):815–822.
3. Globke B, Timmermann L, Klein F et al. Postoperative acute necrotizing pancreatitis of the pancreatic remnant (POANP): A new definition of severe pancreatitis following pancreaticoduodenectomy. *HPB (Oxford)* 2019.
4. Banks PA, Bollen TL, Dervenis C et al. Classification of acute pancreatitis – 2012: Revision of the Atlanta classification and definitions by international consensus. *Gut* 2013;62(1):102–111.
5. Ryska M, Rudis J. Pancreatic fistula and postoperative pancreatitis after pancreatoduodenectomy for pancreatic cancer. *Hepatobiliary Surg Nutr* 2014;3(5):268–275.

# PART 9
# SPLEEN

# 43 Grade 3 Isolated Splenic Laceration with Hemodynamic Instability

*Maria Grazia Sibilla, Sofia Battisti, and Federico Coccolini*

## CONTENTS

## CASE SCENARIO

An 82-year-old man was admitted to the emergency department after sustaining a fall from a height. Initial assessment revealed a hemodynamically unstable patient with a pulse rate of 120 beats/min, blood pressure 80/60 mmHg, respiratory rate of 26 breaths/min, and a Glasgow coma scale of 15. On abdominal examination, the patient was noted to have tenderness in the left upper quadrant with voluntary guard. The focused assessment with sonography for trauma indicated free fluid in the abdomen. Chest X-ray showed left pneumothorax, fractures of the left 4–11th ribs. On the initial arterial blood gas analysis, the base excess was −6 mmol/L and serum lactate was elevated. Fluid resuscitation was initiated which was accompanied with an improvement in blood pressure to 110/60 mmHg. A left tube thoracostomy was positioned. An abdominal computed tomography (CT) scan was performed with evidence of grade III splenic rupture with active arterial blush. During the CT scan, the patient's blood pressure progressively decreased again. He was shifted to the operating room and proximal angioembolization of the splenic artery was performed with a C-arm directly on the operating table. The surgical team was on standby and ready to operate. Following the angioembolization, and transfusion of packed red blood cells, the patient's blood pressure stabilized once again, and he was shifted to the intensive care unit for monitoring. A follow-up contrast-enhanced ultrasound was performed. The recovery of the patient was uneventful. He was discharged home two weeks after admission, after receiving the prescribed vaccinations.

## BACKGROUND OF THE PATHOLOGY

Injury to the spleen is encountered in 30–49% of closed abdominal traumas and in 7–9% of penetrating ones. Splenic hemorrhage is potentially life-threatening and requires prompt management. Splenic injuries may occur in isolation, or in association with other organ injuries. The current existing grading scales used to assess severity are: the American Association for the Surgery of Trauma (AAST) splenic injury scale based on the anatomical extent [1], and the World Society of Emergency Surgery (WSES) classification that takes into account the anatomy as well as the patient's hemodynamic status [2]. The traditional approach to decision making in these patients has been based on hemodynamic status as the primary determinant.

Management of splenic trauma has changed considerably in the last few decades with a paradigm shift in favor of non-operative management [3]. Non-operative management accounts for up to 60% of cases in level 1 trauma centers, and ranges from observation and monitoring alone, to angiography/angioembolization. The aim of non-operative management is to preserve the spleen and its function, and to reduce the morbidity and mortality associated with a negative exploratory laparotomy and often, unwarranted splenectomy. In fact, the immunological function of the spleen and the high risk of overwhelming post-splenectomy infections must be taken into consideration. Operative management of splenic injuries is reserved for a patient regarded to be a non-responder in terms of hemodynamic instability. The gold standard for management of minor lesions (AAST-OIS grade I–II) is non-operative management. However, controversy exists regarding the role of non-operative management for higher grade injuries, especially in multitrauma patients, and in patients with associated severe traumatic brain injuries and spinal cord injuries. The approach to decision making is also determined by the capability of the center to carry out intensive monitoring and the availability of surgeons in case the patient deteriorates and needs an emergency laparotomy. The WSES guidelines recommend the performance of angiography/angioembolization in patients with hemodynamic stability and arterial blush on CT scan irrespective of the injury grade, and in all hemodynamically stable patients with WSES class III lesions (AAST grade IV–V), regardless of the presence of an arterial blush on CT scan.

## APPROACH TO MANAGEMENT

The clinical presentation of a patient with splenic rupture includes left upper quadrant pain, Kehr's sign (shoulder pain secondary to diaphragmatic irritation by the hemoperitoneum), as well as signs of hemodynamic impairment and abdominal tenderness and guard (with signs of peritonism). Hemodynamic instability in adults implies a patient who, at admission, has a systolic blood pressure <90 mmHg and a heart rate of >120 bpm with evidence of skin vasoconstriction (cool, clammy, and decreased capillary refill), altered level of consciousness and/or shortness of breath, or a blood pressure >90 mmHg but requiring bolus infusions/transfusions and/or vasopressor drugs and/or admission base excess >−5 mmol/L and/or shock index >1 and/or transfusion requirement of at least four to six units of packed red blood cells within the first 24 hours. The approach to decision making in a patient in shock is determined by their response to initial fluid resuscitation according to advanced trauma life support criteria that is, initial fluid bolus with 2,000 mL or 29 mg/kg body weight of Ringer's lactate in adults or children over 15–20 minutes. Unstable patients can grossly be divided into two main groups: responders and non-responders. A third subgroup exists and is called transient responders. Transient responders initially recover from hypotension, but may experience subsequent deterioration of perfusion indices with the tapering fluid administration to maintenance levels. A non-responder, on the contrary, does not respond to the initial fluid challenge [2].

Prompt assessment and accurate diagnosis of splenic injury is essential to ensure a favorable outcome in severe blunt abdominal trauma patients. The WSES guidelines suggest, based on a high grade of recommendation, that the choice of diagnostic technique at admission must be determined by the hemodynamic status of the patient [2]. For the initial assessment of patients with blunt splenic trauma, the focused assessment with sonography for trauma examination has been recommended in primary evaluation, together with chest and pelvis X-ray, with sensitivity up to 91% and a specificity up to 96% for free fluid. Studies have shown that focused assessment with

sonography for trauma is an acceptable initial imaging test in hemodynamically unstable patients. Patients presenting with hemodynamic instability with no response or transient response with rapid deterioration after initial fluid challenge and positive focused assessment with sonography for trauma should be transferred to the OR without further secondary radiological imaging [3].

Hypotension in abdominal blunt trauma, however, even when associated to positive focused assessment with sonography for trauma, is not always indicative of active intra-abdominal bleeding. Effective free fluid source identification may require a secondary accurate diagnostic modality with high quality images to plan an adequate treatment strategy, especially in high resource settings. CT has sensitivity and specificity for splenic injury near to 96–100%, but is recommended only in hemodynamically stable or stabilized patients. Proper CT scan evaluation of spleen injuries requires intravenous contrast. Active hemorrhage or parenchymal injury can be accurately diagnosed in the portal venous phase. This may be more sensitive and accurate than the arterial phase in some studies (93 vs 76% and 95 vs 81 %, respectively) [4]. CT scan allows for assessment of splenic injury severity, quantification of hemoperitoneum volume, and may reveal vascular abnormalities such as blush, pseudoaneurysm, or arteriovenous fistula. Furthermore, abdominal CT may also detect other intra-abdominal injuries warranting laparotomy. Contrast extravasation on CT may help in subsequent surgical procedure or in angiography/angioembolization to be more selective.

Hemodynamically unstable patients not responding to fluid resuscitation with a positive focused assessment with sonography for trauma should be transferred to the OR and treated with emergent laparotomy especially in low resource settings.

For hemodynamically unstable patients who are transient responders, the decision whether to perform a CT scan should weigh in the logistical challenges of transporting the patient to the radiology suite, the potential delay in definitive treatment, and a preconceived notion of an inherent increased risk of mortality in patients with active bleeding while the scan is performed. In such cases, the trauma team has to determine the additional value of a CT scan while factoring in the risks and benefits.

In some centers, the hybrid operation room or interventional radiology facilities placed in OR (combined OR) are available. In hybrid operation room, advanced and intensive life support, CT-scan examination, emergency surgery, and interventional radiology (IR) can be carried out promptly and safely on the same table without transferring the patient to different departments. hybrid operation room equipped with CT scanner in the same place of the angiography suite and OR can provide critical real time information in detecting small vessel bleeds even in unstable patients who usually would not undergo CT. The hybrid/combined OR breaks the traditional sequential chain of patient care, whereby a trauma patient is evaluated in the emergency department and resuscitation commenced, considered for imaging within the radiology department, and subsequently tiered to OR or angiography suite for therapeutic intervention.

The management of isolated splenic injuries may change depending on hemodynamic status, clinical presentation, available facilities, surgeon's an interventional radiologist's judgment, and associated injuries.

Splenectomy should be considered in moderate and severe lesions even in stable patients in centers where intensive monitoring cannot be performed and/or when angiography/angioembolization is not readily available [3]. The reported overall hospital mortality for splenectomy in trauma approaches 2%. However, the incidence of postoperative bleeding after splenectomy, ranges from 1.6 to 3%, with an attendant mortality near to 20%. Thus, patients who improve hemodynamically after fluid and blood product resuscitation, even with severe vascular and/or splenic lesions on imaging, should be considered for angiography/angioembolization whenever possible especially in presence of hybrid/combined OR. For patients who respond to resuscitation, there is ample evidence to recommended the use of angiography/angioembolization so long as the CT-scan demonstrated splenic injuries with an arterial blush in the absence of peritonitis and other organ injuries that would merit a laparotomy in themselves. Angioembolization has been widely applied with improved outcome, avoiding OM in several patients who previously would have undergone surgery. non-operative management has the advantage of preservation of splenic function, a lower lifelong risk of overwhelming post splenectomy infections, avoidance of surgery associated morbidity and complications, shorter hospitalization, and a reduction in costs. Deciding between OM, IR, or combined procedures early on is imperative and can potentially change the outcome for the patient.

In centers without hybrid operation room, Teo et al. showed that safe, successful, and cost-effective angioembolization in trauma patients can be carried out using the conventional C-Arm DSA in a standard lead-lined emergency operating room [5]. In centers with such facilities, there is thus a possibility to perform combined treatments between surgeons and interventional radiologists, namely, emergency laparotomy and angiography/angioembolization in patients who are transient responders. Such treatments are done with an aim to preserve the spleen even during trauma laparotomy in very selected cases. The ability to proceed with angiography/angioembolization in a protected environment (operating room) is based on the possibility to proceed with splenectomy at any stage of the angioembolization, should the patient's condition deteriorate. A hybrid/combined operating room broadens the scope and indications for angiography/angioembolization, enabling non-operative management even in patients with a hemodynamic status that would have warranted a splenectomy in all other centers where combined procedures are not available. Severe unstable splenic injuries could ideally benefit from resuscitation in a hybrid/combined operating room with trauma surgeons ready to operate, in order to increase the spleen salvage rate and decrease the trauma laparotomies.

## CONCLUSIONS

The interventional radiological procedures and the modern conception of hybrid and endovascular trauma and bleeding management has led to good results due to a reduction of time needed for emergency resuscitative treatment. It may even increase the rate of patients managed non-operatively, opening new scenarios and options in trauma patient management. The introduction of hybrid/combined operating rooms will progressively change the trauma surgeon's view, at least of the more severe trauma patients, and it will offer the possibility of choosing not to operate in an increasing number of cases.

The non-operative management attempt of transient responder or hemodynamically unstable patients with splenic injuries has gained growing acceptance and is increasingly considered as a viable option in many centers. However, although hybrid/combined suites may significantly minimize time to hemorrhage control, currently they are not widely available as they seriously impact on resources – both, in terms of specialist multidisciplinary teams as well as costs. Last, the practice of non-operative management in transient responders or hemodynamically unstable patients requires teamwork and accurate patient selection.

## KEY MESSAGES

- The approach to decision making in patients in shock with splenic injuries is determined by their response to initial fluid resuscitation according to advanced trauma life support criteria.
- The performance of a contrast-enhanced CT scan allows for assessment of the severity of splenic injury, quantification of hemoperitoneum, and helps reveal or rule out vascular abnormalities and other injuries that may warrant an emergency laparotomy.
- The management of isolated splenic injuries is determined by the patient's hemodynamic status, clinical presentation, available facilities, surgeon's and interventional radiologist's judgment, and associated injuries
- In centers with hybrid/combined operating rooms, there exists the possibility to enforce the indications for non-operative management even in those patients who are hemodynamically unstable or who respond transiently.
- The role of endovascular trauma and bleeding management in hemodynamically unstable splenic trauma patients is evolving and is getting progressively more defined.

## REFERENCES

1. Moore EE, Cogbill TH, Jurkovich GJ et al. Organ injury scaling: Spleen and liver (1994 revision). *J Trauma* 1995;38(3):323–324.
2. Coccolini F, Montori G, Catena F et al. Splenic trauma: WSES classification and guidelines for adult and pediatric patients. *World J Emerg Surg* 2017;12:40.
3. Stassen NA, Bhullar I, Cheng JD et al. A selective nonoperative management of blunt splenic injury: An Eastern Association for the Surgery of Trauma practice management guideline. *J Trauma Acute Care Surg* 2012;73:S294–S300.
4. Boscak AR, Shanmuganathan K, Mirvis SE et al. Optimizing trauma multidetector CT protocol for blunt splenic injury: Need for arterial and portal venous phase scans. *Radiology* 2013;268(1):79–88.
5. Teo LT, Punamiya S, Chai CY et al. Emergency angioembolization in the operating theatre for trauma patients using the C-arm digital substraction angiography. *Injury* 2012;43(9):1492–1496.

# PART 10
# INFERIOR VENA CAVA

# 44  Malignant Inferior Vena Cava Leiomyosarcoma

## Approach to a Tumor Involving the Right Renal Vein

*Richard Smith*

## CONTENTS

## CASE SCENARIO

A 37-year-old woman presented with a painless abdominal mass, several weeks after the birth of her second child. She was an otherwise well woman of Vietnamese origin. She had had an uneventful pregnancy, with a vaginal delivery at term of a healthy girl. As her uterus receded, she noticed a firm mass in the middle section of the right side of the abdomen. She approached her general practitioner who arranged an abdominal computed tomography (CT) scan which revealed a large mass obliterating her inferior vena cava and involving the right kidney, as well as the left renal vein (Figure 44.1). The general practitioner referred her for surgical opinion. After assessing the patient, a core biopsy of the mass was ordered which was suggestive of a high-grade leiomyosarcoma, likely originating in the wall of the inferior vena cava.

## BACKGROUND OF THE PATHOLOGY

Leiomyosarcoma is a mesenchymal malignancy occurring mainly in adults, with its incidence peaking in the sixth decade of life [1] with a slight female preponderance [2]. They occur in the retroperitoneum in about 23% of cases and make up around 19% of all retroperitoneal sarcomas [3]. These may involve the inferior vena cava, intraluminally or extraluminally, or both.

Leiomyosarcomas originate from smooth muscle and are made up of spindle cells with cigar-shaped nuclei. They usually stain for desmin and smooth muscle actin on immunohistochemistry and may show myxoid or epithelioid differentiation. Histologic grade is an important prognostic factor and takes into account differentiation, mitoses, and necrosis. Accordingly, tumors may be regarded as low (grade 1) or high (grade 2 or 3) grade.

Clinically, leiomyosarcomas present with an abdominal mass, abdominal pain, lower limb edema, or as incidental findings [1, 4]. Occasionally patients may have fever and leucocytosis as a result of tumor necrosis invoking an inflammatory response.

Distant metastasis is common in leiomyosarcoma and may occur to the liver from gastrointestinal tumors, and to the lungs from more than 50% of retroperitoneal primaries [5]. They are associated with a high mortality rate.

## APPROACH TO MANAGEMENT

### Investigations

In addition to the basic set of blood tests, including complete blood count, liver and renal function tests and a coagulation profile, once a retroperitoneal sarcoma is suspected, contrast-enhanced (triple phase) computed tomography (CT) scans of the chest (to look for lung metastases), abdomen, and pelvis should be performed. In addition to studying the location and extent of the mass itself, other aspects to be assessed include whether the tumor is involving (or obliterating) the inferior vena cava, as well as the adjacent retroperitoneal structures, particularly the aorta, kidneys and renal vessels, duodenum, and colon.

CT venogram may be helpful to clearly delineate the inferior vena cava and its tributaries, most importantly the renal veins, if

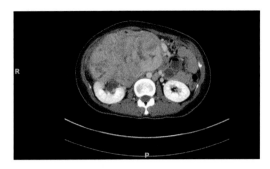

**Figure 44.1** Contrast-enhanced CT scan sections of the abdomen. Axial post-contrast CT section demonstrating a large heterogenous tumor involving the inferior vena cava and right kidney, displacing bowel to the left.

involvement or not remains unclear. It may also demonstrate the presence of collateral veins which can be prominent where the inferior vena cava is obstructed.

Magnetic resonance imaging (MRI) of the abdomen and pelvis may provide better soft tissue definition in cases where invasion is equivocal. However, while this is preferred in sarcomas of the limbs, it is not routinely required for the abdomen.

### Pathology

A percutaneous, CT-guided core biopsy should then be arranged to confirm the diagnosis and grade the tumor. A posterolateral, retroperitoneal approach is preferred, using a co-axial technique to retrieve multiple 14-16G samples. Where the tumor is heterogeneous and partly cystic, suggesting necrosis, multiple solid areas should be targeted.

### Other investigations

Some centers additionally use [18]fluorodeoxy glucose positron emission tomography to complete staging of the whole body. It is useful if there are lesions regarded as equivocal on CT or when the diagnosis or grade is in doubt. It can also be useful before the biopsy to target high [18]fluorodeoxy glucose avidity (high grade) areas.

Other tests to determine fitness for surgery should be arranged as guided by the clinical assessment. Renal function should be assessed where one or both kidneys are at risk, and if reduced, a nuclear medicine renal scan (99mTc-DTPA or MAG3) should be arranged to evaluate differential kidney function.

### TREATMENT

All retroperitoneal sarcomas, and especially those involving critical organs such as the

inferior vena cava, should be referred to an expert sarcoma center and discussed at a multidisciplinary team meeting. This should include review by an expert pathologist with experience in soft tissue tumors.

### Surgical approach

The mainstay of treatment remains complete surgical resection (aiming for microscopically negative R0 margins), so a surgical oncologist must determine whether this is feasible. This is determined based on whether one or both kidneys can be preserved, the involvement of the aorta, or by a retro-hepatic location. Once the decision is made to proceed with surgical exploration, a detailed conversation needs to be held with the patient about the surgery and the risks involved, and informed consent must be obtained.

The preferred surgical approach is through a midline laparotomy. This allows good exposure and maintains the posterior peritoneum as the anterior margin of resection. Clear margins can be difficult to achieve in retroperitoneal sarcomas due to adjacent critical structures. However, in recent years a more aggressive approach to resection with the sacrifice of adjacent organs, such as the kidneys and colon, has shown improved local control and overall survival, albeit only in grade 1 or 2 tumors [6].

In leiomyosarcomas of the inferior vena cava at least part of the wall, if not the entire circumference of the vessel, must be resected. Although inferior vena cava reconstruction with the use of autologous vein or synthetic grafts or patches have been well described [1,4], often no reconstruction is necessary – particularly where the tumor is infrarenal and the lumen has been obstructed preoperatively, as collateral vessels should have already developed. In the patient presented in the Case Scenario both renal veins were involved, however the left kidney was preserved with drainage via a large lumbar vein to the azygous system, and her postoperative renal function remained adequate.

Postoperative drains are not usually necessary unless there is a specific concern, such as a potential pancreatic leak, in which case a 15-Fr or 19-Fr Blake drain may be inserted and connected to gentle suction.

### Adjuvant treatment

Unlike in the extremities, the role of (neo)adjuvant radiotherapy in retroperitoneal sarcoma has not been clearly defined. Retrospective studies have demonstrated improvement in local control [7] and overall survival [8], although a recent presentation of the large, international randomized controlled STRASS trial [9] failed to demonstrate a benefit of preoperative radiotherapy over surgery alone for retroperitoneal sarcomas. Although the low-grade liposarcoma subgroup may benefit, that is a group with a high rate of local recurrence and low rate of distant metastasis, whereas leiomyosarcomas have low rates of local recurrence (~10%) and more frequent distant metastases [3]. This remains a practice in evolution, however based on the above we do not consider radiotherapy beneficial in high-grade leiomyosarcoma.

(Neo)adjuvant chemotherapy is not standard treatment in retroperitoneal leiomyosarcomas, as previous randomized controlled trials looking at all sarcoma subtypes grouped together failed to show a clear benefit. It can be considered in individual cases, however, especially neo-adjuvant treatment in borderline resectable tumors [10]. More often it is reserved for the treatment of distant metastases. The difficulty with sarcoma therapy is the paucity of evidence owing to its rarity and the admixture of subtypes in studies. There is ongoing research around the world to provide clearer guidelines for adjuvant management.

## FOLLOW-UP

There should be a long-term follow-up of patients due to the risk of distant metastases as well as local recurrence. No clear evidence exists to guide surveillance intervals, but the Australian guidelines recommend three to four monthly review for two years where the risk is highest, then six-monthly to five years, then annually to 10 years, with appropriate imaging such as CT chest and abdomen.

## CASE SCENARIO (CONTINUED)

The findings were discussed at the sarcoma multidisciplinary team meeting, following which the patient proceeded to surgery. She underwent a laparotomy via a midline incision along with a resection of the mass including the inferior vena cava, the right kidney, and the right colon, *en bloc* (Figure 44.2). The inferior vena cava and left renal vein were ligated, leaving renal venous drainage via a lumbar collateral. A saline filled spacer was inserted at the time of surgery to facilitate postoperative radiotherapy, however this was removed two weeks postoperatively due to infection and radiotherapy was never administered.

She eventually made a good recovery from the surgery, maintained good renal function, and improved lower limb circulation. She remained disease free until two years postoperatively, when she developed a

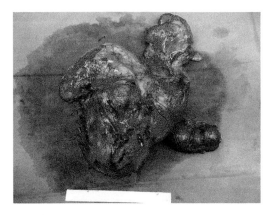

**Figure 44.2** Clinical photograph of the resected tumor including the en bloc resected right kidney, terminal ileum and right colon, and inferior vena cava, with two mersilk sutures marking superior margin of inferior vena cava (left suture with short end) and deep surface (double suture).

left lung metastasis, proven on core biopsy. Metastatectomy was considered but unfortunately not feasible, so she has been referred for palliative chemotherapy.

## KEY MESSAGES

- Leiomyosarcoma of the inferior vena cava is a rare mesenchymal malignancy of smooth muscle origin, presenting in adults as a mass, abdominal pain, or leg swelling.
- Workup imaging involves CT scan of the abdomen and chest (for staging), with or without MRI abdomen and fluorodeoxyglucose-positron emission tomography.
- Diagnosis should be made by CT-guided percutaneous core biopsy.
- All cases should be discussed in a multidisciplinary team meeting at an expert sarcoma center.
- Complete surgical resection is the mainstay of treatment, involving resection of the tumor, inferior vena cava, and adjacent kidney or colon.
- Inferior vena cava reconstruction should be considered but may not be necessary in tumors involving the infra-renal inferior vena cava.
- (Neo)adjuvant chemotherapy or radiotherapy are not routinely offered but may be considered for individual cases.
- Long-term follow-up is necessary due to the high risk of lung metastases.

## REFERENCES

1. Wachtel H, Jackson BM, Bartlett EK et al. Resection of primary leiomyosarcoma of the inferior vena cava (IVC) with reconstruction: A case series and review of the literature. *J Surg Oncol* 2015;111(3):328–333.

2. Mingoli A, Cavallaro A, Sapienza P et al. International registry of inferior vena cava leiomyosarcoma: Analysis of a world series on 218 patients. *Anticancer Res* 1996;16(5B):3201–3205.

3. Gronchi A, Strauss DC, Miceli R et al. Variability in patterns of recurrence After resection of primary retroperitoneal sarcoma (RPS): A report on 1007 patients From the multi-institutional collaborative RPS Working Group. *Ann Surg* 2016;263(5):1002–1009.

4. Ghose J, Bhamre R, Mehta N et al. Resection of the inferior *Vena cava* for retroperitoneal sarcoma: Six cases and a review of literature. *Indian J Surg Oncol* 2018;9(4):538–546.

5. Gronchi A, Miceli R, Allard MA et al. Personalizing the approach to retroperitoneal soft tissue sarcoma: Histology-specific patterns of failure and postrelapse outcome after primary extended resection. *Ann Surg Oncol* 2015;22(5):1447–1454.

6. Gronchi A, Miceli R, Colombo C et al. Frontline extended surgery is associated with improved survival in retroperitoneal low- to intermediate-grade soft tissue sarcomas. *Ann Oncol* 2012;23(4):1067–1073.

7. Kim HJ, Koom WS, Cho J et al. Efficacy of postoperative radiotherapy using modern techniques in patients with retroperitoneal soft tissue sarcoma. *Yonsei Med J* 2018;59(9):1049–1056.

8. Nussbaum DP, Rushing CN, Lane WO et al. Preoperative or postoperative radiotherapy *versus* surgery alone for retroperitoneal sarcoma: A case-control, propensity score-matched analysis of a nationwide clinical oncology database. *Lancet Oncol* 2016;17(7):966–975.

9. Bonvalot S, Gronchi A, Le Pechoux C et al. STRASS (EORTC 62092): A phase III randomized study of preoperative radiotherapy plus surgery *versus* surgery alone for patients with retroperitoneal sarcoma. *J Clin Oncol* 2019;37(15_suppl):11001.

10. Trans-Atlantic, R.P.S.W.G. Management of primary retroperitoneal sarcoma (RPS) in the adult: A consensus approach from the trans-Atlantic RPS Working Group. *Ann Surg Oncol* 2015;22(1):256–263.

# Index

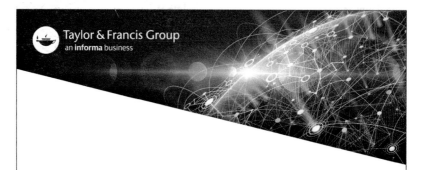